# The Kidney

Donna E. Hansel • Christopher J. Kane
Gladell P. Paner • Sam S. Chang
Editors

# The Kidney

## A Comprehensive Guide to Pathologic Diagnosis and Management

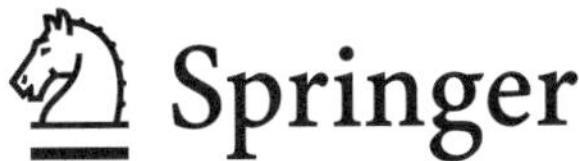

*Editors*
Donna E. Hansel, M.D., Ph.D.
Department of Pathology
University of California at San Diego
San Diego, CA, USA

Gladell P. Paner, M.D.
Department of Pathology and Surgery
Section of Urology
University of Chicago
Chicago, IL, USA

Christopher J. Kane, M.D., F.A.C.S.
Department of Urology
University of California at San Diego
San Diego, CA, USA

Sam S. Chang, M.D., F.A.C.S., M.B.A.
Department of Urologic Surgery
Vanderbilt University Medical Center
Nashville, TN, USA

ISBN 978-1-4939-8012-3     ISBN 978-1-4939-3286-3   (eBook)
DOI 10.1007/978-1-4939-3286-3

Springer New York Heidelberg Dordrecht London
© Springer Science+Business Media New York 2016
Softcover re-print of the Hardcover 1st edition 2016



Printed on acid-free paper

Springer Science+Business Media LLC New York is part of Springer Science+Business Media
(www.springer.com)

# Contents

# Contributors

**Vanesa Bijol, M.D.** Department of Pathology, Brigham and Women's Hospital, Boston, MA, USA

**Anna M. Burgner, M.D.** Division of Nephrology, Department of Medicine, Vanderbilt University Medical Center, Nashville, TN, USA

**Anthony Chang, M.D.** Department of Pathology, University of Chicago Medical Center, Chicago, IL, USA

**Sam S. Chang, M.D., M.B.A.** Department of Urologic Surgery, Vanderbilt University Medical Center, Nashville, TN, USA

**George Chiang, M.D.** Division of Pediatric Urology, Rady Children's Hospital, University of California at San Diego, San Diego, CA, USA

**Peter E. Clark, M.D.** Department of Urologic Surgery, Vanderbilt University Medical Center, Nashville, TN, USA

**Ithaar H. Derweesh, M.D.** Department of Urology, University of California San Diego, San Diego, CA, USA

**John M. DiBianco** Department of Surgery, Section of Urology, Medical College of Georgia – Georgia Regents University, Augusta, GA, USA

**Scott E. Eggener, M.D.** Department of Surgery, Section of Urology, University of Chicago, Chicago, IL, USA

**Christopher P. Filson, M.D., M.S.** Department of Urology, Institute of Urologic Oncology, David Geffen School of Medicine at UCLA, Los Angeles, CA, USA

**Lan L. Gellert, M.D., Ph.D.** Department of Pathology, Microbiology and Immunology, Vanderbilt University Medical Center, Nashville, TN, USA

**Giovanna A. Giannico, M.D.** Department of Pathology, Microbiology and Immunology, Vanderbilt University Medical Center, Nashville, TN, USA

**Edward R. Gould, M.D.** Division of Nephrology, Department of Medicine, Vanderbilt University Medical Center, Nashville, TN, USA

**Charles C. Guo, M.D.** Department of Pathology, MD Anderson Cancer Center, University of Texas, Houston, TX, USA

**Omar Hameed, M.D.** Department of Pathology, Microbiology and Immunology, Vanderbilt University Medical Center, Nashville, TN, USA

Department of Urologic Surgery, Vanderbilt University Medical Center, Nashville, TN, USA

**Donna E. Hansel, M.D., Ph.D.** Department of Pathology, University of California at San Diego, San Diego, CA, USA

**Michelle S. Hirsch, M.D., Ph.D.** Department of Pathology, Brigham and Women's Hospital, Harvard Medical School, Boston, MA, USA

**Jiaoti Huang, M.D., Ph.D.** Department of Pathology and Laboratory Medicine, David Geffen School of Medicine at UCLA, Los Angeles, CA, USA

**Shreyas S. Joshi, M.D.** Department of Urologic Surgery, Vanderbilt University Medical Center, Nashville, TN, USA

**Christopher J. Kane, M.D., F.A.C.S.** Department of Urology, University of California San Diego, San Diego, CA, USA

**Zachary Klaassen, M.D.** Department of Surgery, Section of Urology, Medical College of Georgia – Georgia Regents University, Augusta, GA, USA

**Jamie Koo, M.D.** Department of Pathology and Laboratory Medicine, David Geffen School of Medicine at UCLA, Los Angeles, CA, USA

**Mariah Zampieri Leivo, M.D.** Department of Pathology, University of California at San Diego, San Diego, CA, USA

**Denise M. Malicki, M.D., Ph.D.** Department of Pathology, Rady Children's Hospital San Diego, University of California at San Diego, San Diego, CA, USA

**Jennifer M. McBride, Ph.D.** Cleveland Clinic, Lerner College of Medicine of Case Western Reserve University, Cleveland, OH, USA

**Leili Mirsadraei, M.D.** Department of Pathology, University of California at San Diego, San Diego, CA, USA

**Gladell P. Paner, M.D.** Department of Pathology and Surgery, Section of Urology, University of Chicago Medical Center, Chicago, IL, USA

**Allan J. Pantuck, M.D.** Department of Urology, Institute of Urologic Oncology, David Geffen School of Medicine at UCLA, Los Angeles, CA, USA

**Christian P. Pavlovich, M.D.** Department of Urology, Johns Hopkins University School of Medicine, Johns Hopkins Bayview Medical Center, Baltimore, MD, USA

**Shane M. Pearce, M.D.** Department of Surgery, Section of Urology, University of Chicago, Chicago, IL, USA

**Omer A. Raheem, M.D.** Department of Urology, University of California San Diego, San Diego, CA, USA

**Priya Rao, M.D.** Department of Pathology, MD Anderson Cancer Center, The University of Texas, Houston, TX, USA

**Chad R. Ritch, M.D., M.B.A.** Department of Urology, University of Miami, Miami, FL, USA

**Ahmed Shabaik, M.D.** Department of Pathology, University of California, San Diego Medical Center, San Diego, CA, USA

**Armine K. Smith, M.D.** Department of Urology, Johns Hopkins School of Medicine, Sibley Memorial Hospital, Washington, DC, USA

**Martha K. Terris, M.D.** Department of Surgery, Section of Urology, Medical College of Georgia – Georgia Regents University, Augusta, GA, USA

**Stephen Thomas, M.D.** Department of Radiology, University of Chicago, Chicago, IL, USA

**Michael Yap, M.D.** Division of Pediatric Urology, Rady Children's Hospital, University of California at San Diego, San Diego, CA, USA

# Embryology, Anatomy, and Histology of the Kidney

**1**

Jennifer M. McBride

## Development of the Kidney

During embryonic development, the urinary system emerges from the dorsal body wall as a longitudinal elevation of intermediate mesoderm known as the urogenital ridge (Fig. 1.1a, b). Located along each side of the aorta, the urogenital ridge gives rise to both the urinary system as the nephrogenic cord and the genital system as the gonadal ridge. The following is a description of kidney development from rudimentary nonfunctional structures of the nephrogenic cord to definitive functional organs.

Early in the fourth week, the primitive kidneys or pronephroi appear as elevations along the cervical region of the developing embryo [1]. These transitory structures consist of epithelial buds which extend ventromedially and pronephric ducts which extend caudally to eventually open into the cloaca of the hindgut (Fig. 1.2a). By the end of the fourth week, the pronephroi have degenerated with the pronephric ducts persisting to become incorporated into the second set of kidneys as the mesonephric (Wolffian) duct (Fig. 1.2b).

During the fourth week, the mesonephroi emerge caudal to the pronephroi and function as interim structures until full development of the permanent kidneys around week 9. Along the length of the mesonephric (Wolffian) ducts (formerly pronephric ducts), mesonephric tubules begin to emerge on either side of the vertebral column extending from the upper thoracic region to mid-lumbar levels (Fig. 1.3a, b), with cranial tubules regressing by the end of week 5. The remaining tubules located in the upper three lumbar levels differentiate into cup-like pouches which extend medially to meet loops of capillaries emerging from the aorta (Fig. 1.3c). These structures are collectively referred to as a renal corpuscle and consist of the cup-like glomerular capsule and capillary plexus (Fig. 1.3d). During week 9, the mesonephric ducts regress in the female but persist in the male as part of the genital duct system including the ductus deferens, duct of epididymis, ejaculatory ducts, and seminal vesicles.

During the fifth week, the definitive kidneys or metanephroi begin to develop. Two sources give rise to the definitive kidneys: the ureteric bud (metanephric diverticulum) and the metanephrogenic blastema (metanephric mass of mesenchyme) (Fig. 1.4a). The ureteric buds emerge as outgrowths of the mesonephric ducts adjacent to their entrance into the cloaca. As they elongate, the ureteric buds invade the metanephrogenic blastema which grows from the caudal

J.M. McBride, Ph.D. (✉)
Cleveland Clinic, Lerner College of Medicine of Case
Western Reserve University, Cleveland Clinic/NA24,
9500 Euclid Avenue, Cleveland, OH 44195, USA
e-mail: mcbridj@ccf.org

© Springer Science+Business Media New York 2016
D.E. Hansel et al. (eds.), *The Kidney*, DOI 10.1007/978-1-4939-3286-3_1

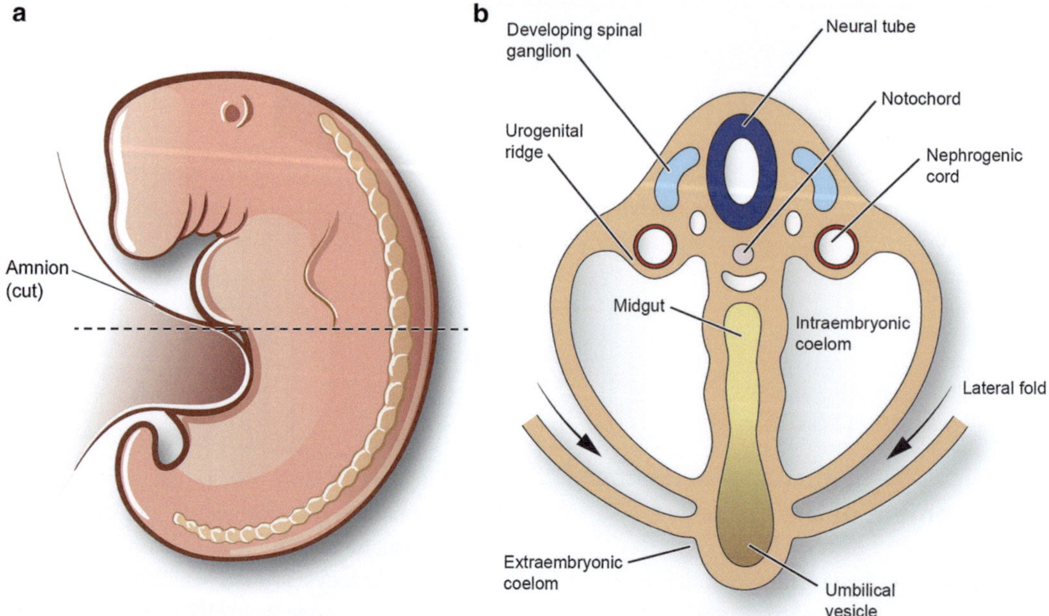



**Fig. 1.1** (**a**) Lateral view of embryo in fourth week. (**b**) Transverse section demonstrating development of the urogenital ridge from the intermediate mesoderm (reprinted with permission, Cleveland Clinic Center for Medical Art & Photography © 2015. All Rights Reserved)

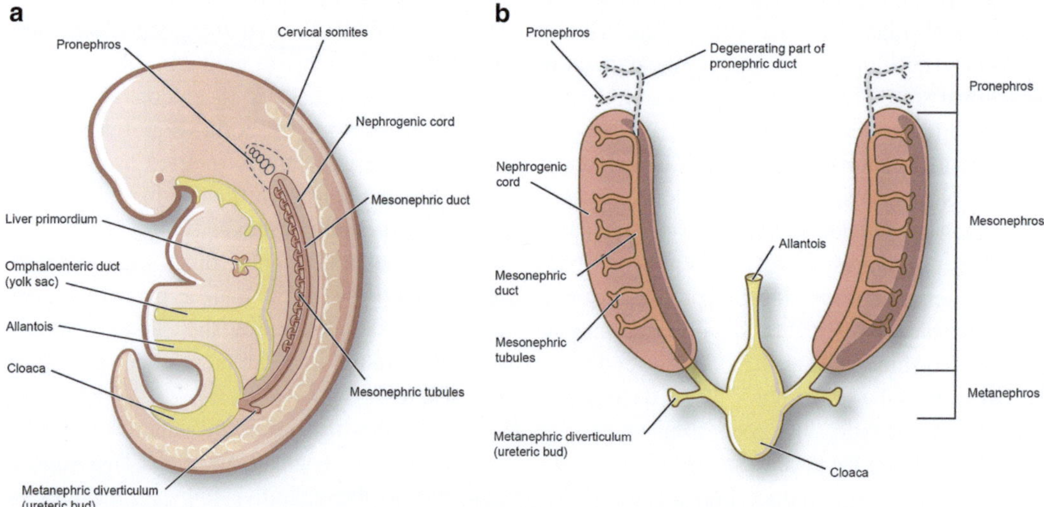



**Fig. 1.2** Depiction of the nephric system transitions from the fourth to fifth week. (**a**) Lateral illustration of embryo in the fifth week with the development of the transitory pronephroi and pronephric ducts which open caudally into the cloaca. (**b**) Ventral view (reprinted with permission, Cleveland Clinic Center for Medical Art & Photography © 2015. All Rights Reserved)

aspect of the nephrogenic cord. Penetration of the metanephric mesenchyme induces the ureteric bud to undergo a series of repetitive branchings, leading to formation of the renal collecting ducts and tubules, calyces, and primitive renal pelvis (Fig. 1.4b–d). Reciprocally, the distal end of the bud induces the metanephric mesenchyme to condense and form metanephric vesicles which

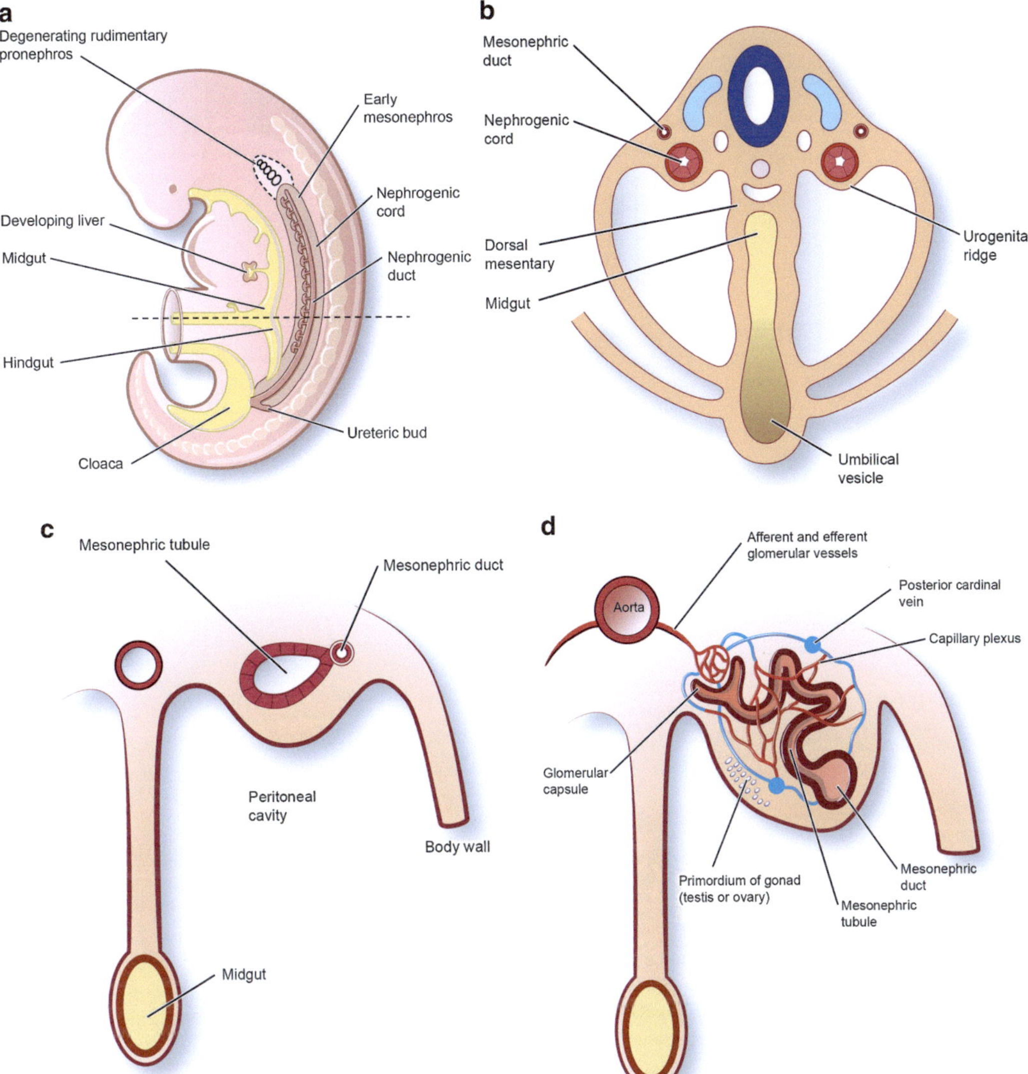



**Fig. 1.3** (**a**) Lateral view indicating degeneration of the pronephros and emergence of the mesonephros. (**b**) Ventral view. (**c**) Sequential development of the mesonephric tubules from weeks 5 to 11. (**d**) The medial aspect of the mesonephric tubules extends to meet loops of capillaries emerging from the aorta (reprinted with permission, Cleveland Clinic Center for Medical Art & Photography © 2015. All Rights Reserved)

will further develop into a series of metanephric tubules (Fig. 1.5a, b). The connection formed between the lumens from these S-shaped metanephric tubules with that of the ureteric duct results in the formation of the definitive uriniferous tubule (Fig. 1.5c). These uriniferous tubules will further differentiate into proximal convoluted tubules, distal convoluted tubules, and the nephron loop including descending and ascending nephron loops (Fig. 1.5d).

During the tenth week, the metanephroi become functional as the distal convoluted and collecting tubules begin to adjoin. In addition, the population of glomeruli further increases during this time up until week 32 of gestation. Nephrons also continue to form with approximately two million nephrons present in each kidney at term.

Between weeks 6 and 9, the kidneys withdraw from the pelvis and ascend along either side of the aorta to reach their permanent location along

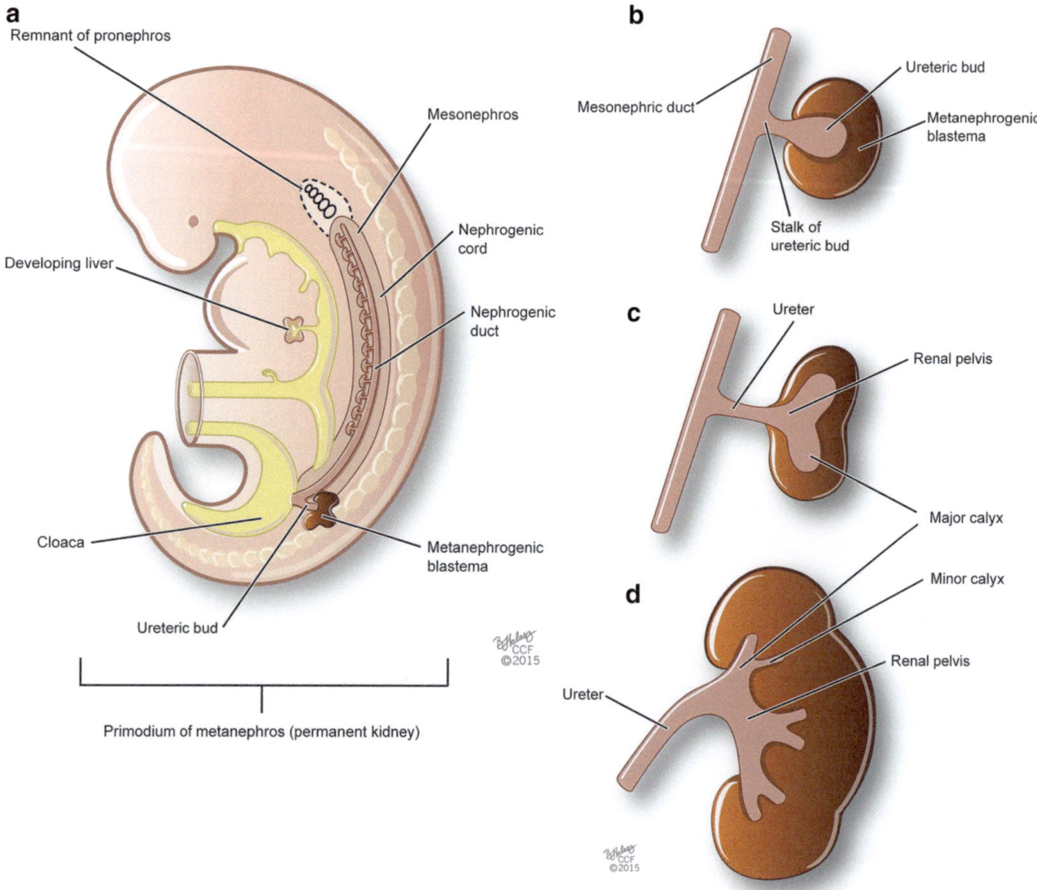



**Fig. 1.4** Metanephros development from the ureteric bud and metanephrogenic blastema. (**a**) Lateral view of an embryo in the fifth week of development. (**b**–**d**) Sequential branching of the ureteric bud as it penetrates the meta- nephric mesenchyme (reprinted with permission, Cleveland Clinic Center for Medical Art & Photography © 2015. All Rights Reserved)

the posterior abdominal wall of the lumbar region (Fig. 1.6a–d). During their ascent, the kidneys' original blood supply from the common iliac arteries disappears with branches from succes- sive levels of the aorta taking their place. After contacting the suprarenal glands, the kidneys become fixed in their position with primary arte- rial supply deriving from the abdominal aorta. Caudal arterial branches may remain as acces- sory renal arteries; typically, these branches arise from the aorta to enter the hilum of the kidney.

## Anatomy of the Kidney

### Overall Structure

The kidneys are reddish-brown bean-shaped structures located retroperitoneally along the pos- terior abdominal wall (Fig. 1.7). While posture and dynamic changes of the diaphragm can mod- ify their relationship to surrounding structures, in the supine position, the kidneys typically extend

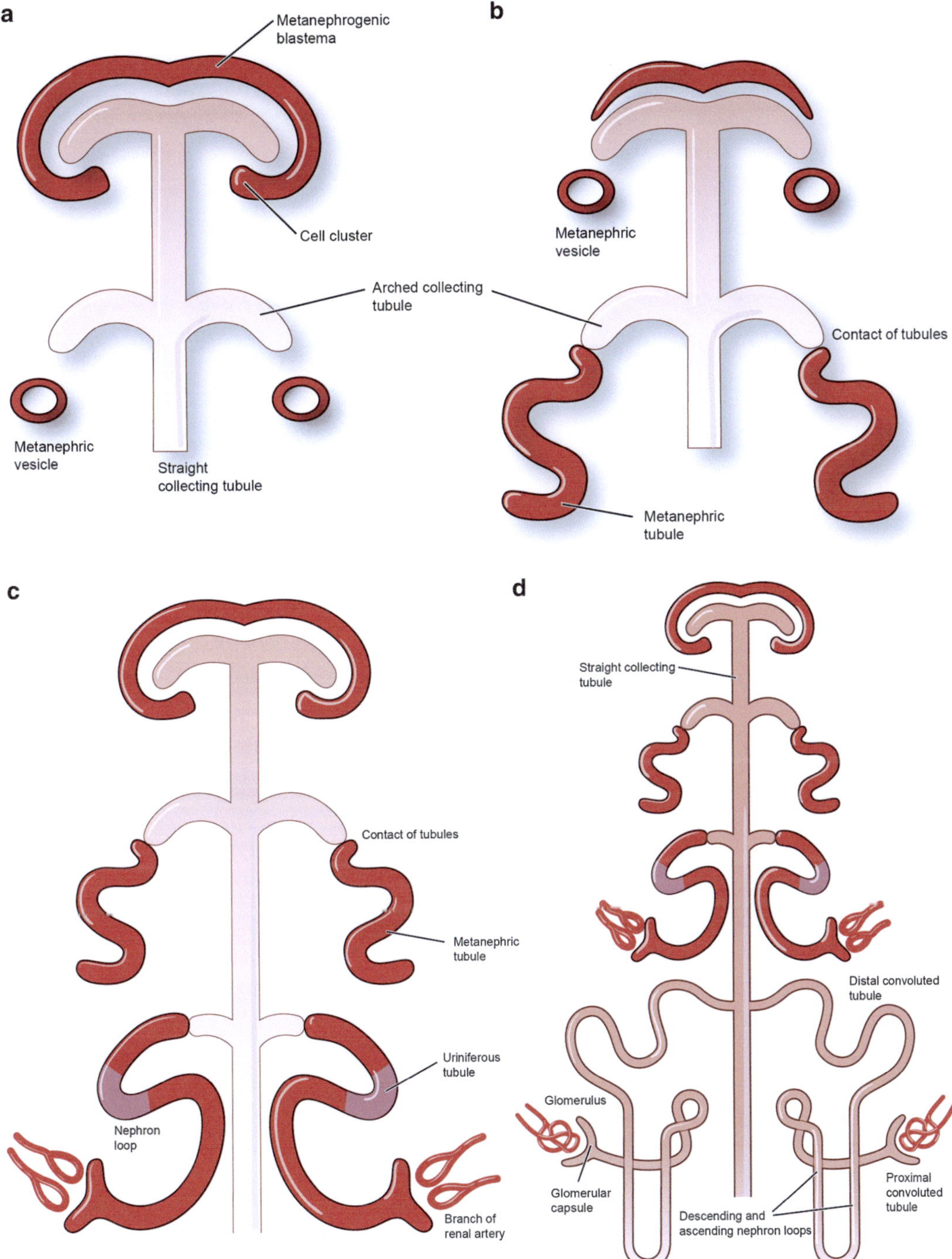


**Fig. 1.5** Development of nephrons. (**a**) The distal end of the ureteric bud develops into a series of metanephric tubules. (**b–d**) These S-shaped structures, along with the ureteric duct, will form the uriniferous tubules (reprinted with permission, Cleveland Clinic Center for Medical Art & Photography © 2015. All Rights Reserved)

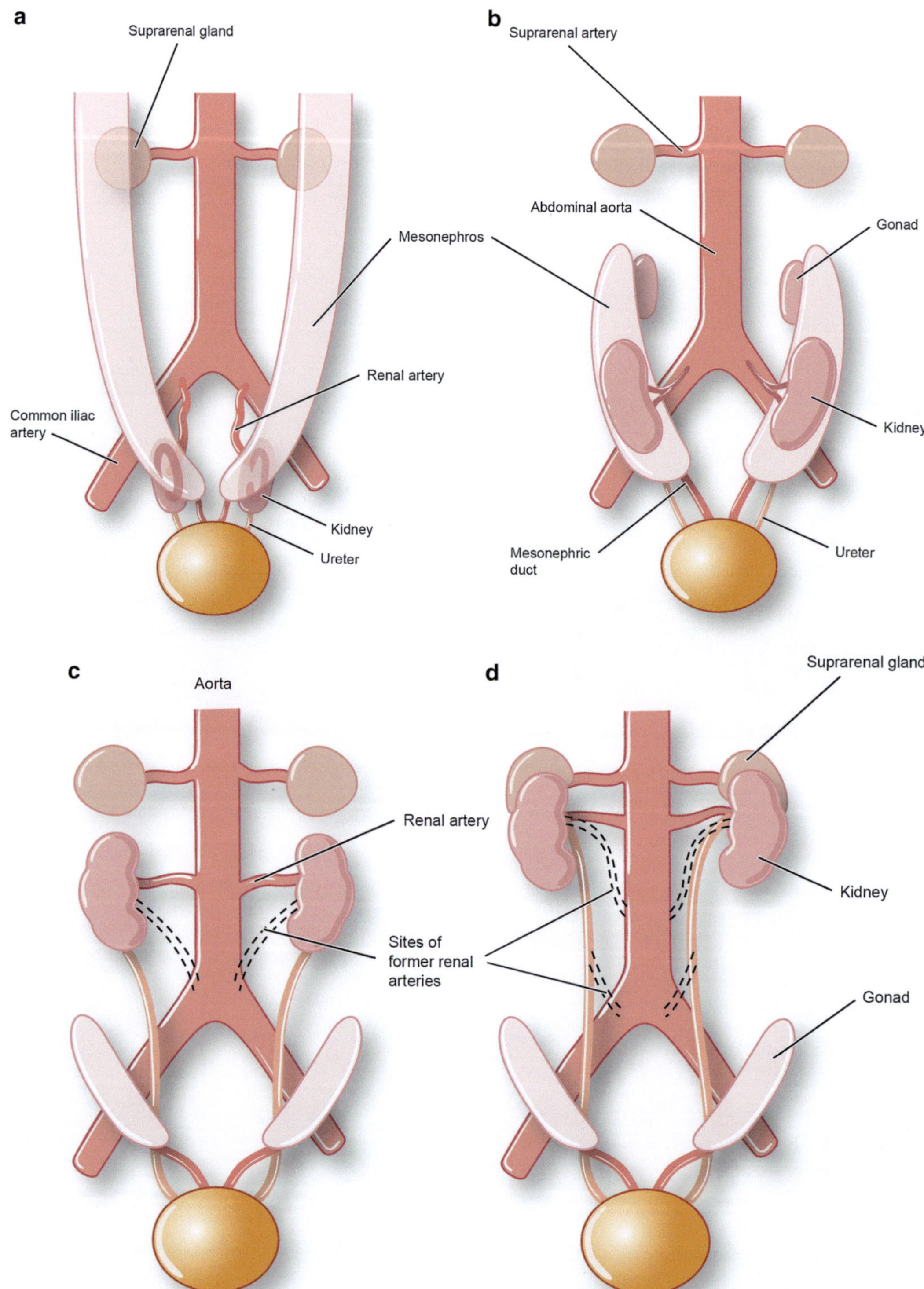


**Fig. 1.6** Ventral abdominopelvic view of embryo from weeks 6 to 9. (**a–d**) The kidneys ascend alongside of the aorta to reach their permanent location in the lumbar region of the posterior abdominal wall (reprinted with permission, Cleveland Clinic Center for Medical Art & Photography © 2015. All Rights Reserved)

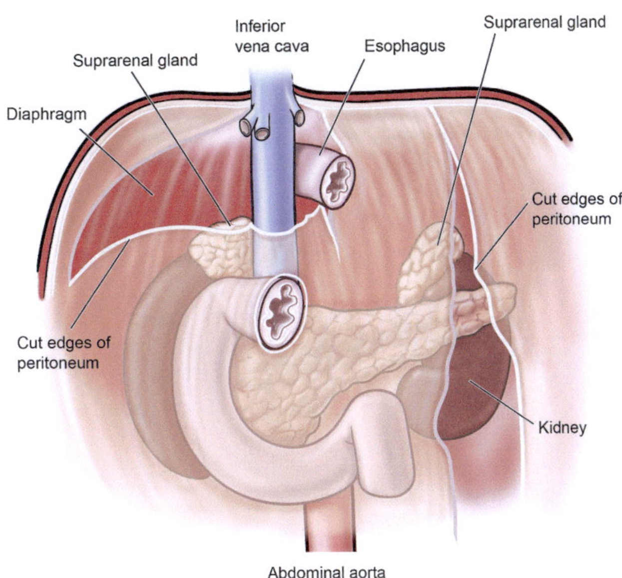


**Fig. 1.7** Retroperitoneal location of the kidneys along the posterior abdominal wall (reprinted with permission, Cleveland Clinic Center for Medical Art & Photography © 2015. All Rights Reserved)

from vertebral levels TXII–LIII. The right kidney occupies a position slightly lower due to its relationship with the liver superiorly. Conversely, the left kidney rests slightly closer to the midline, has a narrower profile, and is somewhat longer. On its medial surface, the kidneys are occupied by blood vessels, nerves, lymphatics, and the renal pelvis entering and exiting the concave-shaped hilum which faces anteriorly and medially.

## Adjacent Structures

Due to their position in the paravertebral gutters along the posterior abdominal wall, the kidneys are in contact with the surfaces of several structures directly or through an intervening layer of peritoneum. Anteriorly, the left kidney is related to the spleen, suprarenal gland, stomach, pancreas, jejunum, descending colon, and left colic flexure (Fig. 1.8a). Alternatively, the anterior surface of the right kidney is related to the liver, suprarenal gland, small intestine, right colic flexure, and descending part of the duodenum. Posteriorly, both kidneys are related to the psoas major muscle, quadratus lumborum muscle, transversus abdominis muscle, diaphragm,

costodiaphragmatic recess, eleventh rib (left kidney only), twelfth rib, subcostal nerve, ilioinguinal nerve, and iliohypogastric nerve (Fig. 1.8b).

## Fascial Contributions

The retroperitoneal connective tissue is organized around the kidneys to form interchanging layers of fascia and adipose tissue. In immediate contact with the kidney is the renal capsule, a fibrous layer which encapsulates the kidney, but it is histologically distinct from the renal parenchyma. Surrounding the renal capsule is the perinephric (perirenal) fat, an accumulation of adipose tissue from the extraperitoneal fatty layer (Fig. 1.9). Adjacent to the anterolateral aspect of the kidney and enclosing the perinephric fat are two layers extending from transversalis fascia that surround the kidney and are referred to as renal (Gerota's) fascia. Towards the midline, the anterior layer of renal fascia adjoins to the connective tissue of the inferior vena cava, aorta, or anterior layer from the opposing side. The posterior layer of renal fascia travels medially to adjoin to the fascia covering the anterior surface of the psoas major muscle. In addition to covering the

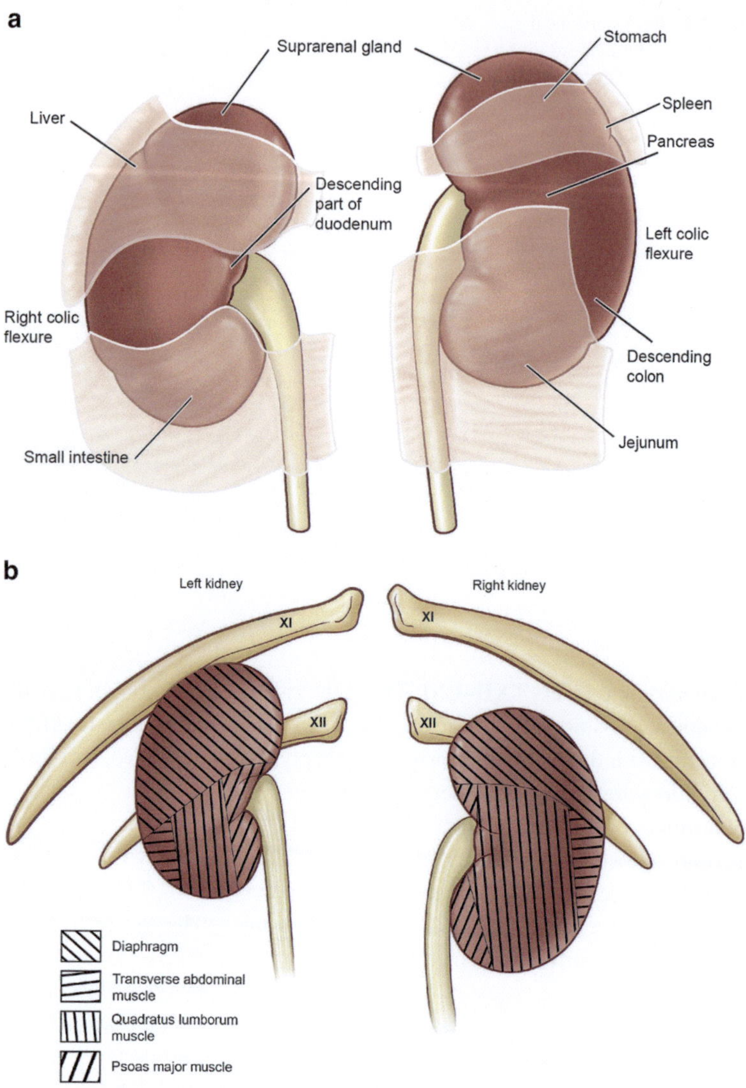



**Fig. 1.8** Relationship of surrounding structures to the kidney. (**a**) Anterior surface. (**b**) Posterior surface (reprinted with permission, Cleveland Clinic Center for Medical Art & Photography © 2015. All Rights Reserved)

kidney, renal fascia also encapsulates the suprarenal gland superiorly; however, an intervening septum ordinarily separates the two structures. A final outermost layer of adipose tissue, paranephric fat, is found posteriorly and lateral to the kidney residing between the posterior layer of renal fascia and transversalis fascia.

## Arterial Supply, Venous Drainage, and Lymphatics

The renal arteries are the primary arterial supply to the kidneys and extend off of the abdominal aorta between vertebral levels LI and LII (Fig. 1.10). Comparatively, the right renal artery emerges from the aorta slightly more superior and passes posterior to the inferior vena cava as it extends towards the kidney. As they course towards the kidney, the renal arteries give off several nonrenal branches which perfuse the adjacent renal capsule, ureters, and suprarenal glands. Just prior to reaching the renal hilum, they divide into five segmental arteries: superior/apical, anterosuperior, anteroinferior, inferior, and posterior. These terminal arteries are responsible for perfusing corresponding regions of the kidney. Clinically, this allows for identification of

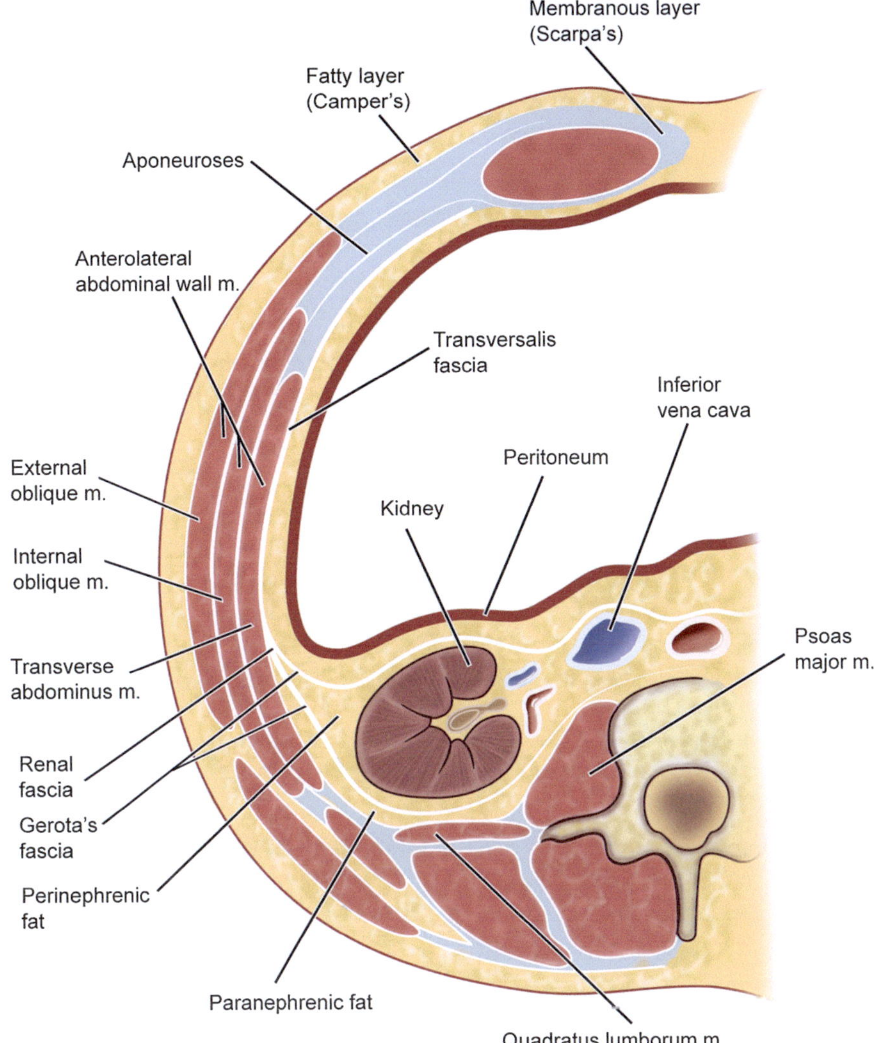



**Fig. 1.9** Illustration of fascia and adipose tissue surrounding the kidney (reprinted with permission, Cleveland Clinic Center for Medical Art & Photography © 2015. All Rights Reserved)

surgically resectable renal segments as the segmental branches exhibit very little anastomotic properties. Accessory renal arteries may also be present, originating directly from the abdominal aorta to enter the hilum or other level (extrahilar arteries) of the kidney.

Positioned anterior to the renal arteries are the renal veins that arise from several small branches exiting the renal hilum. Both veins converge on the inferior vena cava residing just right of mid-line (Fig. 1.11). Due to the positioning of the inferior vena cava, the left renal vein is longer in length and passes anterior to the aorta and posterior to the descending segment of the superior mesenteric artery. This vascular relationship can be significantly compromised with the development of an aneurysm in either the aorta or superior mesenteric artery.

Lymphatic drainage from the kidneys, ureters, and suprarenal glands all coalesce into the left

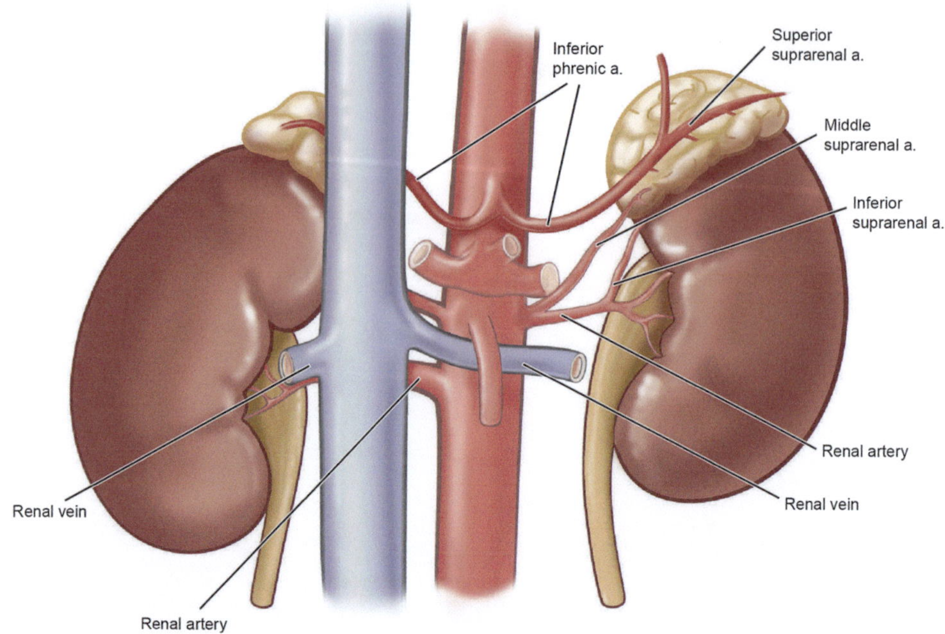


**Fig. 1.10** Arterial supply to the kidney (reprinted with permission, Cleveland Clinic Center for Medical Art & Photography © 2015. All Rights Reserved)

and right lateral lumbar (caval or aortic) nodes (Fig. 1.12). These nodes are located near the source of the renal arteries bilaterally [2].

## Innervation

The kidneys receive nervous system input from the sympathetic nervous system originating from T12 to L1 levels of the spinal cord. These fibers form a renal plexus along the surface of the renal arteries and receive contributions from the celiac plexus, least splanchnic, and first lumbar splanchnic nerves (Fig. 1.13). Upon reaching the kidney, these fibers are responsible for regulating renal blood flow, salt and water reabsorption by the nephron, and glomerular filtration rate. In contrast to sympathetic nerve function, parasympathetic innervation does not appear to play a significant role in regulating kidney function [3].

## Histology of the Kidney

### Renal Capsule

Externally, the kidney is surrounded by the renal capsule, a fibrous connective tissue structure weakly attached to the kidney surface. The capsule includes two discrete layers: an inner layer of myofibroblasts and an outer layer of collagen fibers and fibroblasts [4]. At the hilum, the capsule penetrates the area of the sinus to contribute to the connective tissue covering of the calyces and renal pelvis.

### Parenchyma

#### Overview
When viewing the hemisected kidney, two regions are clearly visible: the centrally located medulla with inner and outer segments and the

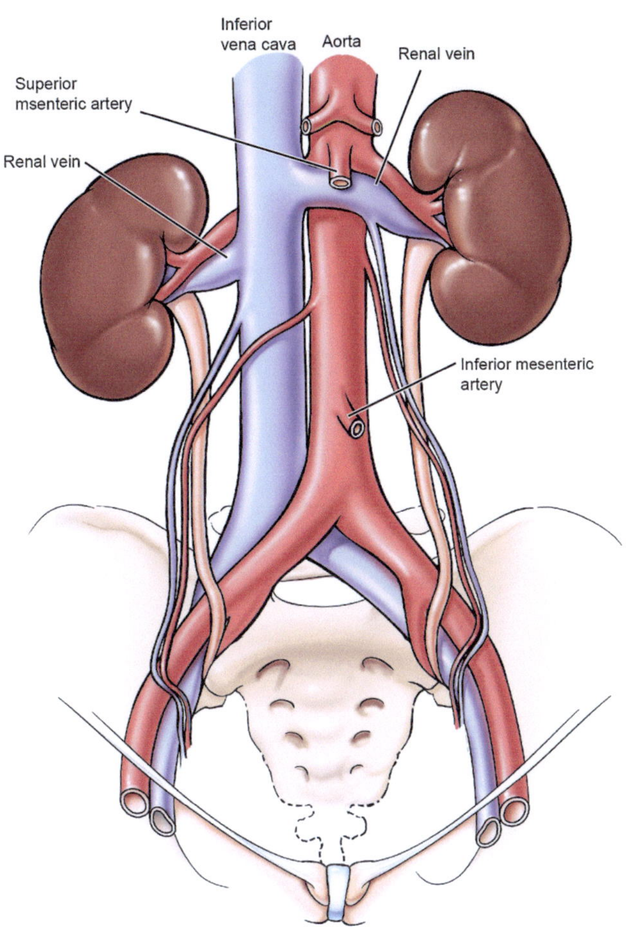



**Fig. 1.11** Venous drainage from the kidney (reprinted with permission, Cleveland Clinic Center for Medical Art & Photography © 2015. All Rights Reserved)

overlying cortex which is subdivided into an outer cortex and a juxtamedullary cortex sitting adjacent to the medullary pyramids (Fig. 1.14). Within each kidney, 8–12 conical-shaped medullary pyramids exist with their bases directed towards the overlying cortex. Between each pyramid, a segment of cortex interjects to form a renal column (of Bertin). The association of the medullary pyramids and their surrounding cortical tissue constitute a renal lobe, with the total number of lobes in the kidney determined by the number of pyramids present. Another level of organization of kidney parenchyma is the lobule which consists of a central medullary ray and the cortical tissue surrounding it. Interstitial tissue throughout the parenchyma is extremely scarce, consisting mostly of reticular tissue and some collagenous fibers which surround blood vessels, large papillary ducts, and glomerular capsules.

## Cortex

In the fresh state, the cortex appears brownish red, a coloring indicative of the extensive blood flow passing through the complex network of vasculature. Every minute, the kidneys receive approximately 20 % of the cardiac output, with 90 % directed towards the cortex and 10 % to the medulla. Populating the cortex are renal corpuscles and various segments of the tubule system including convoluted and straight tubules of the nephron, collecting tubules, and collecting ducts (Fig. 1.15). The renal corpuscle represents the initial, dilated portion of the nephron. Closer examination of this sphere-shaped structure

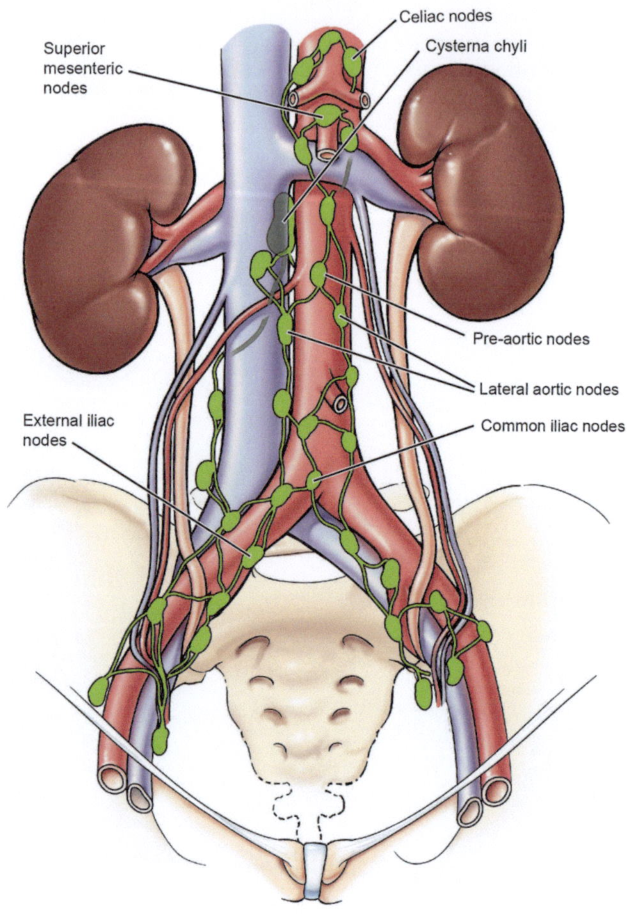



**Fig. 1.12** Lymphatic drainage from the kidneys to the lateral lumbar (caval or aortic) nodes (reprinted with permission, Cleveland Clinic Center for Medical Art & Photography © 2015. All Rights Reserved)

reveals an accompanying capillary system known as the glomerulus. Situated between areas of renal corpuscles and their closely approximated convoluted and collecting tubules are areas of medullary rays which consist of straight tubules of the nephrons and collecting ducts.

## Medulla

The medulla consists of 8–12 conical-shaped medullary pyramids and intervening areas of cortical tissue referred to as renal columns (Fig. 1.14). These structures contain the same cortical structures as described previously but are regarded as part of the medulla. Organizationally, the medullary pyramid and its surrounding cortical tissue constitute a lobe of the kidney, with 8–12 lobes present in a human kidney. Each lobe is further subdivided into lobules which consist of a central medullary ray and surrounding cortical tissue. Within the medullary pyramids are straight tubules and collecting ducts which are accompanied by the vasa recta, a capillary network oriented in parallel to the tubules and ducts. The medullary pyramids are divided into an outer and inner medulla with the inner segment oriented towards the apical end or papilla. Each of these divisions contains specific segments of the nephron. The inner medulla contains the descending thin limbs, ascending thin limbs, and inner medullary collecting ducts. The outer medulla is further subdivided into an outer stripe with proximal straight tubules, distal straight tubules, and outer medullary collecting ducts and an inner stripe with descending thin limbs, distal straight tubules, and outer medullary collecting ducts. The collecting ducts open into a perforated region

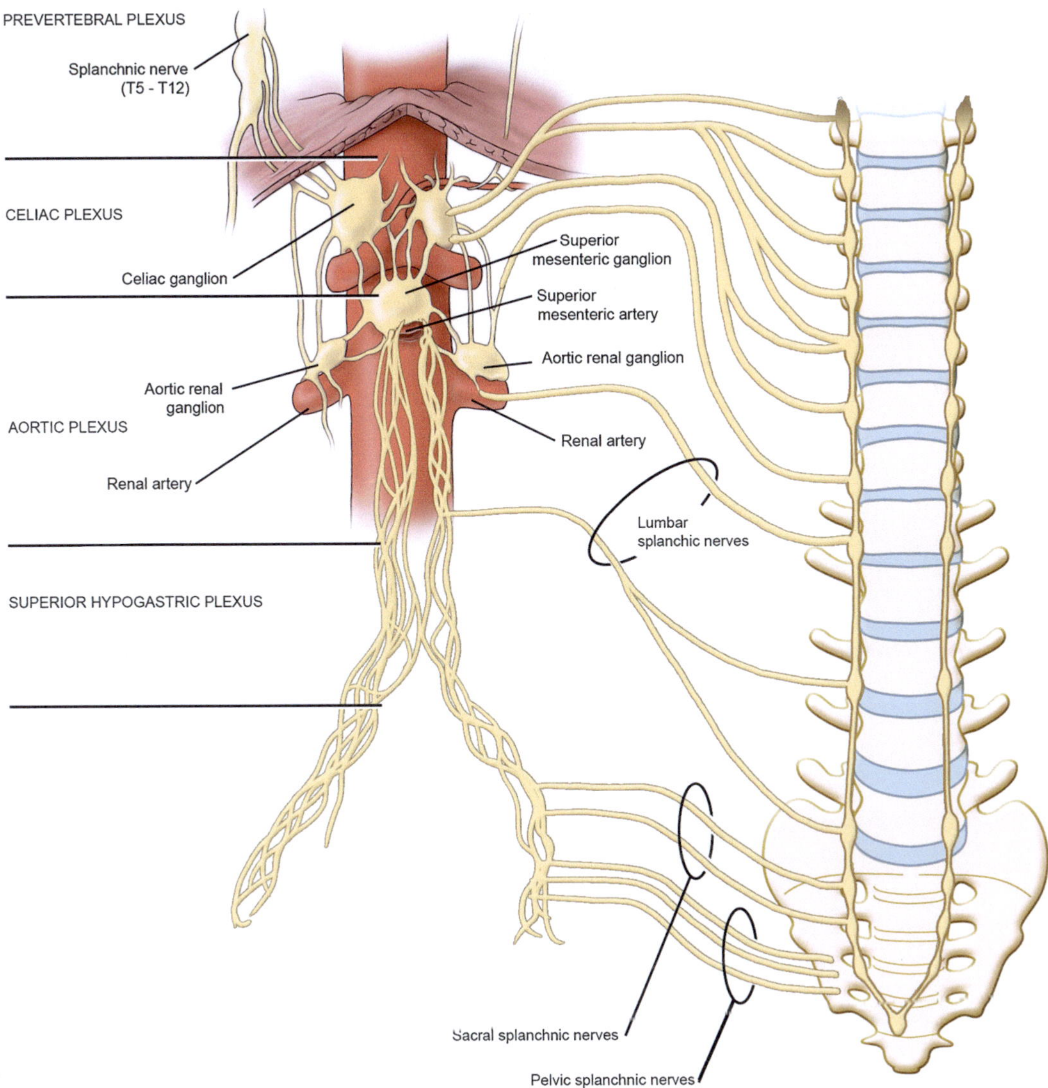


**Fig. 1.13** Sympathetic innervation to the kidneys (reprinted with permission, Cleveland Clinic Center for Medical Art & Photography © 2015. All Rights Reserved)

of the papilla known as the area cribrosa. Each papilla projects into a cup-like minor calyx which is an extension of the renal pelvis.

## Renal Corpuscle

The renal corpuscles consist of a tuft of glomerular capillaries surrounded by the visceral and parietal layers of Bowman's capsule (Fig. 1.16a, b). Each corpuscle has a vascular pole with an afferent and efferent arteriole, as well as a urinary pole in which the proximal tubule arises. Lining the lumen of the capillaries is a layer of fenestrated simple squamous endothelium, with fenestrations spanning 60–100 nm. Immediately adjacent to the basement membrane of the capillary wall is the visceral layer of Bowman's capsule. It is comprised of podocytes or visceral epithelial cells which give off primary processes and then secondary processes called pedicels or foot processes (Fig. 1.17). As the foot processes

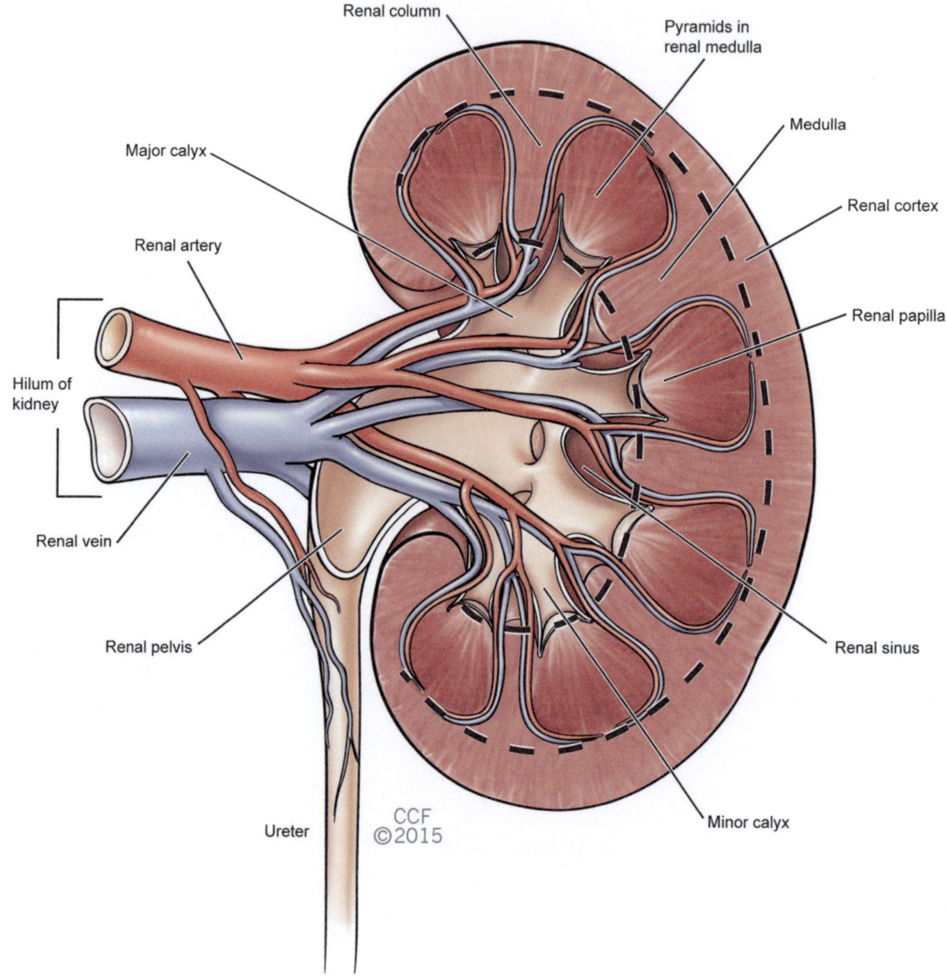



**Fig. 1.14** Depiction of kidney structure in the hemisected kidney (reprinted with permission, Cleveland Clinic Center for Medical Art & Photography © 2015. All Rights Reserved)

interdigitate with one another around the capillary, filtration slits with a diameter of 20–25 nm are formed. Each slit is covered by a filtration slit diaphragm to limit the passage of smaller molecules. Together, the capillary endothelium, glomerular basement membrane, and the visceral layer of Bowman's capsule form the filtration apparatus of the kidney. Surrounding these structures is the external or parietal layer of Bowman's capsule. This layer consists of simple squamous epithelium supported by an indistinct basement membrane.

Between the loops of the glomerular capillaries and around the vascular pole are mesangial cells which play a significant role in maintaining the structure and support of the glomerular filtration barrier. While the primary role of mesangial cells is phagocytosis and structural support, they also proliferate in response to glomerular injury. In addition, these cells retain contractile properties which allow them to regulate glomerular distension in response to increases in blood pressure.

## Nephron

Functionally, the nephron is responsible for the production of urine. In humans, there are approximately two million nephrons present in each kid-

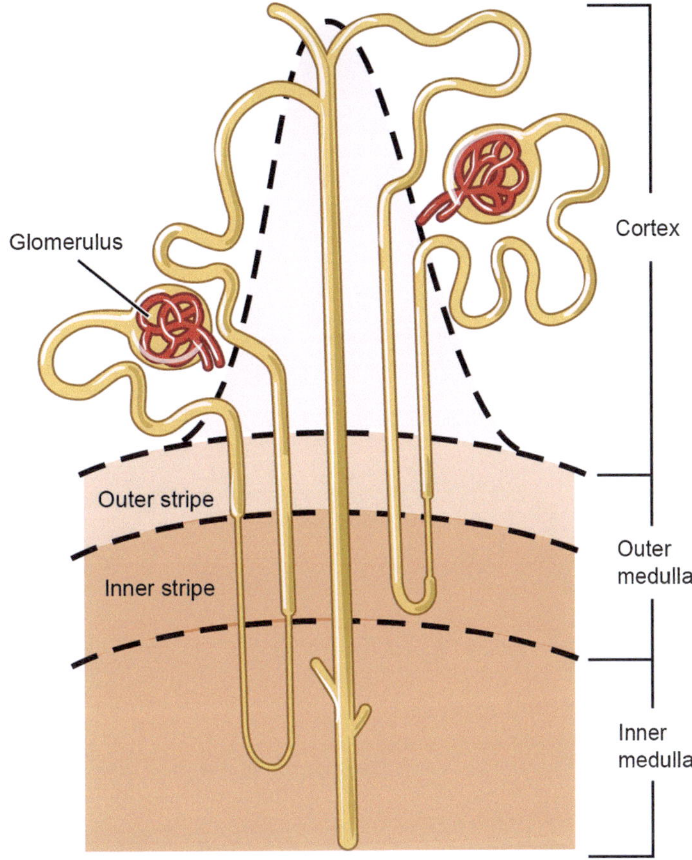



**Fig. 1.15** Diagram of adult kidney indicating the relationship of nephrons to their collecting tubules and ducts within the cortex and medulla (reprinted with permission, Cleveland Clinic Center for Medical Art & Photography © 2015. All Rights Reserved)

ney. The initial segment is comprised of the renal corpuscle with its glomerulus and surrounding renal or Bowman's capsule (Fig. 1.15). Blood entering the glomerular capillary loops passes first through an afferent arteriole and then drains from the efferent arteriole, both of which are located at the vascular pole of Bowman's capsule. On the opposite side of the renal corpuscle is the urinary pole, where the proximal convoluted tubule originates. The remaining tubular segments of the nephron include the proximal thick segment, thin segment, and distal thick segment.

### Nephron Tubules

As mentioned previously, the proximal convoluted tubule represents the initial tubule segment stemming from the urinary pole of the renal corpuscle. This segment takes a tortuous course through the cortex before entering the medullary ray as the proximal straight tubule or thick descending limb of the loop of Henle to enter the medulla (Fig. 1.15). Continuing as the thin descending limb, within the medulla it makes a turn to head back towards the cortex as the thin ascending limb. Entering the medullary ray of the cortex, it transitions into the distal straight tubule or thick ascending limb of the loop of Henle. After leaving the medullary ray, the distal straight tubule makes contact with the vascular pole of its renal corpuscle. The epithelial cells of the tubule near the afferent arteriole of the glomerulus are modified to form the macula densa. After leaving the corpuscle, the tubule becomes the distal convoluted tubule which empties into a collecting duct within the medullary ray by way of an arched collecting tubule or connecting tubule (Fig. 1.15).

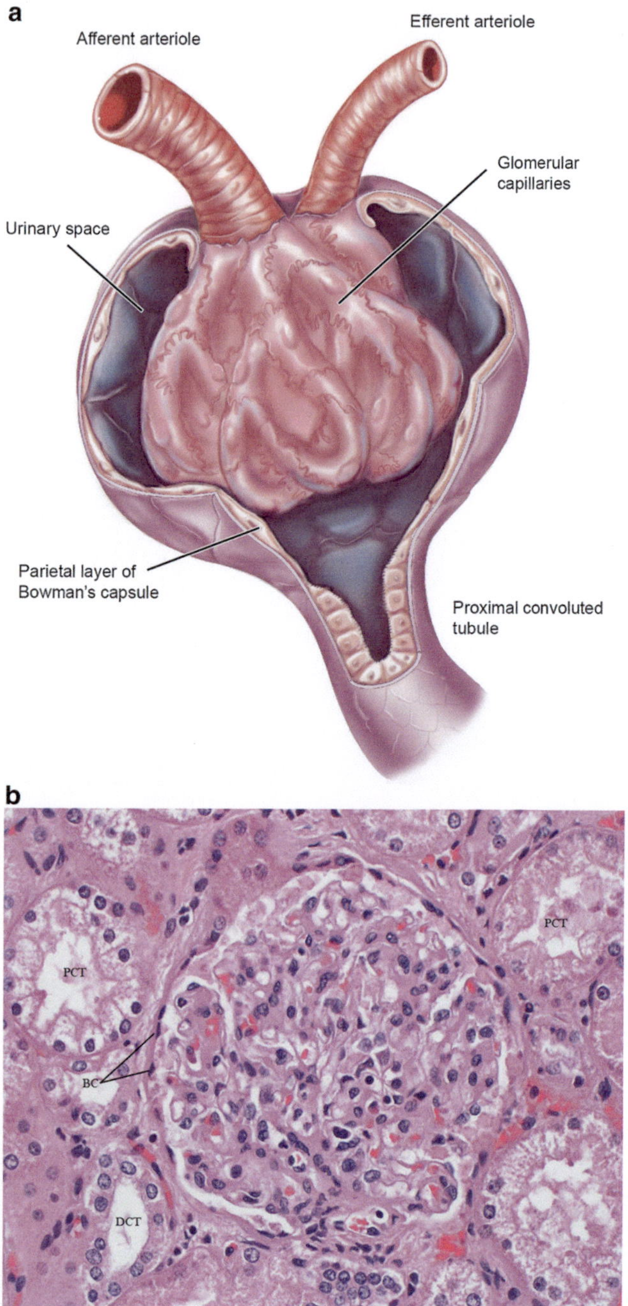



**Fig. 1.16** The renal corpuscle. (**a**) Schematic representation. (**b**) Light micrograph. Note the parietal layer of Bowman's capsule (BC), surrounding proximal convoluted tubules (PCT) and distal convoluted tubules (DCT) (reprinted with permission, Cleveland Clinic Center for Medical Art & Photography © 2015. All Rights Reserved)

## Proximal Convoluted Tubule

The lumen of the proximal convoluted tubule is lined by cuboidal cells with a prominent brush border consisting of apically located microvilli (Fig. 1.16b). Another distinguishing feature is the basal striations, which contain a high concentration of vertically oriented mitochondria. Functionally, the increased surface area offered by the brush border makes this segment of the nephron the primary site of reabsorption, with approximately 65% of the total ultrafiltrate per day being reabsorbed here. With the aid of transmembrane proteins, $Na^+/K^+$-ATPase pumps, and AQP-1, the majority of salts and water

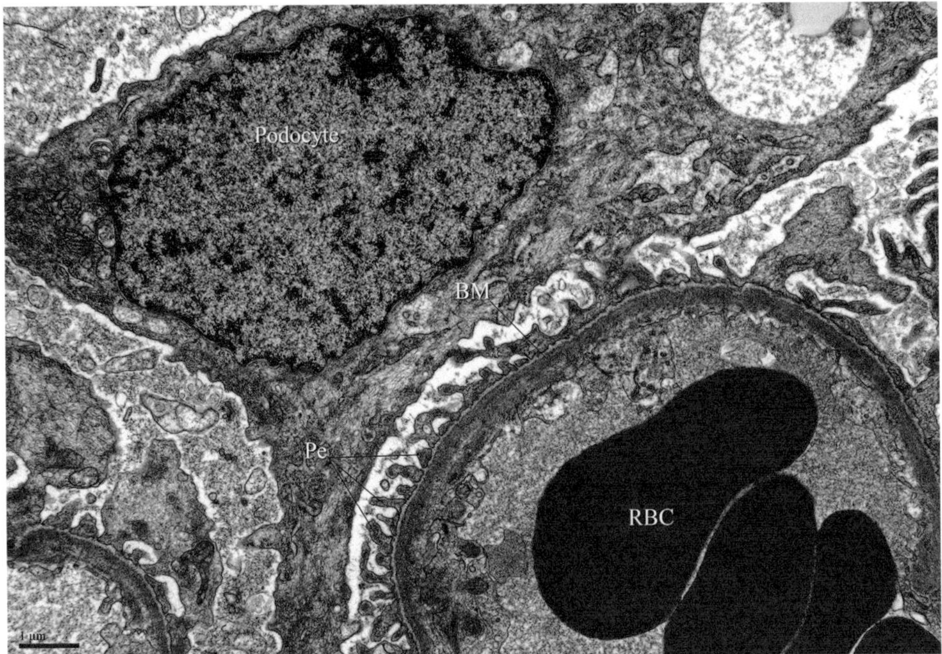


**Fig. 1.17** Transmission electron micrograph of a glomerular capillary and neighboring podocyte. Pedicels (Pe) of the podocyte rest on the basement membrane adjacent to the endothelium of the fenestrated glomerular capillary (courtesy of Jesus Macias, University of California at San Diego)

are absorbed within the proximal convoluted tubule. In addition, the proximal convoluted tubule also reabsorbs glucose, amino acids, and polypeptides.

### Loop of Henle

With a less prominent role in reabsorption, the cuboidal-shaped cells of the proximal straight tubule have a much shorter brush border and smaller, less intricate basal domain and randomly oriented mitochondria. The thin segment is lined with simple squamous epithelium with cells further subdivided at the electron microscopy level into types I–IV based on contact with neighboring cells, abundance of intracellular organelles, as well as the presence and morphology of microvilli. At the level of the descending thin limb, water passively diffuses out to the interstitial space, while a small amount of NaCl and urea enters into the nephron lumen. In contrast, NaCl passively diffuses out to the interstitial space at the level of the thin ascending limb. The thin ascending limb is also impermeable to water.

Transitioning into the distal straight tubule, the cells lining the lumen exhibit a cuboidal shape, fewer microvilli, extensive basolateral plications, and numerous basal located mitochondria. At this level, NaCl is actively pumped out of the nephron lumen and into the medullary interstitium. Near the vascular pole, the cells of the straight tubule take on a columnar shape and are more numerous. As the cells appear crowded and somewhat overlapping, this area is referred to as the macula densa, a component of the juxtaglomerular apparatus. The distal convoluted tubule is the continuation of the distal straight tubule within the cortical labyrinth. It is similar in structure and appearance. Exchange of $Na^+$ and $K^+$ at this level is mediated through aldosterone secreted by the adrenal glands. Under this influence, $Na^+$ is reabsorbed and $K^+$ is secreted.

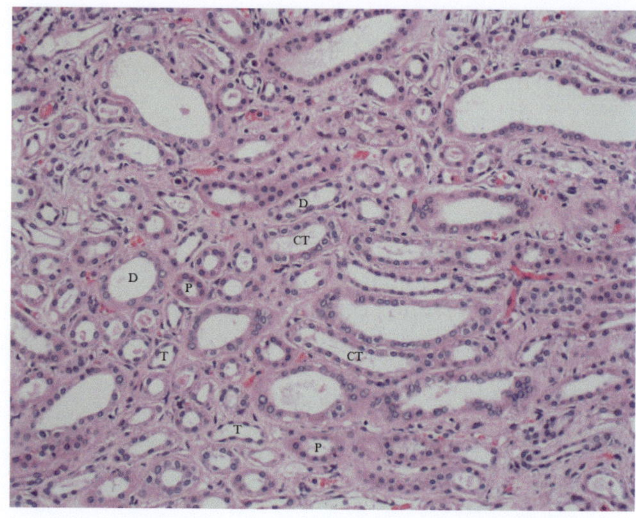

**Fig. 1.18** Light micrograph from the outer potion of the medulla region. Note the presence of proximal straight tubules (P), distal straight tubules (D), collecting tubules (CT), and thin segments (T)



## Collecting Tubules and Ducts

Connecting to the distal convoluted tubules are collecting tubules (Fig. 1.18) which then transition into collecting ducts. Both of these structures are comprised of simple epithelium. In general, the cells of the collecting ducts transition from squamous to cuboidal in nature as they pass from outer to inner medulla and become columnar near the renal papilla. The two principal cell types in the collecting tubules and collecting ducts are light cells or collecting duct cells and dark cells or intercalated cells. The collecting duct cells are greater in number and are identified by their pale-staining cytoplasm and sparse microvilli. These cells possess several aquaporin channels and thus play a role in water permeability in the collecting ducts. In contrast, the intercalated cells are less abundant and exhibit a dark staining cytoplasm. These cells secrete $H^+$ or bicarbonate and thus play an important role in acid–base balance.

## References


1. The urogenital system. In: Moore KL, Persaud TVN, editors. The developing human: clinically oriented embryology. 9th ed. Philadelphia: Saunders; 2013. p. 245–53.
2. Abdomen. In: Drake RL, Vogl AW, Mitchell AWM, editors. Gray's anatomy for students. 3rd ed. Philadelphia: Churchill Livingstone; 2015. p. 373–97.
3. Structure and function of the kidneys. In: Koeppen BM, Stanton BA, editors. Renal physiology. 4th ed. Philadelphia: Mosby; 2007. p. 19–30.
4. Urinary system. In: Ross MH, Pawlina W, editors. Histology a text and atlas: with correlated cell and molecular biology. 6th ed. Philadelphia: Lippincott Williams & Wilkins; 2011. p. 698–739.

# Polycystic Kidney Disease

Shreyas S. Joshi, Gladell P. Paner, and Sam S. Chang

## Autosomal Dominant Polycystic Kidney Disease

### Background

Autosomal dominant polycystic kidney disease (ADPKD) is a common heritable form of renal cystic disease with an incidence of up to 1 in 400 live births [1, 2]. It is one of the most common monogenetic disorders in the USA and is also the most common heritable cause of renal failure, accounting for up to 15 % of all patients receiving hemodialysis [2–4]. Its genetic pattern of inheritance has been extensively studied and generally transmits in the expected autosomal dominant fashion. Although up to 10 % of cases present sporadically, the presence of other contributory loci is the focus of ongoing investigation [5–7]. The age of onset of ADPKD is predictably in the 4th or 5th decade of life, with penetrance approaching 100 % for all patients who live long enough. Rare cases in infants and children do occur and tend to portend a more aggressive form of the disease; but for the stereotypical adult patient, progression to serious manifestations, like renal failure, rarely occurs before the 4th decade of life [8]. ADPKD is a heterogeneous disease once it manifests. Associated anomalies are commonly co-expressed, including cysts of the liver, pancreas, spleen, seminal vesicles, arachnoid membrane, and lungs. Noncystic lesions include berry aneurysms (vascular aneurysms of the circle of Willis), colonic diverticula, aortic aneurysms, and mitral valve prolapse [9].

### Genetics/Pathogenesis

Almost all ADPKD cases are the result of mutations in either *PDK1* or *PDK2* genes located on the short arm of chromosome 16 and the long arm of chromosome 4, respectively [10–12]. The resultant gene products, polycystin-1 and polycystin-2, are both part of a complex of molecules that regulate cell proliferation and cyst formation. These proteins are thought to interact as part of the same pathway; thus, a mutation in either can lead to similar disease manifestations [13]. The presence of a third specific locus, *PDK3*, has been evaluated as the cause of disease in a very small subset of patients, though recent reanalysis

S.S. Joshi, M.D. (✉) • S.S. Chang, M.D., M.B.A.
Department of Urologic Surgery, Vanderbilt University Medical Center, A-1302 Medical Center North, Nashville, TN 37232, USA
e-mail: shreyas.joshi@vanderbilt.edu; sam.chang@vanderbilt.edu

G.P. Paner, M.D.
Department of Pathology and Surgery, Section of Urology, University of Chicago Medical Center, Chicago, IL 60637, USA
e-mail: gladell.paner@uchospitals.edu

© Springer Science+Business Media New York 2016
D.E. Hansel et al. (eds.), *The Kidney*, DOI 10.1007/978-1-4939-3286-3_2

of this locus in designated families failed to demonstrate its existence [6].

The progression of disease appears to differ based on which of the two genes is deficient. 85 % of ADPKD is accounted for by mutations in *PDK1*. These patients generally develop more aggressive disease, with 90 % of patients demonstrating cysts by age 20 and ESRD occurring by the 5th decade. *PDK2* mutations result in slower disease progression, with ESRD typically not occurring until the 7th decade, though there is extensive phenotypic variability even within groups with similar mutations [14].

Polycystin-1 and polycystin-2 are believed to form a functional transmembrane protein complex within the cilia of renal tubular cells; and when functioning properly, inhibit cell proliferation [7, 13, 15–17]. Polycystin-2 is required for the proper conformational maturation of polycystin-1, after which the complex acts in tandem to react to calcium-rich urine that passes through the renal tubules. The $Ca^{2+}$ channel contained on polycystin-2 is induced open by polycystin-1, initiating a process within the renal tubular cell that regulates cell proliferation. Multiple signaling pathways are then activated (including cAMP, MAPK/ERK, Src, among others), many of which have become therapeutic targets to interfere with cyst proliferation and disease progression [18, 19]. Intact, appropriately functioning cilia appear to be required for cyst growth in many cystic kidney diseases, but mutations altering appropriate cilia formation lead to abnormally activated cell proliferation. Thus, when mutated polycystins impede proper ciliary function, proliferative pathways go unopposed.

The formation of cysts occurs by secretion of fluid from the tubular epithelium lining the cyst wall. Fluid absorption occurs slower than secretion, causing the amount of cystic fluid to increase over time. This appears to be driven by certain cAMP pathways, but is directly the result of secondary active chloride transport [19].

Since ADPKD is genetically inherited, all cells will have the same mutation, though only a small percentage of glomerular units will ever be affected by cyst formation. Hence, although the disease is transmitted in an autosomal dominant fashion, it appears that a "second hit" to the complementary allele of *PDK1* or *PDK2* on the non-

diseased chromosome may be required for cyst formation [9, 20].

ADPKD can be inherited in conjunction with other systemic diseases, on the basis of its known genetic origins. For example, tuberous sclerosis is usually caused by a disruption of the *TSC2* gene, which happens to be proximally related to the *PDK1* locus on chromosome 16. Large mutations in this chromosomal neighborhood therefore affect both genes and lead to the renal cystic manifestations often seen in patients with tuberous sclerosis [9].

## Pathology

Grossly, the kidneys in the early stage of disease are normal in size and interrupted by occasional small cystic formations [21]. Fully affected kidneys in adults can be massively enlarged and diffusely involved by innumerable medullary and cortical cysts (Fig. 2.1). The cysts are rounded,

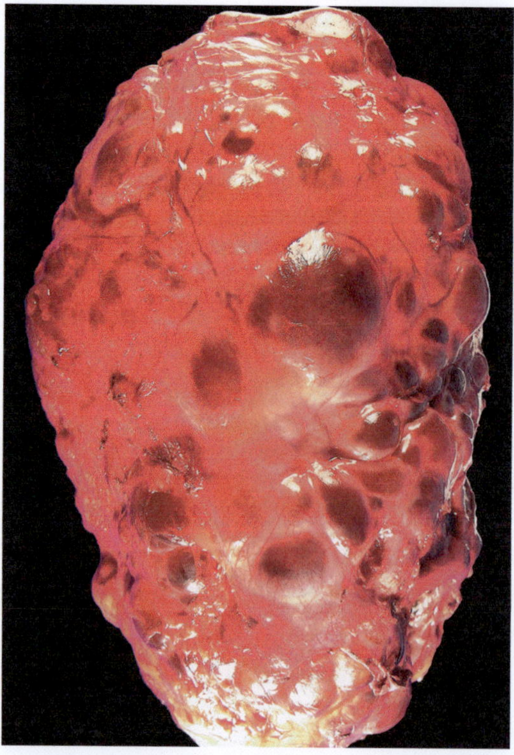

**Fig. 2.1** Autosomal dominant polycystic kidney disease. The kidney is massively enlarged with innumerable cysts

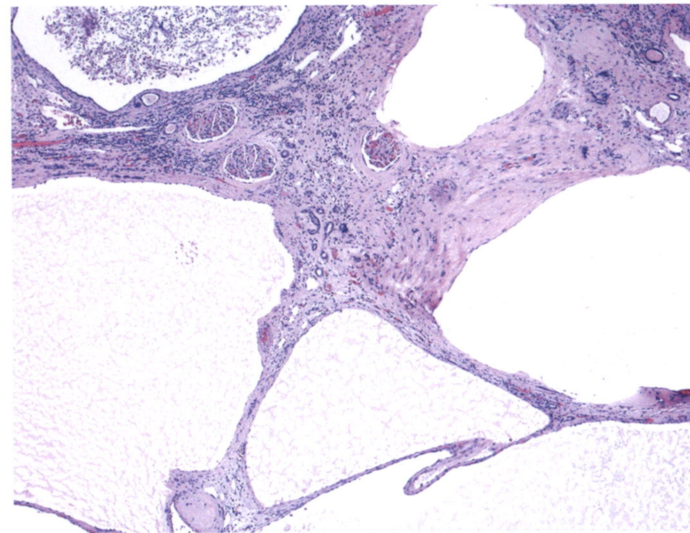

**Fig. 2.2** The cysts in ADPKD are unilocular with simple flat to cuboidal epithelial lining. The renal parenchyma exhibits interstitial fibrosis and chronic inflammation

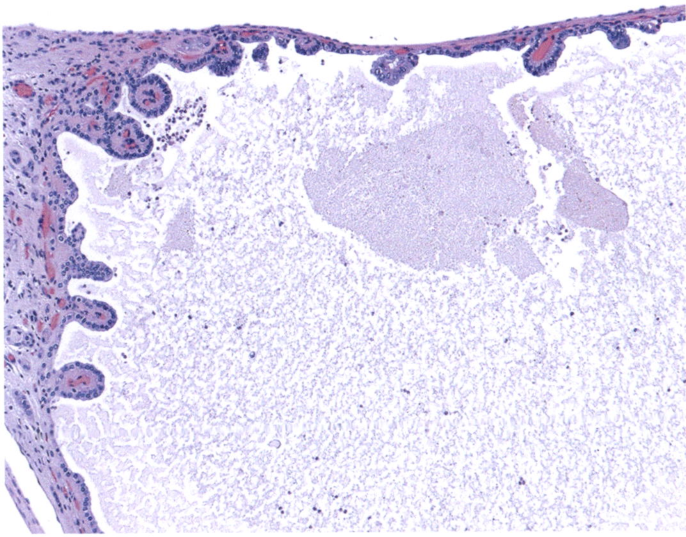

**Fig. 2.3** Simple papillary formations in the cyst lining of ADPKD

unilocular, and expansile, some up to several cm in size. The cysts have thin translucent walls and contain clear to yellowish or hemorrhagic fluid. Uncommonly, inflammatory abscess may form and calculi can be present. In about 1–5 % of resected ADPKD kidneys, a non-cystic or minimally-cystic mass of renal cell carcinoma is encountered [22]. The renal pelvis and ureter show no histoanatomic abnormality.

Histologically, the cysts are lined by a single layer of cuboidal or flattened epithelial cells (Fig. 2.2). Focal cellular proliferations and small papillary formations may develop along the cysts lining (Fig. 2.3). The intervening renal parenchyma in the early stages of cyst formations can be normal. Both tubular and glomerular cysts can be present [23]. In the advanced stage, the parenchyma is attenuated in between cysts and exhibits interstitial fibrosis, tubular atrophy, glomerular sclerosis, calcifications, and lymphocytic infiltrates. About two-thirds of the rare renal tumors arising in ADPKD exhibit a papillary phenotype (Fig. 2.4).

## Clinical Presentation

The phenotype of ADPKD can be highly variable despite the known genetic inheritance patterns

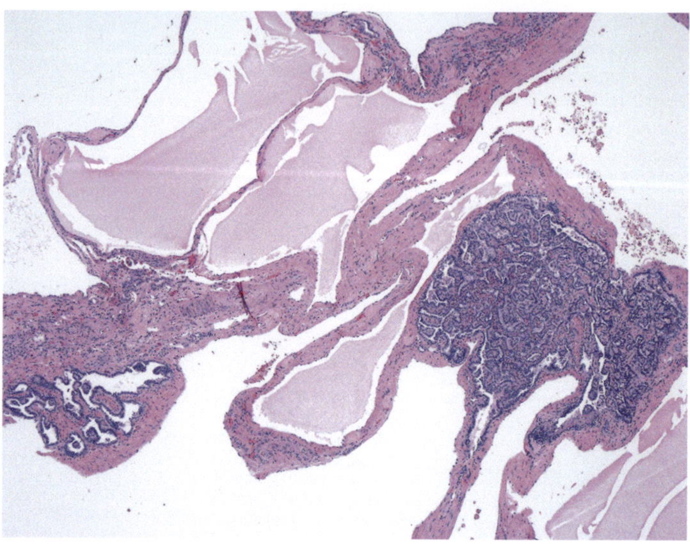

**Fig. 2.4** Papillary adenomas arising in ADPKD

caused by mutations in *PDK1/PDK2*. Aside from the "second-hit" theory of cyst formation, the genetic, hormonal, and environmental backgrounds of patients with ADPKD appear to affect disease manifestation. Characterization of these external factors is the subject of ongoing research [24].

Disease signs and symptoms usually begin between the 3rd and 5th decades of life for those with the *PDK1* gene mutation. The main presenting symptoms include flank pain, microscopic and/or gross hematuria, gastrointestinal discomfort, renal colic, and hypertension [25–28]. Up to 43 % of patients experience at least one episode of gross hematuria and 25 % report more than six episodes. Recurrent episodes of gross hematuria have been associated with an accelerated decline in renal function [29].

Pain is the most common presenting symptom, and its etiology is multifactorial. The size of the cysts and the location of the cysts with relation to other organs, the abdominal wall, and the renal collecting system can affect the type of pain a patient experiences. In full-blown ADPKD, each kidney can weigh several kilograms and occupy a large volume within the abdomen, displacing other organs. Furthermore, complications such as hemorrhage into cysts, infected cysts, urinary tract infections, and nephrolithiasis can make appropriate diagnosis and treatment

challenging. Up to 30 % of patients with ADPKD develop nephrolithiasis, though identifying obstruction and hydronephrosis can be difficult when multiple large cysts are present [30–32].

Hypertension is almost universally present in patients with ADPKD [28]. About half of all patients in their 2nd or 3rd decade will have hypertension with normal renal function, with an increasing incidence to 100 % by the time they acquire ESRD [33]. Several mechanisms have been proposed to explain the high prevalence of hypertension in this population, most of which involve the renin-angiotensin-mediated pathway activated by ischemic glomerular units. It is postulated that cyst growth causes stretching of intrarenal arteries and subsequent ischemia of the zones dependent on this vasculature [26]. As further ischemia occurs, renal dysfunction ensues and leads to worsening hypertension, which in turn leads to vascular remodeling and further decline in renal function.

Diagnosing ADPKD just from declining renal function is rare, as most renal function is preserved until the 4th–6th decade of life. However, the presence of enlarging cysts and/or enlarging kidneys is proportionately related to the decline in renal function. As such, monitoring kidney size may help alert clinicians of impending functional decline [34].

## Extrarenal Manifestations

Hepatic cysts are the most common extrarenal manifestation of ADPKD, and virtually all patients will exhibit some hepatic cyst formation by their 5th decade [35]. The hormonal influence of estrogen has been found to increase cyst formation and growth; the incidence of hepatic cysts is therefore higher in females than males [31, 36]. Although usually asymptomatic, hepatic cysts can rarely be responsible for mass effects, cyst hemorrhage, and portal hypertension from hepatic fibrosis, though portal hypertension is almost uniquely a finding of ARPKD [37].

Intracranial aneurysms (ICAs), or berry aneurysms, can be an immediately life-threatening extrarenal manifestation of ADPKD. 10–30 % of ADPKD patients exhibit ICAs, and the risk of aneurysm rupture increases significantly with poorly controlled hypertension [38, 39]. There is an increasing incidence with age; hence, it is proposed (though not universally practiced) that all patients older than 45 years of age get regular screening for ICAs [40]. ICAs form relatively quickly and are caused by a defect in the elastic lamina of vessel walls, allowing outward bulging that either ruptures or stabilizes due to collagenous remodeling. It is thought that ICAs <7 mm are less likely to grow or rupture, but since ADPKD results in wall protein deficiency (polycystins 1 and 2 are expressed in vascular smooth-muscle cells), the regular rules for ICAs may not apply [41]. ICA formation is a hypertension-independent event; thus, proper control of blood pressure is critical in preventing rupture [42]. The role of MRI screening for berry aneurysms is somewhat controversial, but evidence does seem to suggest that patients with a positive family history of ruptured ICAs and those with a *PDK1* genotype are at highest risk of mortality and should therefore be considered for earlier screening. Coronary and abdominal aortic aneurysms have also been associated with ADPKD; screening should be considered, especially for those on hemodialysis [43].

Seminal vesicle cysts (rare), arachnoid membrane cysts (5 %), pineal cysts (rare), pancreatic (10 %), and splenic cysts (5 %) may also be seen. Other abnormalities such as mitral valve prolapsed (26 %) and colonic diverticula (80 %) are also associated with ADPKD [44, 45].

## Diagnosis/Evaluation

Most patients will present after their 2nd or 3rd decade, but as mentioned previously, pediatric cases do arise. In these cases, radiographic characteristics may mimic ARPKD, and it may take time for macrocysts to appreciably develop. In these patients, an evaluation of family history is critical to making the correct diagnosis. Genetic testing should be discussed with members of the patient's family who are at risk for carrying the disease. All the usual implications of genetic counseling apply in ADPKD. The benefits of allowing for family planning and early intervention should be carefully weighed against the harms of psychological and psychosocial stress induced by knowing the diagnosis. Of particular interest in family genetic counseling is identifying related individuals who do not have the disease and can act as living-related organ donors. Pregnancy in patients with ADPKD can also potentially lead to more rapid progression toward ESRD and enlargement of hepatic cysts from estrogen effects. However, fertility itself is preserved, especially if renal function is normal [45].

In the index patient, one can use simple radiographic findings to guide the diagnosis. Renal ultrasound can be used with high sensitivity to guide diagnosis using the following criteria: the presence of at least two renal cysts (unilateral or bilateral) in individuals at risk and younger than 30, the presence of at least two cysts in each kidney for patients aged 30–59, and the presence of at least four cysts in each kidney in those above the age of 60 [46]. This results in a sensitivity of 100 % for those older than 30 years of age. However, caution should be exercised in patients younger than 30 with suspected *PDK2* mutations because ultrasound is only about 67 % sensitive in these cases; hence, further DNA linkage analysis would be prudent [47]. Occasionally, patients will present with predominantly extrarenal manifestations or with incidentally discovered cysts

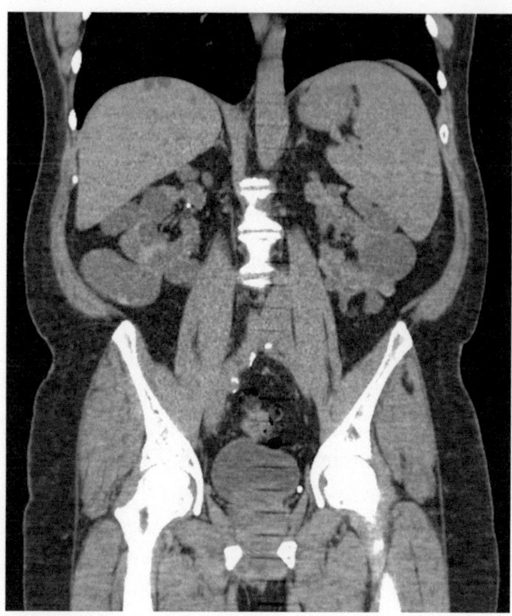

**Fig. 2.5** Coronal CT scan view of a patient with ADPKD. Note the derangement of normal renal architecture by innumerable large renal cysts. Some small liver cysts are also noted on this view

without a family history of disease. The diagnosis of ADPKD can be established with the presence of two or more renal cysts along with a polycystic liver, an ICA, or pancreatic cysts [45].

The use of axial imaging is not strictly necessary to diagnose ADPKD. However, CT and MRI can be useful adjuncts in the monitoring of disease progression or for assisting in the diagnosis of complicated presentations (Fig. 2.5). Contrasted CT imaging is useful in assessing hemorrhage within a cyst by demonstrating a predictable rise in contrast density [30]. Newer advances in MRI computing technology have the ability to segment individual renal cysts in ADPKD kidneys and provide a quantitative indicator of severity in early and moderate stages of disease [48]. MRI can also be an important tool to evaluate cystic lesions or hemorrhage in patients with advanced renal dysfunction who cannot receive the contrast load required for appropriate CT imaging.

Nocturia can sometimes be an early sign of decreased renal concentrating ability, and non-nephrotic proteinuria is present in ~33 % of patients with ADPKD. Recent advances in urinary proteomics have identified patterns that can aid in diagnosis and risk stratification with a sensitivity of 85 % and specificity of 94 %, with some biomarkers able to predict height-adjusted total kidney volume [49]. Assessing total kidney volume (TKV) is an important step in evaluating and monitoring these patients, as TKV has been confirmed as a clinically meaningful surrogate marker in ADPKD [50]. This metric was established by the Consortium for Radiological Imaging in Studies of Polycystic Kidney Disease (CRISP Study), which helped identify markers of disease progression. It was found that patients with higher rates of kidney enlargement and overall larger TKV have a more rapid decline in kidney function and should be monitored more closely [51].

In patients with a family history of ruptured ICAs, cranial MRI is appropriate to identify asymptomatic patients with ICAs. Some authors recommend screening all ADPKD patients above the age of 45 due to a prevalence of ICAs of up to 22 % in this age group. Older patients generally have an increased risk of rupture, especially in the setting of poorly controlled hypertension [40]. Although ICA rupture is considerably rarer in younger patients, identification and early management of an ICA in a younger patient would lead to the greatest benefit in life expectancy. However, it remains unclear if the natural history of aneurysm formation, growth, and rupture-risk parallels that of the general population; and thus more data are still required before definitive radiographic guidelines can be established to screen for ICAs [41, 52].

In some patients with recurrent upper tract or cyst infections, prompt treatment is imperative but can be hindered by difficulty in evaluation. Definitive diagnosis requires evaluation of cyst fluid, but a probable diagnosis can be made if all four of the following criteria are met: temperature >38C for >3 days, loin or liver tenderness, C-reactive protein plasma level of >5 mg/dL, and no evidence for intracystic bleeding on CT. Positron-emission tomography (PET) after intravenous injection of 18-fluorodeoxyglucose (PET/CT) has also been studied as a more reliable imaging modality when evaluating for the presence of pyocysts [53].

## Sequelae

Cyst infections, UTIs, nephrolithiasis, chronic pain, hematuria, progression to ESRD, and a possible increased risk of renal malignancy are all sequelae for which these patients should be monitored and counseled.

The progression to end-stage renal disease (ESRD) is an important clinical outcome that must be evaluated in all patients once the diagnosis of ADPKD is established. eGFR declines rapidly in the decade preceding ESRD, at a rate of 4.4–5.9 ml/min/year; and a 30-year retrospective analysis from the United Kingdom demonstrated that a decline in eGFR can be seen as early as 20 years prior to ESRD, affording an earlier ability to stratify for patients that will have a more aggressive decline in renal function [54]. A combination of serum chemistries and radiographic follow-up is the ideal method to monitor this decline, and management by Nephrology is mandatory to preserve renal function for as long as possible. About half of patients with ADPKD will eventually progress to ESRD.

There is a small risk of hepatic dysfunction in these patients, though the mechanism is likely not directly related to ADPKD. Hepatic cysts are usually asymptomatic; but in rare cases, such as women in whom cyst growth can be greater, direct compression of the portal vein can result in portal hypertension [37]. Portal hypertension can also be a symptom of primary hepatic fibrosis. Unlike in the autosomal recessive disease, ADPKD is not thought to be directly associated with primary hepatic fibrosis. Nonetheless, there can be a concomitant diagnosis of hepatic fibrosis, especially with a perinatal diagnosis of ADPKD.

The incidence of renal cell carcinoma (RCC) in patients with ADPKD has been a matter of debate in the literature. The incidence of renal adenomas is 1 in 4–5 patients, similar to the incidence seen in patients with cystic disease related to dialysis [9]. The combination of ADPKD and dialysis is thought to raise the incidence of RCC up to 2–3 times the frequency seen in ESRD patients without ADPKD [22, 55]. However, ADPKD patients without ESRD appear to have a similar RCC incidence as the general population.

In a retrospective analysis of 240 ADPKD patients who underwent renal surgeries, 12 (5 %) patients presented with malignant lesions. Two-thirds of these patients had undergone dialysis prior to surgery. Of the malignant tumors identified, 63 % were papillary RCC, 31 % were clear cell RCC, and 6 % had papillary noninvasive urothelial carcinoma [22]. Other characteristics associated with ADPKD patients who develop RCC include diagnosis at a younger age, bilateral tumors (12 % vs. 1–5 % in the general population), multicentric tumors (28 % vs. 6 % in the general population), and sarcomatoid histologic features (33 % vs. 1–5 % in the general population) [56].

Importantly, retrospective series studying the incidence of RCC in ADPKD patients are limited by the small numbers of patients who actually develop malignant lesions. However, it seems apparent that the combination of ADPKD and ESRD with at least 1 year of dialysis does confer a greater risk of developing malignant lesions [55]. Unfortunately, a variety of clinical features of the disease may mask or prevent diagnosis of malignant lesions, including cystic distortion impairing imaging quality, cystic hemorrhage, and proteinaceous debris, all of which are common findings in regular ADPKD kidneys.

## Treatments

The common theme for all treatments is to prevent secondary or downstream effects of the disease, such as hypertension, pain, infection, and ESRD. Appropriately controlling hypertension is likely the most important factor in preventing future morbidity. As discussed, uncontrolled hypertension is a harbinger for rapidly declining renal function, unstable berry aneurysms, and significant cardiovascular disease. The use of antihypertensives, specifically ACE inhibitors, appears to be the most effective way to manage blood pressure, especially when considering that hypertension from ADPKD is most likely a renin-based phenomenon. The recently published HALT-PKD study evaluated the combined use of renin-angiotensin agents and blood pressure targets on total kidney volume growth, estimated GFR, and urinary albumin excretion [19, 57]. Findings suggest that the combination of an ACE inhibitor (lisinopril) + angiotensin receptor blocker (telmisartan) had no significant benefit versus standard blood pressure management, which normally includes just an ACE inhibitor. Interestingly, the lower blood pressure group (95/60 to 110/75 mmHg), as compared to the standard blood pressure group (120/70 to 130/80 mmHg) had a slower increase in total kidney volume and greater reduction in urinary albumin secretion, but did not affect estimated GFR [58]. These findings seem to suggest that tight blood pressure regulation in ADPKD patients may slow the progression of disease.

Many patients will inevitably require dialysis for ESRD. Obviously, patients who require unilateral or bilateral nephrectomy, such as for mass effect or tumors, are at highest risk for needing renal replacement. However, a gradual progression to ESRD can be predicted for many symptomatic patients, and early planning and discussion with patients can help when decisions are required regarding renal replacement. Guidelines for renal transplant vary by geographic location, but should be considered when appropriate.

Clinicians should be aggressive in treating stones and infections. Patients with ADPKD almost universally have chronic pain, which can complicate the diagnosis and clinical presentation of treatable pathologies. Although these patients almost universally have chronic pain, there should be a high risk of suspicion for obstruction (from stones or cyst compression) when patients present with acute pain. Prompt treatment of the offending pathology can help save renal function. Pain should be managed carefully in this population, since opioid dependence is common and even surgical intervention may not completely alleviate symptoms. Nephrotoxins such as nonsteroidal anti-inflammatories (NSAIDs) should be avoided as much as possible.

The prevalence of kidney stones in this patient population appears to be greater than in the general population. ADPKD patients more prone to stone formation are those with lower eGFR and more/larger renal cysts. Metabolic evaluation in ADPKD stone formers tends to demonstrate lower urinary volumes and lower levels of urinary phosphate, magnesium, potassium, and citrate. Prevention of stone formation in these patients requires attention to metabolic factors (increasing stone inhibitors such as water, magnesium, and citrate) and structural factors (preventing large cyst formation) [32].

Some patients, especially women, are at high risk of developing upper tract infections and should be treated aggressively with IV antibiotics for pyelonephritis. Occasionally, infections can be harbored in noncommunicating cysts and will need to be surgically drained or percutaneously aspirated.

Very large cysts causing clinical symptoms can be managed in a variety of ways. They occasionally require surgical unroofing (usually done laparoscopically) or percutaneous aspiration with chemical ablation [59]. Nephrectomy may be an appropriate step in patients with severe pain who have already developed ESRD [60]. Open surgical excision via a lumbodorsal or abdominal midline incision has been described as an effective way to remove very large kidneys. However, improvements in laparoscopic techniques have allowed laparoscopic surgeons to effectively and safely perform a nephrectomy on many of these patients [61].

There are a variety of medical therapies being tested to control the primary disease process. Many of these treatments are aimed at decreasing intracellular cAMP, which is produced as a result of overproduction of vasopressin in ADPKD patients [62–65]. cAMP contributes to cyst and kidney enlargement and subsequent renal dysfunction. Tolvaptan, a V2 receptor antagonist that downregulates cAMP production, was shown to slow the increase in TKV, but unfortunately did not improve eGFR [66].

Somatostatin analogs, such as octreotide, have been found to inhibit cAMP pathways that lead to fluid secretion into cysts. A randomized clinical trial studying the effectiveness of somatostatins showed that it slowed kidney and liver growth, improved patient health perception, and was well tolerated [67].

The mammalian target of rapamycin (mTOR)inhibitors sirolimus and everolimus have each been studied in RCTs [68, 69]. Both had a relatively short follow-up period (~2 years), making it difficult to determine the long-term effect of mTOR inhibition. Nonetheless, everolimus did appear to decrease total kidney growth compared to placebo, though the effect on eGFR decline was unclear [68, 70]. Several antineoplastic drugs have been tested, including lonidamine and curcumin, with the idea that abnormal proliferative pathways in ADPKD kidneys can be generically targeted. Though these drugs have met with limited experimental success, it awaits to be seen if they play a role in the medical management of ADPKD in the future. Other possible therapies have focused on the cystoprotein complexes involved in aberrant signaling cascades, such as the Src pathway. Metformin, a commonly used oral diabetic agent, may activate AMP-activated protein kinase, thereby inhibiting CFTR and mTOR pathways that are responsible for downstream cyst formation [19]. Inhibition of HSP90 has been shown to induce degradation of many ADPKD-relevant genes in mouse models. This was associated with a decrease in cyst formation and improved renal function, which is a promising lead for future investigation [7].

Unfortunately, no current medical therapies have shown a significant effect on the overall progression of disease. For this reason, it is essential that patients be monitored for secondary effects of the disease, such as hypertension and other above-mentioned pathologies that can decrease the severity of consequent morbidity.

## Prognosis

Though the disease has a very heterogeneous phenotypic presentation, patients who are managed appropriately can have excellent long-term health. In a 30-year natural-history retrospective analysis of patients with ADPKD, investigators were able to demonstrate that the rate of eGFR change can predict progression to ESRD as much as 10 years before onset. It is therefore critical to continually assess renal function once the diagnosis of ADPKD is established. The analysis also showed that the rate of eGFR change can be predicted by mean kidney length and patient's age at the time of diagnosis [54]. Patients diagnosed at a later age have a slower rate of renal function decline than do patients who are diagnosed young, which supports the idea that early manifestation of the disease may indicate more aggressive clinical progression.

Monitoring for hypertension, infections, and, in select patients, intracranial vascular aneurysms is key to long-term health. A multidisciplinary approach should be used when managing these patients, including a primary care physician, Nephrologist, and Urologist. Patient education about the disease process and prognosis can greatly aid in early identification of treatable pathologies.

## Autosomal Recessive Polycystic Kidney Disease

### Background

Autosomal recessive polycystic kidney disease (ARPKD) is a rare but severe congenital hepatorenal disease that affects an estimated 1 in 20,000 live births [71]. It is a neonatal disease characterized by symmetric, massively enlarged kidneys and congenital hepatic fibrosis that presents with varying clinical severity. Typical disease presentation occurs in neonates and includes fetal oligohydramnios, massively enlarged kidneys, and "Potter" sequence abnormalities, such as pulmonary hypoplasia and severe respiratory insufficiency [72]. Perinatal death occurs in 30–50 % of affected newborns [73, 74]. For those who survive the perinatal period, long-term survival depends on the degree of renal and hepatic dysfunction. One-year survival has been reported as high as 92–95 % for those who survive the first month of life [72]. Systemic hypertension, pulmonary hypertension, impaired nutrition from GI mass effect, pulmonary insufficiency, and neurocognitive dysfunction are all sequelae that can greatly affect the morbidity associated with the disease in survivors [75].

ARPKD is thought to be in a similar class as a host of other hepatorenal fibrocystic diseases, such as ADPKD, Joubert syndrome, Bardet-

Biedl syndrome, glomerulocystic disease, renal-hepatic-pancreatic dysplasia, and Zellweger syndrome, just to name a few [75]. The common thread is that they all have defects localized to primary cilia/basal body structures, which in turn appears to result in similar hepatorenal dysfunction.

The implicated gene, *PKHD1*, is now required for the diagnosis of ARPKD, especially given its overlap with other syndromes. The recent discovery of this gene has allowed clinicians to better understand the heterogeneity of disease presentation, and is helping elucidate better molecular targets for future treatments [76, 77]. The improved genetic understanding of the disease has also changed the psychosocial impact the diagnosis has on families. Since families can now be tested for the implicated gene mutations, they can face difficult decisions with regard to future reproduction. As such, a multidisciplinary approach to disease management is critical when a patient is diagnosed with ARPKD.

## Genetics/Pathogenesis

ARPKD is transmitted in the usual autosomal recessive pattern. Although newer genetic testing can identify the majority of mutant alleles for diagnostic purposes, appropriate pedigrees should be constructed for at least three generations to identify the carriers of the diseased alleles. ARPKD is caused by mutations to *PKHD1*, a large gene with a very complex splicing pattern that is located on chromosome 6p21.1-p12 [76, 77]. The gene product is fibrocystin/polyductin (FPC), a transmembrane protein that is expressed predominantly in renal collecting ducts, the thick ascending loops of Henle, pancreatic tissues, and hepatic bile duct epithelia [4, 76, 78].

Although the exact function of FPC is unclear, it is known to localize to ciliary/basal body structures and apical membranes, which associates it with other diseases caused by ciliary defects that manifest in hepatorenal fibrocystic disease. The exact molecular mechanism of pathogenesis is unclear, though the complex does interact with polycystin-2, one of the ADPKD genes.

*PKHD1* is a long gene that is susceptible to a large variety of mutations along its entire length, the majority of which are missense mutations or truncations. Over 300 mutations are currently known, though there are likely more that spontaneously form [75]. Given the heterogeneity of mutations, most patients with ARPKD are actually compound heterozygotes and carry two different mutant alleles, contributing to the large variation in disease phenotypes. Many patients are found to have novel mutations when genetic analysis is completed, making interpretation and prognostication of disease severity difficult.

## Pathology

Both kidneys in lethal neonatal form are massively enlarged although their reniform configuration is generally maintained [79, 80]. Numerous cysts derived from the collecting ducts are present in the medulla and inner cortex that impart a spongy appearance. These cysts in neonates are elongated (in contrast to the rounded cysts in ADPKD) and are characteristically oriented perpendicular to the renal cortex ("radial rays"). The cysts are lined by small cuboidal epithelial cells. Most cysts represent ectatic collecting ducts, although glomerular cysts may also be present [23]. In infantile and childhood cases, the involved kidneys can be smaller with variable round to elongated cysts that are more consistent in the medulla than in the cortex. The intervening renal parenchyma is usually normal, but those in older patients may have interstitial fibrosis, tubular atrophy, and glomerular sclerosis. Due to the variable cysts and parenchymal changes, some childhood ARPKD may histologically resemble ADPKD. The renal pelvis and ureter are normal. In the liver, the portal tracts characteristically exhibit bile duct proliferation and irregular anastomosis associated with fibrosis.

## Clinical Presentation

Patients may present with prenatal oligohydramnios from poor renal function and subsequent pulmonary hypoplasia with severe respiratory compromise. Prenatal ultrasounds will usually detect bilateral, massively enlarged, echogenic kidneys, though normal-appearing kidneys do not rule out the presence of disease. Many infants are born with "Potter" facies and limb deformities. Perinatal death is usually secondary to respiratory compromise or uremia [81]. Though ARPKD has considerable phenotypic variability, patients diagnosed at an earlier age generally have more severe and life-threatening disease burden. All patients will have histologic biliary abnormalities and hepatic fibrosis [82].

Initial presentation in some infants will include kidneys so large that they impede delivery or quickly cause pulmonary compromise by preventing diaphragmatic excursion. Impaired nutrition from GI compression can also occur, and a small proportion of patients will require early unilateral or bilateral nephrectomy to improve ventilation and/or nutrition. Given the severity of early complications and the potential need for early life-saving interventions, it is advisable to involve palliative-care providers and/or medical ethicists soon after diagnosis to assist providers and family members with the difficult decisions required after the birth of an affected neonate.

Most patients will progress to ESRD, and the age at ARPKD diagnosis is a significant predictor of the rate of renal functional decline. The consequences of chronic renal insufficiency from ARPKD are similar to any other disease-causing renal insufficiency in children. Common findings in surviving patients include growth failure, anemia, osteodystrophy, and renal calcifications. Obviously, many of these findings become more evident as the child ages.

Systemic hypertension can cause considerable morbidity in children and is usually severe enough to require multidrug therapy for control [72]. Some studies have indicated an intrarenal renin-angiotensin-pathway activation, thus leading to the reliance on ACE inhibitors and angiotensin receptor blockers for appropriate blood pressure management.

Hyponatremia from inadequate urine dilution is common in early infancy, though the prevalence of this varies by cohort. There does appear to be an increased risk of urinary tract infections in children with ARPKD, which may be a result of urinary stasis in the cystic collecting duct units.

Hepatobiliary manifestations are universal and are developmentally referred to as "ductal plate malformations" [83]. The ciliary and epithelial defects in the portal tree lead to progressively dilated intrahepatic bile ducts that eventually become cysts. Portal tract fibrosis will lead to portal hypertension and its associated complications, such as hypersplenism and variceal dilation. In a large cohort of 73 patients with ARPKD, 70 % had clinically relevant biliary abnormalities. Platelet count was found to be the best predictor of portal hypertension severity, which can be a useful clinical tool to monitor surviving patients [84]. Interestingly, liver enzymes tend to remain normal and are generally not well correlated with the degree of hepatic fibrosis or portal hypertension.

Ascending cholangitis in these patients can be severe and life threatening. Unresponsive, recurrent cholangitis can be an indication to proceed to liver transplantation when antibiotic suppression repeatedly fails [85].

## Diagnosis/Evaluation

Prenatal ultrasound findings will usually identify symmetrically enlarged, echogenic kidneys with a loss of corticomedullary differentiation [86]. Hyperechogenicity is owed to the microscopic cysts that are formed from the tightly compacted and dilated collecting ducts throughout the kidney. This causes innumerable interfaces that produce their characteristic ultrasonographic appearance (Fig. 2.6). Because of this echogenicity, the ability to differentiate cortex from medulla also becomes obscured, as does the ability to predict the health of the kidneys in utero. Some variants of severe ADPKD can also present with similarly hyperechoic-appearing neonatal kidneys, and the correct diagnosis requires genetic confirmation of the diseased gene. Unlike ARPKD, however, ADPKD more typically presents with larger cysts and asymmetric kidney sizes at birth. Rarely ARPKD kidneys can develop macrocysts, though usually less than 1 cm [87]. Further complicating the diagnosis, hepatic fibrosis has been known to occur in ADPKD patients and brain aneurysms have been reported in ARKPD patients [88, 89].

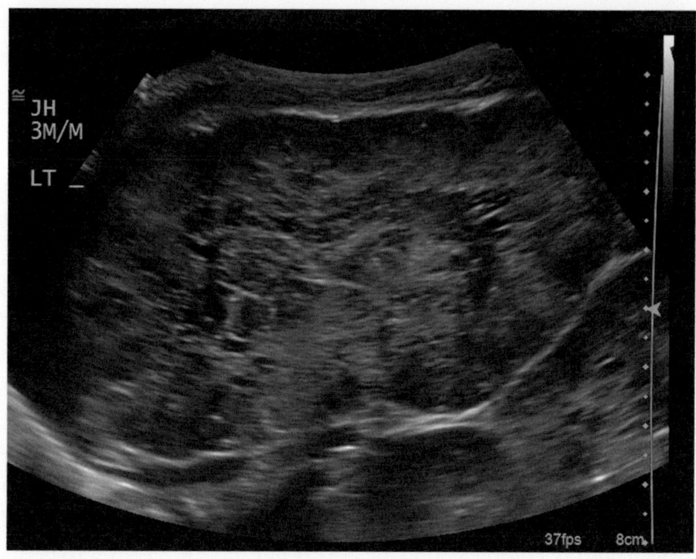

**Fig. 2.6** Longitudinal view of left kidney. Note enlarged, echogenic kidney with loss of corticomedullary differentiation. There are innumerable dilated renal tubules and macrocysts present within the renal parenchyma

Perinatal ultrasound is useful for initially helping make the diagnosis of ARPKD, but no imaging modality has been shown to reliably monitor the progression of disease. Kidney size is not clearly correlated with function in ARPKD, unlike in patients with ADPKD. Portal ultrasounds can be useful in determining the degree of portal hypertension present, including the presence of hypersplenism and variceal dilatation. MRI of abdominal structures may also be useful in some cases, but this modality has limited prognostic value.

For those patients that survive the neonatal period, monitoring renal function and blood pressure is critical to preventing long-term morbidity and early mortality. The goal of therapy in these patients is to preserve renal and hepatic function for as long as possible. Complications from portal hypertension can be managed conservatively, though many patients with progressive hepatic fibrosis will eventually need liver transplantation when older.

## Treatment/Prognosis

No cure exists for ARPKD. However, for the subset of patients who are lucky to survive the perinatal period, medical management can now allow many to survive into adulthood. Patients that are diagnosed beyond the neonatal period may have primarily hepatic manifestations of the disease and are sometimes managed quite differently than the stereotypical ARPKD patient. For all patients surviving past the 1st month of life, several important systemic manifestations of the disease must be identified and treated aggressively. These include growth impairment, hypertension, and neurocognitive delays. Of course, the mainstay of treatment consists of early and appropriate management of renal impairment and minimizing the sequelae of hepatic dysfunction/portal hypertension.

Hypertension management starts early in life for most patients. The probability of requiring antihypertensive treatment for those surviving the 1st month of life is roughly 39 % at 1 year and 60 % at 15 years [73]. However, when followed closely, multidrug regimens consisting of drugs that target the renin-angiotensin pathway can effectively manage systemic hypertension throughout childhood.

Portal hypertension, recurrent cholangitis, severe Caroli disease (dilatation of intra- and/or extrahepatic bile ducts), hypersplenism, cholestasis, and bleeding gastroesophageal varices can be managed in a variety of fashions. The early use of decompressive procedures, such as splenorenal shunts, can extend the lifespan of a patient's native liver function. Esophageal varices can be managed with endoscopic sclerotherapy or, in severe cases, gastric section and reanastamosis. Rarely, patients will progress to end-stage liver disease before progressing to ESRD. Many patients will eventually fit the criteria to receive both renal and liver transplants. The decision to perform a renal transplant alone versus a combined renal/liver transplant poses a particularly challenging clinical dilemma; experts have helped objectify this process by creating decision trees to assist clinicians when determining the type of transplant a patient should receive [85]. Promisingly, studies of patients with ARPKD who underwent combined transplants have reported patient survival rates of 70–100 %, demonstrating that transplants in carefully selected patients can be a safe and effective therapy [90, 91].

Unilateral or bilateral nephrectomy is often necessary due to mass effect early in life. However, this must clearly be weighed against the morbidity associated with dialysis and can be a difficult decision for parents and clinicians to make. The decision to perform nephrectomy should be guided by clinical necessity rather than as primary treatment for the disease.

Progression to ESRD in patients able to preserve their kidneys appears to be dependent on age at diagnosis. In one large cohort of neonatal survivors, renal survival (lack of need for dialysis/transplantation) was 86 % at 5 years, but decreased to 42 % by 20 years [92]. Another cohort demonstrated that the renal survival rate 20 years after diagnosis was 36 % if ARPKD was diagnosed before the age of 1, but was as high as 80 % for those diagnosed after the age of 1 [93]. Hemodialysis can be effectively performed in older patients, but peritoneal dialysis may be preferable in younger children (though peritoneal disruption from prior surgery can complicate this).

Growth impairment occurs in a large percentage of ARPKD children, likely as a consequence of combined renal dysfunction and nutritional deficiencies. These children have been successfully treated with growth hormone, similar to treatment regimens given to children with other forms of CKD [94]. Neurocognitive and behav-

ioral issues are common in ARPKD patients. The combination of CKD and severe hypertension during important neurodevelopmental periods put these children at significant risk of abnormal neurocognitive development. Early behavioral therapy and psychosocial referrals are necessary to maintain appropriate neurological and psychological development as these patients age.

Ongoing translational research is trying to identify molecular targets that can blunt the effects of the disease. ARPKD and ADPKD share multiple molecular pathways that lead to pathogenesis, including mTOR pathway activation [95]. Upregulation of cAMP production by vasopressin V2 receptor activation has also been shown to play a role in both disease states. Tolvaptan, a V2 receptor antagonist, has been shown to slow the rate of renal enlargement in ADPKD patients but has not been tested yet on human ARPKD patients. Somatostatin analogs have shown some benefit in slowing kidney and liver cyst growth in ADPKD and are a potential avenue for clinical trials in ARPKD patients. Improved understanding of the gene mutations and dysregulated molecular pathways will hopefully allow new therapies to slow disease progression in the future. Greater understanding of the FPC protein will also hopefully define better targets to help monitor disease progression.

Lastly, clinicians caring for ARPKD patients should be mindful of the psychosocial ramifications for affected families. Suspicion of ARPKD by prenatal ultrasound may be necessary information for families who choose to pursue genetic testing when considering possible pregnancy termination. Genetic counselors, ethicists, social workers, and psychologists can all be helpful in assisting families with these difficult decisions. Some carrier families may also choose to undergo preimplantation genetic diagnosis as a means to select for embryos that do not carry the mutant *PKHD1* allele(s). Surviving children are at risk for severe renal and hepatic disease that impairs their health-related quality of life and can place heavy burdens on caretakers. Early multidisciplinary care of the patient and his/her caretakers should be coordinated by the primary medical provider.

## References


1. Iglesias CG, Torres VE, Offord KP, Holley KE, Beard CM, Kurland LT. Epidemiology of adult polycystic kidney disease, Olmsted County, Minnesota: 1935–1980. Am J Kidney Dis. 1983;2(6):630–9.
2. Grantham JJ. The etiology, pathogenesis, and treatment of autosomal dominant polycystic kidney disease: recent advances. Am J Kidney Dis. 1996;28(6):788–803.
3. Hildebrandt F. Genetic renal diseases in children. Curr Opin Pediatr. 1995;7(2):182–91.
4. Wilson PD. Polycystic kidney disease: new understanding in the pathogenesis. Int J Biochem Cell Biol. 2004;36(10):1868–73.
5. Gabow PA. Polycystic kidney disease: clues to pathogenesis. Kidney Int. 1991;40(6):989–96.
6. Paul BM, Consugar MB, Ryan Lee M, Sundsbak JL, Heyer CM, Rossetti S, Kubly VJ, Hopp K, Torres VE, Coto E, et al. Evidence of a third ADPKD locus is not supported by re-analysis of designated PKD3 families. Kidney Int. 2013;85:383–92.
7. Seeger-Nukpezah T, Proia DA, Egleston BL, Nikonova AS, Kent T, Cai KQ, Hensley HH, Ying W, Chimmanamada D, Serebriiskii IG, et al. Inhibiting the HSP90 chaperone slows cyst growth in a mouse model of autosomal dominant polycystic kidney disease. Proc Natl Acad Sci U S A. 2013;110(31):12786–91.
8. Proesmans W, Van Damme B, Casaer P, Marchal G. Autosomal dominant polycystic kidney disease in the neonatal period: association with a cerebral arteriovenous malformation. Pediatrics. 1982;70(6):971–5.
9. Wein AJ, Kavoussi LR, Novick AC, Partin AW, Peters CA (2011) Campbell-Walsh urology tenth edition, 10th revised ed. Elsevier, Philadelphia.
10. Breuning MH, Reeders ST, Brunner H, Ijdo JW, Saris JJ, Verwest A, van Ommen GJ, Pearson PL. Improved early diagnosis of adult polycystic kidney disease with flanking DNA markers. Lancet. 1987;2(8572):1359–61.
11. Reeders ST, Breuning MH, Davies KE, Nicholls RD, Jarman AP, Higgs DR, Pearson PL, Weatherall DJ. A highly polymorphic DNA marker linked to adult polycystic kidney disease on chromosome 16. Nature. 1985;317(6037):542–4.
12. Ryynanen M, Dolata MM, Lampainen E, Reeders ST. Localisation of a mutation producing autosomal dominant polycystic kidney disease without renal failure. J Med Genet. 1987;24(8):462–5.
13. Qian F, Watnick TJ, Onuchic LF, Germino GG. The molecular basis of focal cyst formation in human autosomal dominant polycystic kidney disease type I. Cell. 1996;87(6):979–87.
14. Hateboer N, van Dijk MA, Bogdanova N, Coto E, Saggar-Malik AK, San Millan JL, Torra R, Breuning M, Ravine D. Comparison of phenotypes of polycystic kidney disease types 1 and 2. European PKD1-PKD2 Study Group. Lancet. 1999;353(9147):103–7.
15. Braun WE. Autosomal dominant polycystic kidney disease: emerging concepts of pathogenesis and new treatments. Cleve Clin J Med. 2009;76(2):97–104.
16. Nauli SM, Alenghat FJ, Luo Y, Williams E, Vassilev P, Li X, Elia AE, Lu W, Brown EM, Quinn SJ, et al. Polycystins 1 and 2 mediate mechanosensation in the primary cilium of kidney cells. Nat Genet. 2003;33(2):129–37.
17. Oatley P, Talukder MM, Stewart AP, Sandford R, Edwardson JM. Polycystin-2 induces a conformational change in polycystin-1. Biochemistry. 2013;52:5280–7.
18. Pazour GJ. Intraflagellar transport and cilia-dependent renal disease: the ciliary hypothesis of polycystic kidney disease. J Am Soc Nephrol. 2004;15(10):2528–36.
19. Steinman TI. Polycystic kidney disease: a 2011 update. Curr Opin Nephrol Hypertens. 2012;21(2):189–94.
20. Knudson Jr AG. Mutation and cancer: statistical study of retinoblastoma. Proc Natl Acad Sci U S A. 1971;68(4):820–3.
21. Bisceglia M, Galliani CA, Senger C, Stallone C, Sessa A. Renal cystic diseases: a review. Adv Anat Pathol. 2006;13(1):26–56.
22. Jilg CA, Drendel V, Bacher J, Pisarski P, Neeff H, Drognitz O, Schwardt M, Glasker S, Malinoc A, Erlic Z, et al. Autosomal dominant polycystic kidney disease: prevalence of renal neoplasias in surgical kidney specimens. Nephron Clin Pract. 2013;123(1–2):13–21.
23. Lennerz JK, Spence DC, Iskandar SS, Dehner LP, Liapis H. Glomerulocystic kidney: one hundred-year perspective. Arch Pathol Lab Med. 2010;134(4):583–605.
24. Rossetti S, Harris PC. Genotype-phenotype correlations in autosomal dominant and autosomal recessive polycystic kidney disease. J Am Soc Nephrol. 2007;18(5):1374–80.
25. Delaney VB, Adler S, Bruns FJ, Licinia M, Segel DP, Fraley DS. Autosomal dominant polycystic kidney disease: presentation, complications, and prognosis. Am J Kidney Dis. 1985;5(2):104–11.
26. Gabow PA. Autosomal dominant polycystic kidney disease. N Engl J Med. 1993;329(5):332–42.
27. Milutinovic J, Fialkow PJ, Agodoa LY, Phillips LA, Rudd TG, Bryant JI. Autosomal dominant polycystic kidney disease: symptoms and clinical findings. Q J Med. 1984;53(212):511–22.
28. Zeier M, Geberth S, Ritz E, Jaeger T, Waldherr R. Adult dominant polycystic kidney disease – clinical problems. Nephron. 1988;49(3):177–83.
29. Gabow PA, Duley I, Johnson AM. Clinical profiles of gross hematuria in autosomal dominant polycystic kidney disease. Am J Kidney Dis. 1992;20(2):140–3.
30. Choyke PL, Glenn GM, Walther MM, Patronas NJ, Linehan WM, Zbar B. von Hippel-Lindau disease: genetic, clinical, and imaging features. Radiology. 1995;194(3):629–42.
31. Fick GM, Johnson AM, Gabow PA. Is there evidence for anticipation in autosomal-dominant polycystic kidney disease? Kidney Int. 1994;45(4):1153–62.

32. Grampsas SA, Chandhoke PS, Fan J, Glass MA, Townsend R, Johnson AM, Gabow P. Anatomic and metabolic risk factors for nephrolithiasis in patients with autosomal dominant polycystic kidney disease. Am J Kidney Dis. 2000;36(1):53–7.

33. Kelleher CL, McFann KK, Johnson AM, Schrier RW. Characteristics of hypertension in young adults with autosomal dominant polycystic kidney disease compared with the general U.S. population. Am J Hypertens. 2004;17(11 Pt 1):1029–34.

34. Gabow PA, Chapman AB, Johnson AM, Tangel DJ, Duley IT, Kaehny WD, Manco-Johnson M, Schrier RW. Renal structure and hypertension in autosomal dominant polycystic kidney disease. Kidney Int. 1990;38(6):1177–80.

35. Bae KT, Zhu F, Chapman AB, Torres VE, Grantham JJ, Guay-Woodford LM, Baumgarten DA, King Jr BF, Wetzel LH, Kenney PJ, et al. Magnetic resonance imaging evaluation of hepatic cysts in early autosomal-dominant polycystic kidney disease: the Consortium for Radiologic Imaging Studies of Polycystic Kidney Disease cohort. Clin J Am Soc Nephrol. 2006;1(1):64–9.

36. Sherstha R, McKinley C, Russ P, Scherzinger A, Bronner T, Showalter R, Everson GT. Postmenopausal estrogen therapy selectively stimulates hepatic enlargement in women with autosomal dominant polycystic kidney disease. Hepatology. 1997;26(5):1282–6.

37. Campbell GS, Bick HD, Varco RL, Paulsen EP, Lober PH, Watson CJ. Bleeding esophageal varices with polycystic liver: report of three cases. N Engl J Med. 1958;259(19):904–10.

38. Ryu SJ. Intracranial hemorrhage in patients with polycystic kidney disease. Stroke. 1990;21(2):291–4.

39. Wakabayashi T, Fujita S, Ohbora Y, Suyama T, Tamaki N, Matsumoto S. Polycystic kidney disease and intracranial aneurysms. Early angiographic diagnosis and early operation for the unruptured aneurysm. J Neurosurg. 1983;58(4):488–91.

40. Niemczyk M, Gradzik M, Niemczyk S, Bujko M, Golebiowski M, Paczek L. Intracranial aneurysms in autosomal dominant polycystic kidney disease. AJNR Am J Neuroradiol. 2013;34(8):1556–9.

41. Klein JP. On the role of screening for intracranial aneurysms in autosomal dominant polycystic kidney disease. AJNR Am J Neuroradiol. 2013;34(8):1560–1.

42. Huston 3rd J, Torres VE, Sulivan PP, Offord KP, Wiebers DO. Value of magnetic resonance angiography for the detection of intracranial aneurysms in autosomal dominant polycystic kidney disease. J Am Soc Nephrol. 1993;3(12):1871–7.

43. Kato A, Takita T, Furuhashi M, Maruyama Y, Hishida A. Abdominal aortic aneurysms in hemodialysis patients with autosomal dominant polycystic kidney disease. Nephron. 2001;88(2):185–6.

44. Scheff RT, Zuckerman G, Harter H, Delmez J, Koehler R. Diverticular disease in patients with chronic renal failure due to polycystic kidney disease. Ann Intern Med. 1980;92(2 Pt 1):202–4.

45. Martinez JR, Grantham JJ. Polycystic kidney disease: etiology, pathogenesis, and treatment. Dis Mon. 1995;41(11):693–765.

46. Ravine D, Gibson RN, Walker RG, Sheffield LJ, Kincaid-Smith P, Danks DM. Evaluation of ultrasonographic diagnostic criteria for autosomal dominant polycystic kidney disease 1. Lancet. 1994;343(8901):824–7.

47. Nicolau C, Torra R, Badenas C, Vilana R, Bianchi L, Gilabert R, Darnell A, Bru C. Autosomal dominant polycystic kidney disease types 1 and 2: assessment of US sensitivity for diagnosis. Radiology. 1999;213(1):273–6.

48. Bae K, Park B, Sun H, Wang J, Tao C, Chapman AB, Torres VE, Grantham JJ, Mrug M, Bennett WM, et al. Segmentation of individual renal cysts from MR images in patients with autosomal dominant polycystic kidney disease. Clin J Am Soc Nephrol. 2013;8(7):1089–97.

49. Kistler AD, Serra AL, Siwy J, Poster D, Krauer F, Torres VE, Mrug M, Grantham JJ, Bae KT, Bost JE, et al. Urinary proteomic biomarkers for diagnosis and risk stratification of autosomal dominant polycystic kidney disease: a multicentric study. PLoS One. 2013;8(1):e53016.

50. Higashihara E, Nutahara K, Okegawa T, Shishido T, Tanbo M, Kobayasi K, Nitadori T. Kidney volume and function in autosomal dominant polycystic kidney disease. Clin Exp Nephrol. 2013;18:157–65.

51. Grantham JJ, Torres VE, Chapman AB, Guay-Woodford LM, Bae KT, King Jr BF, Wetzel LH, Baumgarten DA, Kenney PJ, Harris PC, et al. Volume progression in polycystic kidney disease. N Engl J Med. 2006;354(20):2122–30.

52. Pirson Y, Chauveau D, Torres V. Management of cerebral aneurysms in autosomal dominant polycystic kidney disease. J Am Soc Nephrol. 2002;13(1):269–76.

53. Jouret F, Lhommel R, Devuyst O, Annet L, Pirson Y, Hassoun Z, Kanaan N. Diagnosis of cyst infection in patients with autosomal dominant polycystic kidney disease: attributes and limitations of the current modalities. Nephrol Dial Transplant. 2012;27(10):3746–51.

54. Thong KM, Ong AC. The natural history of autosomal dominant polycystic kidney disease: 30-year experience from a single centre. QJM. 2013;106(7):639–46.

55. Hajj P, Ferlicot S, Massoud W, Awad A, Hammoudi Y, Charpentier B, Durrbach A, Droupy S, Benoit G. Prevalence of renal cell carcinoma in patients with autosomal dominant polycystic kidney disease and chronic renal failure. Urology. 2009;74(3):631–4.

56. Keith DS, Torres VE, King BF, Zincki H, Farrow GM. Renal cell carcinoma in autosomal dominant polycystic kidney disease. J Am Soc Nephrol. 1994;4(9):1661–9.

57. Torres VE, Chapman AB, Perrone RD, Bae KT, Abebe KZ, Bost JE, Miskulin DC, Steinman TI, Braun WE, Winklhofer FT, et al. Analysis of baseline parameters in the HALT polycystic kidney disease trials. Kidney Int. 2012;81(6):577–85.

58. Schrier RW, Abebe KZ, Perrone RD, Torres VE, Braun WE, Steinman TI, Winklhofer FT, Brosnahan G, Czarnecki PG, Hogan MC, et al. Blood pressure in early autosomal dominant polycystic kidney disease. N Engl J Med. 2014;371(24):2255–66.

59. Lee YR, Lee KB. Ablation of symptomatic cysts using absolute ethanol in 11 patients with autosomal-dominant polycystic kidney disease. Korean J Radiol. 2003;4(4):239–42.

60. Lee DI, Clayman RV. Hand-assisted laparoscopic nephrectomy in autosomal dominant polycystic kidney disease. J Endourol. 2004;18(4):379–82.

61. Eng M, Jones CM, Cannon RM, Marvin MR. Hand-assisted laparoscopic nephrectomy for polycystic kidney disease. JSLS. 2013;17(2):279–84.

62. Mangoo-Karim R, Uchic M, Lechene C, Grantham JJ. Renal epithelial cyst formation and enlargement in vitro: dependence on cAMP. Proc Natl Acad Sci U S A. 1989;86(15):6007–11.

63. Belibi FA, Wallace DP, Yamaguchi T, Christensen M, Reif G, Grantham JJ. The effect of caffeine on renal epithelial cells from patients with autosomal dominant polycystic kidney disease. J Am Soc Nephrol. 2002;13(11):2723–9.

64. Gattone 2nd VH, Wang X, Harris PC, Torres VE. Inhibition of renal cystic disease development and progression by a vasopressin V2 receptor antagonist. Nat Med. 2003;9(10):1323–6.

65. Wang X, Gattone 2nd V, Harris PC, Torres VE. Effectiveness of vasopressin V2 receptor antagonists OPC-31260 and OPC-41061 on polycystic kidney disease development in the PCK rat. J Am Soc Nephrol. 2005;16(4):846–51.

66. Torres VE, Chapman AB, Devuyst O, Gansevoort RT, Grantham JJ, Higashihara E, Perrone RD, Krasa HB, Ouyang J, Czerwiec FS. Tolvaptan in patients with autosomal dominant polycystic kidney disease. N Engl J Med. 2012;367(25):2407–18.

67. Hogan MC, Masyuk TV, Page LJ, Kubly VJ, Bergstralh EJ, Li X, Kim B, King BF, Glockner J, Holmes 3rd DR, et al. Randomized clinical trial of long-acting somatostatin for autosomal dominant polycystic kidney and liver disease. J Am Soc Nephrol. 2010;21(6):1052–61.

68. Walz G, Budde K, Mannaa M, Nurnberger J, Wanner C, Sommerer C, Kunzendorf U, Banas B, Horl WH, Obermuller N, et al. Everolimus in patients with autosomal dominant polycystic kidney disease. N Engl J Med. 2010;363(9):830–40.

69. Serra AL, Poster D, Kistler AD, Krauer F, Raina S, Young J, Rentsch KM, Spanaus KS, Senn O, Kristanto P, et al. Sirolimus and kidney growth in autosomal dominant polycystic kidney disease. N Engl J Med. 2010;363(9):820–9.

70. He Q, Lin C, Ji S, Chen J. Efficacy and safety of mTOR inhibitor therapy in patients with early-stage autosomal dominant polycystic kidney disease: a meta-analysis of randomized controlled trials. Am J Med Sci. 2012;344(6):491–7.

71. Zerres K, Mucher G, Becker J, Steinkamm C, Rudnik-Schoneborn S, Heikkila P, Rapola J, Salonen R, Germino GG, Onuchic L, et al. Prenatal diagnosis of autosomal recessive polycystic kidney disease (ARPKD): molecular genetics, clinical experience, and fetal morphology. Am J Med Genet. 1998;76(2):137–44.

72. Guay-Woodford LM, Desmond RA. Autosomal recessive polycystic kidney disease: the clinical experience in North America. Pediatrics. 2003;111(5 Pt 1):1072–80.

73. Roy S, Dillon MJ, Trompeter RS, Barratt TM. Autosomal recessive polycystic kidney disease: long-term outcome of neonatal survivors. Pediatr Nephrol. 1997;11(3):302–6.

74. Kaplan BS, Fay J, Shah V, Dillon MJ, Barratt TM. Autosomal recessive polycystic kidney disease. Pediatr Nephrol. 1989;3(1):43–9.

75. Hartung EA, Guay-Woodford LM. Autosomal recessive polycystic kidney disease: a hepatorenal fibrocystic disorder with pleiotropic effects. Pediatrics. 2014;134(3):e833–45.

76. Onuchic LF, Furu L, Nagasawa Y, Hou X, Eggermann T, Ren Z, Bergmann C, Senderek J, Esquivel E, Zeltner R, et al. PKHD1, the polycystic kidney and hepatic disease 1 gene, encodes a novel large protein containing multiple immunoglobulin-like plexin-transcription-factor domains and parallel beta-helix 1 repeats. Am J Hum Genet. 2002;70(5):1305–17.

77. Ward CJ, Hogan MC, Rossetti S, Walker D, Sneddon T, Wang X, Kubly V, Cunningham JM, Bacallao R, Ishibashi M, et al. The gene mutated in autosomal recessive polycystic kidney disease encodes a large, receptor-like protein. Nat Genet. 2002;30(3):259–69.

78. Al-Bhalal L, Akhtar M. Molecular basis of autosomal recessive polycystic kidney disease (ARPKD). Adv Anat Pathol. 2008;15(1):54–8.

79. Bisceglia M, Galliani CA, Senger C, Stallone C, Sessa A. Renal cystic diseases: a review. Adv Anat Pathol. 2006;13(1):26–56.

80. Rajanna DK, Reddy A, Srinivas NS, Aneja A. Autosomal recessive polycystic kidney disease: antenatal diagnosis and histopathological correlation. J Clin Imaging Sci. 2013;3:13.

81. Capisonda R, Phan V, Traubuci J, Daneman A, Balfe JW, Guay-Woodford LM. Autosomal recessive polycystic kidney disease: outcomes from a single-center experience. Pediatr Nephrol. 2003;18(2):119–26.

82. Habib R, Bois E. Heterogeneity of early onset nephrotic syndromes in infants (nephrotic syndrome "in infants"). Anatomical, clinical and genetic study of 37 cases. Helv Paediatr Acta. 1973;28(2):91–107.

83. Wen J. Congenital hepatic fibrosis in autosomal recessive polycystic kidney disease. Clin Transl Sci. 2011;4(6):460–5.

84. Gunay-Aygun M, Font-Montgomery E, Lukose L, Tuchman Gerstein M, Piwnica-Worms K, Choyke P, Daryanani KT, Turkbey B, Fischer R, Bernardini I, et al. Characteristics of congenital hepatic fibrosis in a large cohort of patients with autosomal recessive

polycystic kidney disease. Gastroenterology. 2013;144(1):112–21. e112.

85. Telega G, Cronin D, Avner ED. New approaches to the autosomal recessive polycystic kidney disease patient with dual kidney-liver complications. Pediatr Transplant. 2013;17(4):328–35.

86. Reuss A, Wladimiroff JW, Niermeyer MF. Sonographic, clinical and genetic aspects of prenatal diagnosis of cystic kidney disease. Ultrasound Med Biol. 1991;17(7):687–94.

87. Avni FE, Guissard G, Hall M, Janssen F, DeMaertelaer V, Rypens F. Hereditary polycystic kidney diseases in children: changing sonographic patterns through childhood. Pediatr Radiol. 2002;32(3):169–74.

88. Cobben JM, Breuning MH, Schoots C, ten Kate LP, Zerres K. Congenital hepatic fibrosis in autosomal-dominant polycystic kidney disease. Kidney Int. 1990;38(5):880–5.

89. Neumann HP, Krumme B, van Velthoven V, Orszagh M, Zerres K. Multiple intracranial aneurysms in a patient with autosomal recessive polycystic kidney disease. Nephrol Dial Transplant. 1999;14(4):936–9.

90. Chapal M, Debout A, Dufay A, Salomon R, Roussey G, Burtey S, Launay EA, Vigneau C, Blancho G, Loirat C, et al. Kidney and liver transplantation in patients with autosomal recessive polycystic kidney disease: a multicentric study. Nephrol Dial Transplant. 2012;27(5):2083–8.

91. Brinkert F, Lehnhardt A, Montoya C, Helmke K, Schaefer H, Fischer L, Nashan B, Bergmann C, Ganschow R, Kemper MJ. Combined liver-kidney transplantation for children with autosomal recessive polycystic kidney disease (ARPKD): indication and outcome. Transpl Int. 2013;26(6):640–50.

92. Bergmann C, Senderek J, Windelen E, Kupper F, Middeldorf I, Schneider F, Dornia C, Rudnik-Schoneborn S, Konrad M, Schmitt CP, et al. Clinical consequences of PKHD1 mutations in 164 patients with autosomal-recessive polycystic kidney disease (ARPKD). Kidney Int. 2005;67(3):829–48.

93. Adeva M, El-Youssef M, Rossetti S, Kamath PS, Kubly V, Consugar MB, Milliner DM, King BF, Torres VE, Harris PC. Clinical and molecular characterization defines a broadened spectrum of autosomal recessive polycystic kidney disease (ARPKD). Medicine. 2006;85(1):1–21.

94. Lilova M, Kaplan BS, Meyers KE. Recombinant human growth hormone therapy in autosomal recessive polycystic kidney disease. Pediatr Nephrol. 2003;18(1):57–61.

95. Fischer DC, Jacoby U, Pape L, Ward CJ, Kuwertz-Broeking E, Renken C, Nizze H, Querfeld U, Rudolph B, Mueller-Wiefel DE, et al. Activation of the AKT/mTOR pathway in autosomal recessive polycystic kidney disease (ARPKD). Nephrol Dial Transplant. 2009;24(6):1819–27.

# Nonneoplastic Disease Presenting as a Renal Lesion

3


Shane M. Pearce, Priya Rao, Stephen Thomas, and Scott E. Eggener


## Introduction

Renal neoplasms are relatively common and typically diagnosed by routine imaging. However, less commonly, nonneoplastic processes (Table 3.1) can clinically and radiographically mimic a renal mass, thus raising suspicion for malignancy. This may cause delays in diagnosis and appropriate treatment, placing the patient at risk for increased morbidity and mortality. In this chapter, we will review a subset of nonneoplastic entities that mimic renal masses or that can otherwise distort normal renal anatomy and include focal pyelonephritis, renal abscess, xanthogranulomatous pyelonephritis, and malakoplakia. Other rare infectious processes that may mimic a renal mass include renal aspergillosis, renal echinococcus, and upper tract fungal infections.

## Inflammatory and Infectious Lesions

### Focal (Localized) Pyelonephritis

Focal pyelonephritis refers to the infection of a single lobe of the kidney which, in contrast to more diffuse infection, can mimic a renal mass on imaging, especially in the setting of soft tissue extension of the inflammatory process (Fig. 3.1) [1]. Contrast-enhanced computed tomography (CT) is the gold standard for diagnosis of focal pyelonephritis when suspected. On CT, the lesion will appear as a hypoattenuating, poorly circumscribed, or wedge-shaped lesion. Ultrasound may provide a useful ancillary imaging modality and may demonstrate generalized renal enlargement with or without an ill-defined focal lesion [2, 3].

Focal pyelonephritis typically occurs in children and immunocompromised patients, and the diagnosis should be suspected in patients with fever, chills, or flank pain (Table 3.2). Other findings such as nausea, vomiting, and lower urinary tract symptoms (frequency, urgency, or dysuria) can occur. Physical exam may reveal abdominal pain and/or costovertebral angle tenderness in association with fever [4]. Leukocytosis and an elevated C-reactive protein are frequently


S.M. Pearce, M.D. (✉) • S.E. Eggener, M.D.
Department of Surgery, Section of Urology, University of Chicago, 5841 South Maryland Avenue, MC 6038, Chicago, IL 60637, USA
e-mail: pearce.shane@gmail.com; seggener@surgery.bsd.uchicago.edu

P. Rao, M.D.
Department of Pathology, MD Anderson Cancer Center, The University of Texas, Houston, TX 77030, USA
e-mail: prao@mdanderson.org

S. Thomas, M.D.
Department of Radiology, University of Chicago, Chicago, IL 60637, USA
e-mail: sthomas@radiology.bsd.uchicago.edu



© Springer Science+Business Media New York 2016
D.E. Hansel et al. (eds.), *The Kidney*, DOI 10.1007/978-1-4939-3286-3_3

demonstrated on laboratory evaluation and urine, and blood cultures are commonly positive. The vast majority of responsible pathogens are gram-negative bacteria, and *E. coli* is the most commonly isolated organism [5]. As pyuria may be absent in 50–70 % of patients, a normal urinalysis does not exclude the diagnosis in the appropriate clinical setting [5, 6]. Biopsy is not typically required in the setting of classic symptoms; however, in instances in which a biopsy is performed, a mixed acute and chronic inflammatory infiltrate may be seen. However, giant cells are not typical.

Diagnosis and aggressive treatment is critical in these cases, as the outpatient therapy typically used for acute uncomplicated pyelonephritis is rarely effective in these cases. Furthermore, hospitalizations may be prolonged due to persistent fever. The recommended duration of intravenous and oral antimicrobial treatment is at least 3 weeks [7].

**Table 3.1** Nonneoplastic renal masses

| **Infectious conditions** |
| --- |
| Focal pyelonephritis |
| Renal abscess |
| Xanthogranulomatous pyelonephritis |
| Malakoplakia |
| Aspergillosis |
| Echinococcus |
| Upper tract fungal infection |
| **Cystic lesions** |
| Acquired cystic kidney disease |
| Polycystic kidney disease |
| **Miscellaneous lesions** |
| Renal-adrenal fusion |
| Ectopic adrenal tissue |
| Splenorenal fusion |
| Extramedullary hematopoiesis |

**Table 3.2** Symptoms and signs of infectious process

| **Symptoms** |
| --- |
| Fevers |
| Chills |
| Flank or abdominal pain |
| Nausea, vomiting |
| Lower urinary tract symptoms (dysuria, frequency) |
| Malaise |
| Fatigue |
| Anorexia |
| **Signs** |
| Fever |
| Tachycardia |
| Diaphoresis |
| Abdominal tenderness |
| Costovertebral angle tenderness |
| Weight loss |
| Palpable mass |
| Fistulous tract |
| Skin infection |

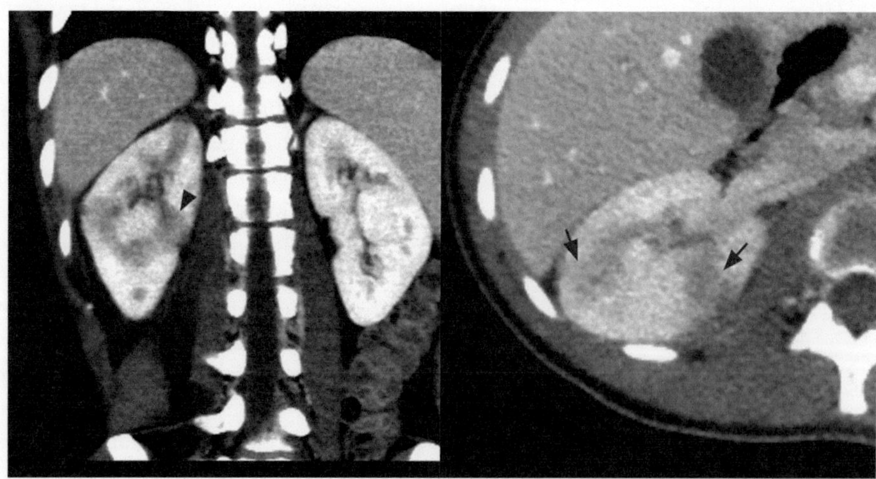

**Fig. 3.1** Focal pyelonephritis. Contrast-enhanced CT of the right kidney shows geographic areas of poor cortical enhancement (*black arrows*) that has a wedge-shaped configuration (*black arrow head*)

## Renal Abscess

Renal abscess refers to a discrete collection of purulent material originating from the renal parenchyma. This is in contrast to focal pyelonephritis, which but does not present with a collection of fluid and/or debris within the renal parenchyma. While this condition can present at any age, most published literature examines the pediatric experience. The majority of cases occur secondary to ascending infection of the urinary tract, although spread to the kidney may also occur via a hematogenous route. The clinical presentation is similar to focal pyelonephritis with fever, chills, and flank pain (Table 3.2); laboratory evidence of infection, including leukocytosis and positive blood cultures, is evident [8, 9]. Common etiologic pathogens include *E. coli*, *P. mirabilis*, and *S. aureus*, although other less common bacteria have also been documented [1, 10].

On imaging, these lesions have variable characteristics dependent on the phase of infection (early vs. late) and the amount of solid debris within the abscess (Fig. 3.2). Ultrasound and CT are the most commonly utilized imaging modalities to evaluate these lesions. The margins of the abscess are difficult to distinguish in the acute phase, and large amounts of cellular debris may result in a solid appearing mass, which is difficult to differentiate from a tumor. Historically, surgical exploration was employed to distinguish between renal abscess and renal carcinoma [11]. As the abscess coalesces, renal ultrasound will more reliably demonstrate a fluid-filled hypoechoic mass surrounded by a thick wall. Air within the abscess will produce a strong echo and posterior shadowing on ultrasonographic imaging. Angiography can also help differentiate abscess from tumor by demonstrating a hypovascular or avascular interior surrounded by a hypervascular rim, although this technique has the disadvantage of being more invasive [12].

Given some of the limitations of ultrasound and angiography, CT is currently the most widely utilized imaging modality for this lesion, as it is noninvasive and provides the most accurate anatomic information [13]. In the acute phase of infection, CT may simply reveal an enlarged, enhancing mass, leading to an incorrect diagnosis of a neoplastic process [14]. Most abscesses will appear as low-density masses with rim enhancement; the presence of intralesional gas is pathognomonic for renal abscess [13]. Once the diagnosis is made, a variety of treatment approaches can be successful that include intravenous antibiotics alone in an abscess less than 3 cm or percutaneous drainage and/or surgical intervention for larger abscesses [15].

In the modern era, most renal abscesses are managed without surgical resection and are generally not seen in surgical pathology suites. However, renal abscesses may be seen at the time of autopsy and appear as yellow-brown infarcted regions within the renal cortex or medulla. An acute abscess may show the presence of purulent material on transection (Fig. 3.3).

## Xanthogranulomatous Pyelonephritis (XGP)

XGP is an uncommon, chronic pyelonephritis resulting from an atypical, partial immune response to a subacute bacterial infection. XGP is usually seen in conjunction with renal obstruction

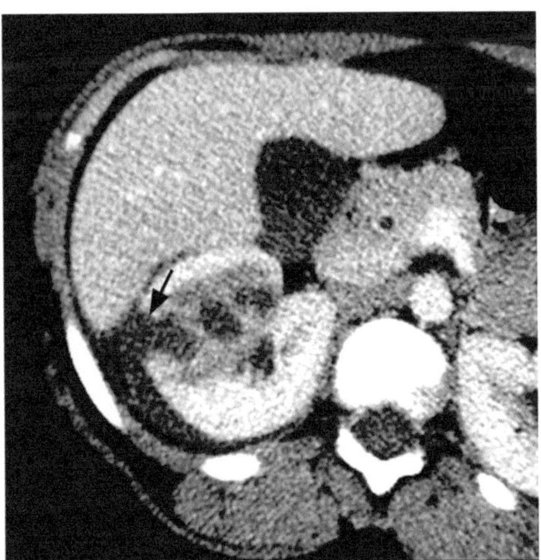

**Fig. 3.2** Renal abscess. Contrast-enhanced CT of the right kidney shows area of poor perfusion in the right kidney and focal area of cortical disruption (*black arrow*) and crescentic pus collection around the right kidney

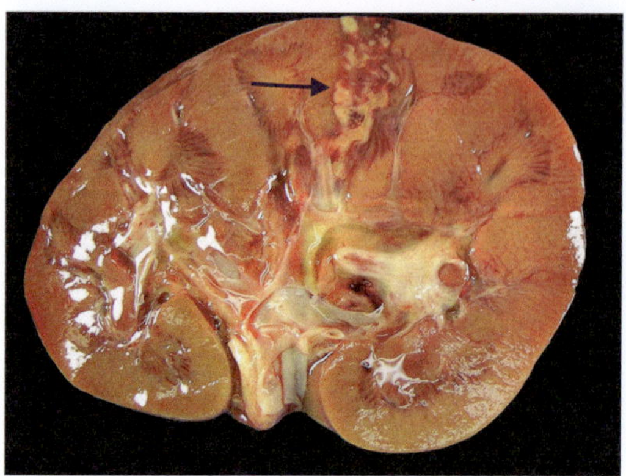

**Fig. 3.3** Renal abscess on gross pathology. Gross image demonstrating the presence of a renal cortical abscess that is extending down to the medulla. The lesion grossly appears as a *yellow*, *hemorrhagic area* that may resemble a focus of infarction

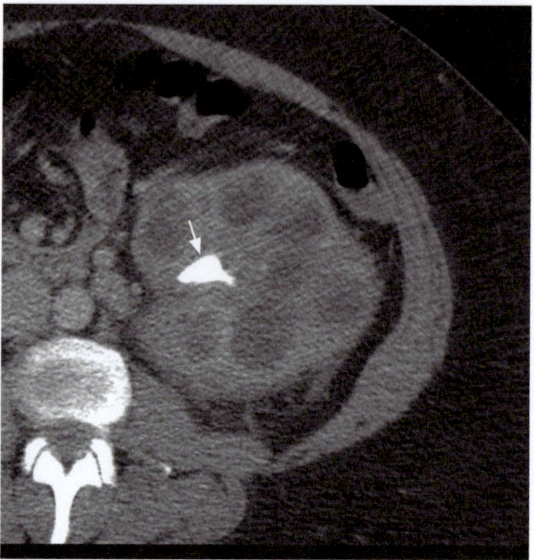

**Fig. 3.4** Xanthogranulomatous pyelonephritis (XGP). Contrast-enhanced CT shows an enlarged left kidney with a staghorn calculus (*white arrow*) in the renal pelvis with multiple hypodense surrounding areas representing hydronephrotic calyces and abscess cavities

and staghorn calculi in approximately 80 % of cases [16]. Common pathogens implicated include *E. coli*, *P. mirabilis*, *S. aureus*, *Pseudomonas aeruginosa*, and *Klebsiella pneumoniae* [17, 18]. XGP usually presents in middle-aged women, but can be seen in men. Diabetes is an established risk factor. The typical clinical presentation includes fever, chills, and flank or abdominal pain (Table 3.2). XGP may masquerade as a malignant process due to the frequent presence of nonspecific constitutional complaints including malaise, fatigue, and weight loss [19, 20]. As with other infectious processes involving the renal parenchyma, urinalysis is not specific. Blood work may reveal leukocytosis, anemia, abnormal liver function tests, hypoalbuminemia, hypergammaglobulinemia, and hyperuricosemia [19, 21].

Two distinct forms of XGP include the diffuse form in 85 % of cases and the localized form in 15 % of cases. Imaging studies commonly show nephromegaly, renal function impairment, and urinary obstruction secondary to calculi (Fig. 3.4) [22]. Ultrasound findings include diffuse renal enlargement, multiple hypoechoic areas, and echogenic foci with posterior acoustic shadowing suggesting calculi (Table 3.3). CT is the most useful imaging modality as it can define the extent of the inflammatory process and aid in surgical planning. Findings on CT that suggest XGP include renal enlargement, calcification of the

**Table 3.3** Imaging findings suggestive of XGP

| **Ultrasound** |
| --- |
| Diffuse renal enlargement |
| Multiple hypoechoic masses |
| Hyperechoic foci with posterior acoustic shadowing |
| Hydronephrosis/pyonephrosis |
| Perirenal/psoas abscess |
| **CT scan** |
| Diffuse renal enlargement |
| Hydronephrosis/pyonephrosis |
| Renal calculus |
| Parenchymal thinning |
| Nonfunctioning kidney |
| Multiple hypodense areas |
| Areas of fat accumulation |
| Cutaneous fistula |
| Abscess |
| **Suggest focal XGP** |
| Isolated pseudo-cystic mass |
| Solitary calyceal dilation with calculus |
| Adherent Gerota's fascia |
| Normal kidney function |

renal pelvis, and multiple hypodense areas representing hydronephrotic calyces and abscess cavities (Table 3.3) [22, 23]. Contrast enhancement

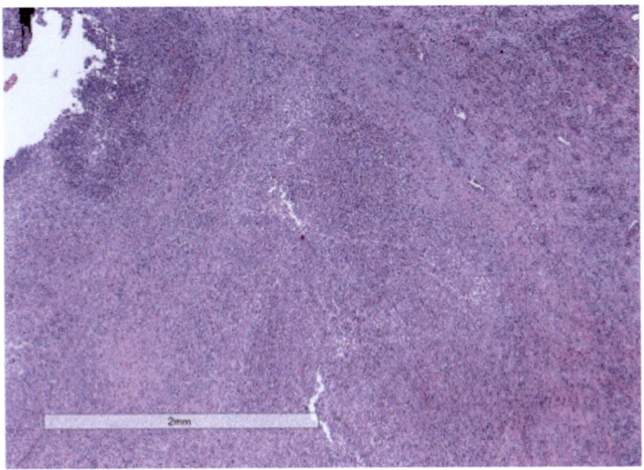

**Fig. 3.5** Xanthogranulomatous pyelonephritis (XGP). Low-power view showing the architecture of the kidney being effaced by a mixed inflammatory infiltrate

may additionally show wall enhancement, cortical thinning with reduced contrast excretion, and areas of fat attenuation due to lipid-rich xanthomatous tissue [23]. There are also rare case reports describing XGP associated with renal vein or caval thrombus and lymphadenopathy, further complicating the diagnostic picture [24, 25]. Given the more limited nature of localized XGP, a renal neoplasm is common in the differential diagnosis [26].

XGP reflects up to 19 % of the final diagnoses in cases of end-stage pyelonephritis [27] While nephrectomy remains the mainstay of treatment for XGP, optimal management likely includes appropriate antibiotic therapy, percutaneous drainage of associated abscesses, and possible percutaneous nephrostomy-tube drainage prior to surgical intervention [23]. While a laparoscopic approach may be attempted in cases of suspected XGP, it is associated with a high complication and conversion rate [27, 28]. Partial nephrectomy can be successful in cases of focal XGP [23, 29]. Additionally, if the diagnosis can be confirmed with percutaneous needle biopsy, there are rare reported cases of resolution of focal XGP with percutaneous drainage and antibiotics alone [30, 31].

On gross evaluation, the kidney is usually enlarged and shows a thickened capsule. The parenchymal surface may contain multiple, bright, yellow nodules. Necrosis of the renal parenchyma and dilatation of the renal pelvis secondary to renal calculi may also be seen.

Microscopic sections show a granulomatous process (Fig. 3.5) that contains a mixed inflammatory infiltrate associated with a prominence of lipid-laden macrophages containing foamy cytoplasm (xanthoma cells) (Fig. 3.6). Surrounding fibrosis of the region may be seen. XGP may represent a diagnostic pitfall especially on frozen section evaluation, as foamy macrophages may be mistaken for clear cells associated with clear cell renal cell carcinoma. On permanent section, the presence of diffuse immunoreactivity for CD68 in the foamy macrophages and absence of immunoreactivity for epithelial markers in the lesion can aid in the diagnosis [32].

Fine needle aspiration (FNA) may be used as an adjunct in preoperative diagnosis and will show xanthomatous cells with round vesicular nuclei that lack prominent nucleoli [32, 33]. The diagnosis on FNA can be especially challenging due to significant morphologic overlap with clear cell renal cell carcinoma. Immunohistochemistry can prove to be a useful adjunct in arriving at the correct diagnosis [34].

## Renal Malakoplakia

Renal malakoplakia is a rare, chronic inflammatory disease that can affect any organ system but most commonly involves the urinary tract. While it shows a predilection for the urinary bladder,

**Fig. 3.6** Xanthogranu-
lomatous pyelonephritis
(XGP). High-power view
showing a prominent
mixed infiltrate
composed of lipid-laden
macrophages or so-called
xanthoma cells,
lymphocytes, neutrophils,
and eosinophils.
Xanthoma cells may
represent a diagnostic
challenge, especially on
frozen section, and may
be mistaken for clear cell
renal cell carcinoma

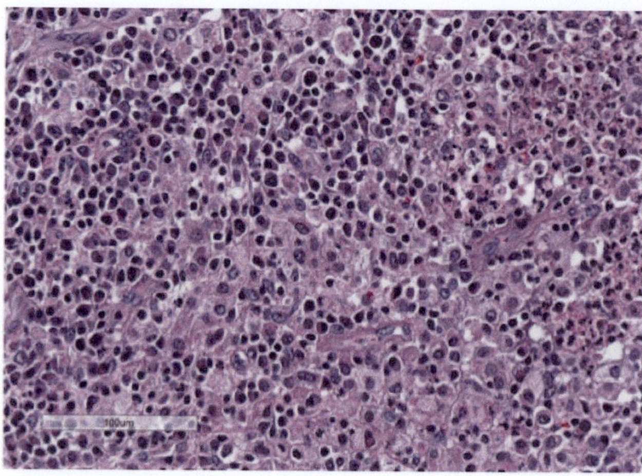

it may occur anywhere in the urinary tract including the upper tract and renal parenchyma. Malakoplakia has a predilection for immuno-compromised patients and is also frequently seen in middle-aged women with a history of chronic urinary tract infections. Renal failure is also common at presentation [35]. Common symptoms include fever, dysuria, and urinary frequency and urgency [36, 37]. Gram-negative bacteria are often associated with malakoplakia, with *E. coli* and *Proteus* species accounting for the vast majority of cases [38]. The pathogenesis is thought to be secondary to an impaired host immune response to infection, likely abnormal macrophage function, that results in the formation of mass-like lesions in the urinary tract. While the process is usually multifocal, a single lesion can be seen in up to 25 % of cases [38]. Most cases with renal parenchymal involvement are unilateral, although there are reports of bilateral disease at this location [39].

The radiographic appearance of malakoplakia can vary and the findings are nonspecific. Malakoplakia may appear as a unilateral enlarged kidney due to diffuse infiltrative disease, as multiple parenchymal lesions, or as a solitary low-attenuation mass. Solitary lesions are particularly difficult to diagnose because they can mimic solid renal masses. Ultrasound may demonstrate a diffusely enlarged kidney with poorly defined hypoechoic masses and distorted renal architecture. CT scan may show multiple low-attenuation areas of various sizes, which may coalesce into a single larger mass [1, 40]. The diagnosis can be confirmed by endoscopic, percutaneous, or open biopsy. The treatment of malakoplakia varies depending on the extent of disease and the overall condition of the patient. Bilateral or multifocal disease can be treated with antibiotics with the addition of bethanechol, which helps correct the macrophage lysosomal defect. Surgical excision is the standard of care for unifocal disease [38].

Histology shows a granulomatous process associated with the presence of characteristic targetoid bodies called "Michaelis–Gutmann" bodies (Fig. 3.7). Michaelis–Gutmann bodies are thought to result from incompletely digested bacteria within phagolysosomes and the deposition of calcium and iron [41, 42]. Several stains including iron, calcium and PAS stains can highlight Michaelis–Gutmann bodies (Fig. 3.8, PAS shown).

## Cystic Lesions of the Kidney

In this section, we will discuss autosomal dominant and recessive forms of polycystic kidney disease, as well as acquired renal cystic disease. Renal dysplasia, which may demonstrate cyst formation, is discussed in Chap. 11.

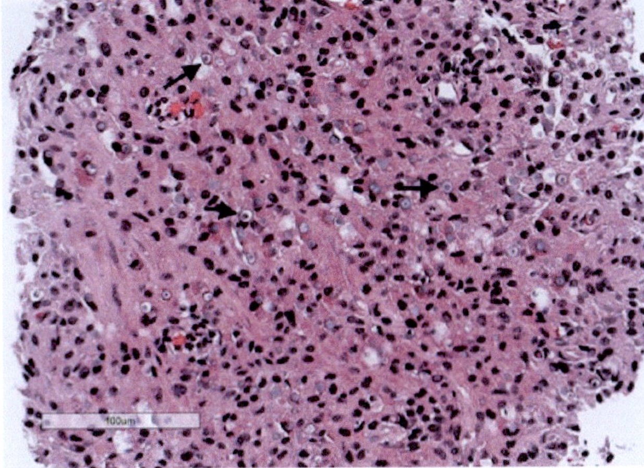

**Fig. 3.7** Renal malakoplakia. Renal biopsy showing a granulomatous infiltrate in the background, with numerous targetoid "Michaelis-Gutmann" bodies (*arrows*)

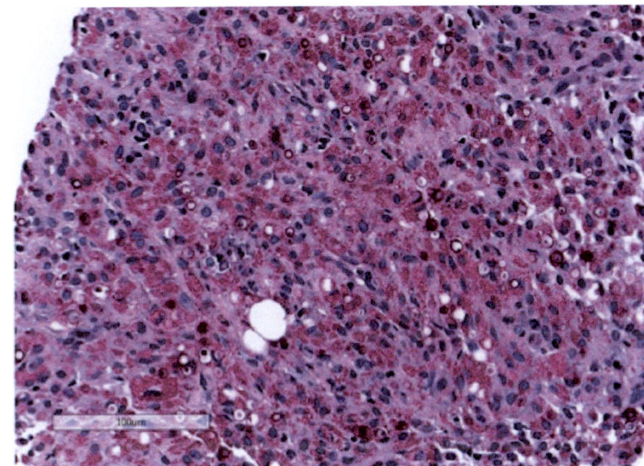

**Fig. 3.8** Renal malakoplakia. Periodic acid-Schiff (PAS) stain highlights Michaelis-Gutmann bodies that are believed to occur due to deposition of calcium and incompletely digested bacteria within phagolysosomes

## Autosomal Dominant Polycystic Kidney Disease (ADPKD)

Autosomal dominant polycystic kidney disease (ADPKD) has an incidence of 1/500–1000 persons in the general population and results from a germline mutation in the *PKD1* or *PKD2* genes [43]. It is the most common inherited disease of the kidney and accounts for ~5 % of cases of end-stage renal disease (ESRD) in the United States [44]. ADPKD is a systemic disorder with clinical manifestations in many locations including the liver, seminal vesicles, pancreas, and intracranial circulation. Due to the autosomal dominant pattern of inheritance, there is a 50 % probability that the child of an affected parent will inherit the disease. The progressive loss of nephrons as a

result of cyst formation usually does not become clinically significant until the third or fourth decade of life [45]. While most patients are asymptomatic, some may present early with abdominal or flank pain, hematuria, or urinary tract infections. Pain is the most frequent symptom of ADPKD, while hypertension is the most common sign of the disease [45, 46].

Patients with a family history of ADPKD should be screened after the age of 18 years; if ADPKD is diagnosed, the patient's first-degree relatives should be screened as well [47]. ADPKD is diagnosed on imaging (Fig. 3.9) based on well-established criteria (Table 3.4) [48, 50]. Although CT and magnetic resonance imaging (MRI) are more sensitive for identification of renal cysts, ultrasound is the preferred imaging modality for

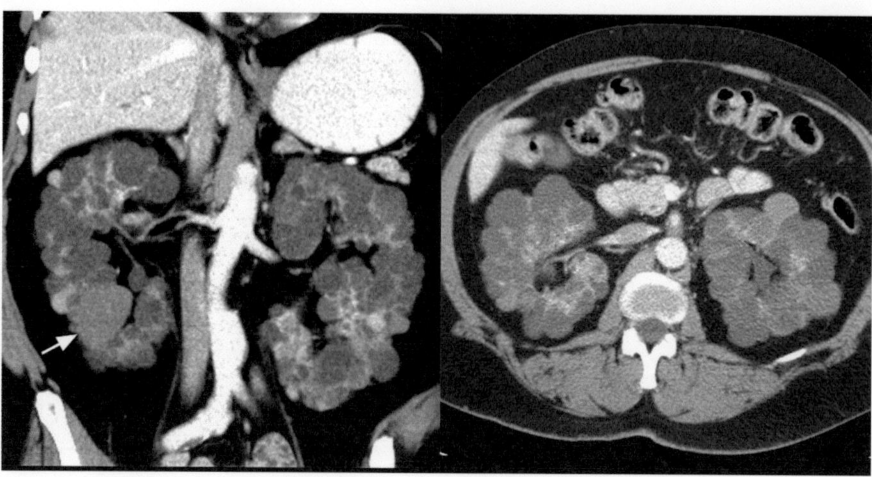

**Fig. 3.9** Autosomal dominant polycystic kidney disease (ADPKD). Axial and coronal contrast-enhanced CT of the kidneys showing bilateral enlarged kidneys with the parenchyma replaced by multiple cysts, some that are hyperdense (*white arrow*)

**Table 3.4** Imaging-based diagnostic criteria for ADPKD [48, 49]

| Age (years) | Criteria |
| --- | --- |
| *Ultrasonography (if 50 % risk of disease)* | |
| 15–39 | ≥3 cysts (unilateral or bilateral) |
| 40–59 | ≥2 in each kidney |
| 60+ | ≥4 in each kidney |
| *Magnetic resonance imaging (if at risk)* | |
| <30 | ≥5 in each kidney |
| 30–44 | 6 in each kidney |
| 45–59 (female) | >6 in each kidney |
| 45–59 (male) | >9 in each kidney |

screening as it is low cost and lacks radiation exposure. Genetic testing is not routinely recommended for ADPKD, but can be useful on a case-by-case basis [49].

Initial treatment approaches are aimed at preserving renal function and managing symptoms through pain medication, antibiotics, and antihypertensive agents. Symptomatic relief can also be obtained with cyst aspiration or laparoscopic cyst decortication [51]. Relative indications for total nephrectomy include pain, fullness, early satiety, cyst hemorrhage, uncontrolled hypertension, infections, nephrolithiasis, and space considerations prior to transplant. Nephrectomy has been successfully performed laparoscopically, even for very large kidneys [52, 53]. Development of targeted therapeutics that can slow the rate of cyst formation and growth and potentially preserve renal function has become an area of great interest. There are currently numerous preclinical and clinical trials investigating the role of mTOR inhibitors, vasopressin V2 receptor antagonists, somatostatin, and other agents in slowing disease progression [45].

There may be an association between ADPKD and renal cell carcinoma (RCC) with the prevalence of RCC reported to be anywhere from 5 to 12 % in ADPKD nephrectomy specimens [54]. However, ADPKD as a risk factor for RCC is controversial because these patients are frequently on dialysis for ESRD, which is also a known risk factor for RCC development. Diagnosis of RCC in ADPKD patients using CT or MRI is challenging due to distorted renal anatomy and architecture, making small, solitary lesions difficult to detect.

On gross evaluation, ADPKD kidneys are markedly enlarged and diffusely involved by large cysts that are filled with clear fluid and blood (Fig. 3.10). In later stages of disease, the normal renal parenchyma is often unidentifiable and replaced with fibrosis (Fig. 3.11). Rarely, ADPKD manifests in infancy and shows pathognomonic "glomerular cysts," which are characterized by normal-sized glomeruli with an enlarged Bowman's space and marked dilatation of the tubules [55, 56].

## Autosomal Recessive Polycystic Kidney Disease (ARPKD)

In contrast to ADPKD, autosomal recessive polycystic kidney disease (ARPKD) is very rare, with an incidence of 1/10,000–40,000 live births [57]. ARPKD involves a defect in the *PKHD1* gene. The classic presentation is in neonates with a history of oligohydramnios, massively enlarged kidneys, and the "Potter" sequence with pulmonary hypoplasia. Perinatal death occurs in

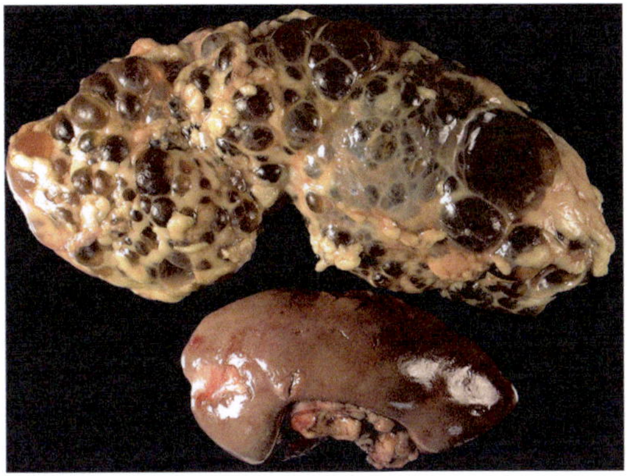

**Fig. 3.10** Autosomal dominant polycystic kidney disease (ADPKD). Example of a kidney affected by ADPKD (*above*) which shows a markedly enlarged kidney as compared to an unaffected kidney (*below*). Grossly, the affected kidney is extensively replaced by large cysts of varying sizes, with virtually no identifiable normal renal parenchyma

~30 % of affected neonates, although improved supportive care over the last several decades has increased survival [58]. This increased longevity has allowed a broader range of disease manifestations to now be recognized. These children frequently progress to ESRD, although the time required to progression is highly variable. Other ARPKD disease associations include liver disease, systemic hypertension, and neurocognitive dysfunction [59]. The most common renal phenotype in ARPKD is symmetrically enlarged, echogenic kidneys with fusiform dilation of the collecting ducts and loss of corticomedullary differentiation (Fig. 3.12). The renal parenchyma is echogenic in ARPKD due to the innumerable microscopic cysts. Discrete cysts may also be observed, although this is less common. ARPKD can be distinguished from ADPKD by the finding of increased corticomedullary differentiation in ADPKD [60]. It is important to note that a single normal prenatal sonogram does not exclude the diagnosis of ARPKD, because abnormalities may not be appreciated until the end of the second trimester or later [60]. Genetic testing can confirm the diagnosis [61].

Initial management in the perinatal period is supportive in nature. While associated pulmonary hypoplasia can contribute to respiratory problems, massively enlarged kidneys also impair ventilation by limiting diaphragmatic

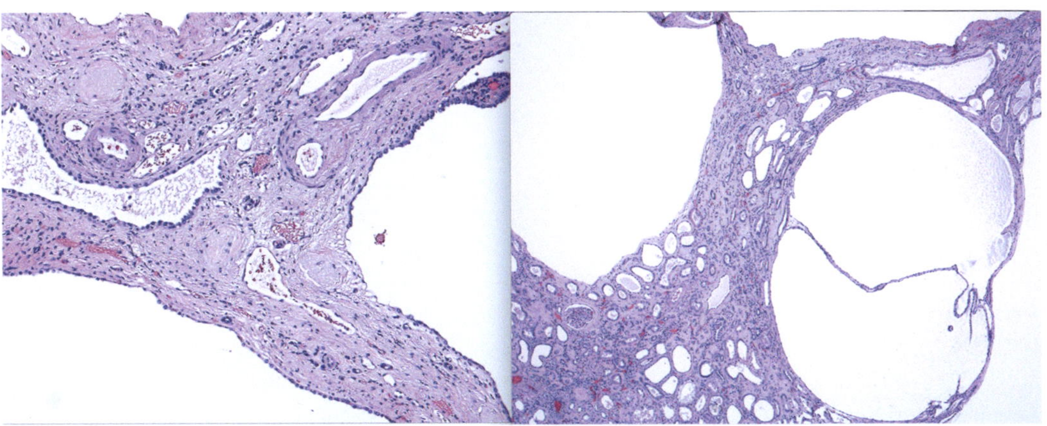

**Fig. 3.11** Autosomal dominant polycystic kidney disease (ADPKD). Microscopically, the affected kidneys show the presence of diffuse involvement by large cysts with little to no normal intervening renal parenchyma (*left*). Microscopically, cysts are lined by flattened epithelium with no cytologic atypia. In late stages, the kidney may be entirely fibrotic with virtually no identifiable normal renal parenchyma microscopically

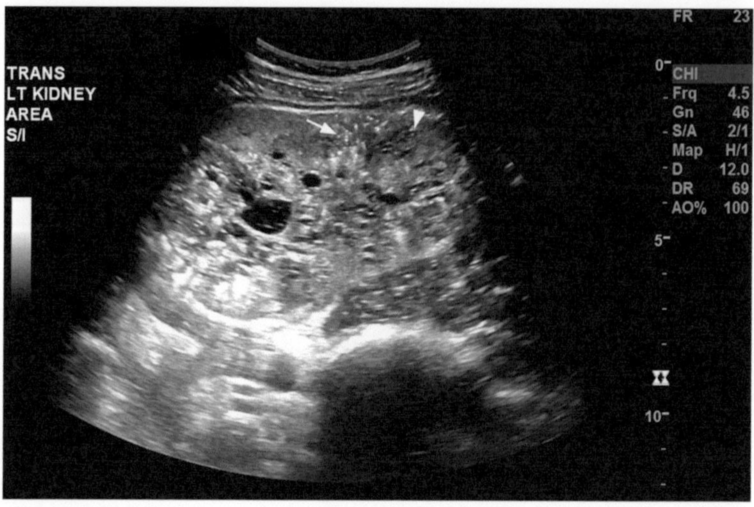



**Fig. 3.12** Autosomal recessive polycystic kidney disease (ARPKD). Ultrasonography of the kidney in a child shows an enlarged kidney, which is echogenic. There are bright echogenic foci with comet tail artifact (*white arrow*) and dilated tubules (*arrow head*)

excursion. The enlarged kidneys can also cause nutritional deficiencies through compression of the gastrointestinal tract [45]. Optimal surgical management is not clear; however, unilateral and/or bilateral nephrectomy has helped improve ventilation and nutrition in small case series [62–64]. The decision to perform nephrectomy must be weighed against the risks of surgery and the potential need for earlier renal replacement therapy.

On gross examination, kidneys affected by ARPKD show bilateral, symmetrical involvement. The kidneys are markedly enlarged with a bosselated surface. The cysts in ARPKD, in contrast to those of ADPKD, are small and uniform, usually 1–2 mm in diameter. In utero, the cysts are typically radially arranged and elongated with little intervening normal parenchyma. Microscopically, cysts are lined by flattened to cuboidal epithelium without any nuclear atypia [65, 66].

## Acquired Cystic Kidney Disease (ACKD)

Acquired cystic kidney disease (ACKD) refers specifically to bilateral renal cystic changes that can occur in chronic kidney disease. Contrary to previous understanding, cysts do not occur as a consequence of dialysis [67, 68]. While the mechanism of cyst formation remains unclear, the etiology may be secondary to accumulation of growth factors and systemic toxins among patients with impaired renal function. Of note, cystic changes have been shown to regress after renal transplant [69]. Acquired cystic disease occurs in 7–22 % of patients with a serum creatinine >3 ng/mL who are not yet on dialysis [68]. The incidence of ACKD does increase with duration of dialysis, ranging from 35 % in patients on dialysis for 2 years to 92 % in patients on dialysis for >8 years [68].

In contrast to ADPKD and ARPKD, there is a well-established association between renal cell carcinoma and ACKD. There is a 50-fold increased risk of renal cell carcinoma in these patients compared to the general population [70]. Screening for ACKD and renal cell carcinoma is recommended and should be initiated approximately 3 years after beginning dialysis, with renal ultrasounds every 1–2 years thereafter. Complex cystic lesions on ultrasound can then be further characterized with CT or MRI (Fig. 3.13) [68]. ACKD tends to be an asymptomatic disease process; however, symptoms combined with the specific clinical scenario should guide any intervention or treatment.

On gross examination, the affected kidney typically shows multiple variably sized cysts

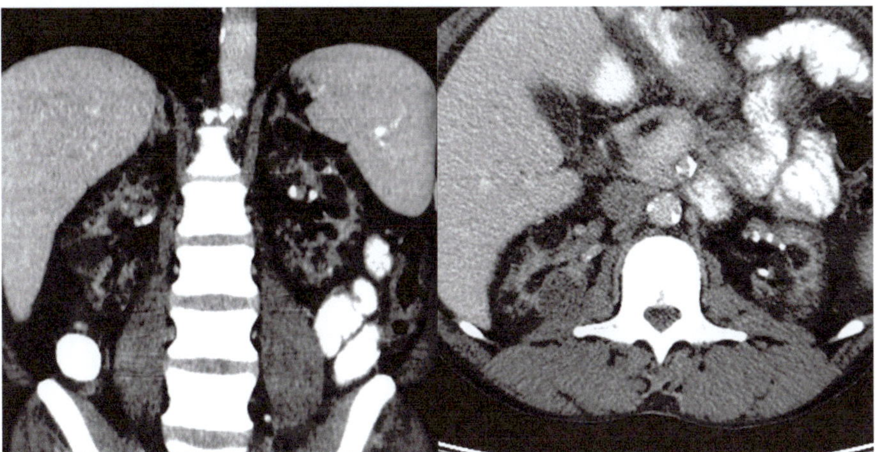

**Fig. 3.13** Acquired cystic kidney disease (ACKD). Axial and coronal contrast-enhanced CT of the kidneys showing bilateral atrophic kidneys with numerous cortical cysts in a patient on chronic hemodialysis

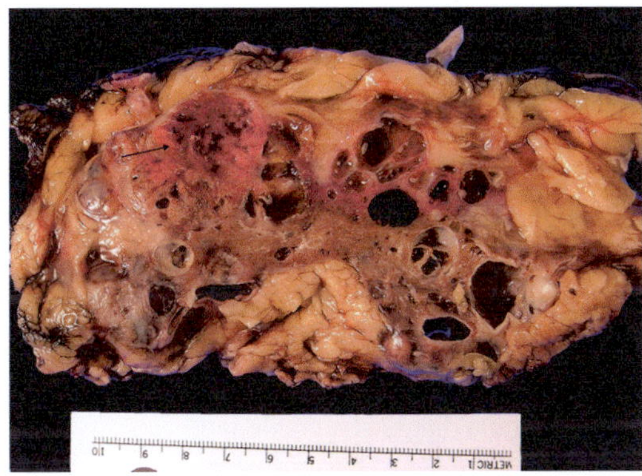

**Fig. 3.14** Acquired cystic kidney disease (ACKD). A case of renal cell carcinoma in a patient with ACKD. The kidney is diffusely involved by cysts of varying sizes that involve both the renal cortex and medulla. Patients are also prone to develop renal cell carcinoma which occurs as solid mass lesions (*arrow*) that are easily visualized by imaging studies and gross examination, when they are large enough

(Fig. 3.14) [71]. These cysts are lined by non-stratified epithelium with occasional papillary tufting. Any cysts lined by abundant clear cells should raise the suspicion for clear cell renal cell carcinoma in this setting. In addition, multiple forms of renal cell carcinoma may occur in this setting, including both conventional subtypes (discussed in Chap. 5) and ACKD-associated renal cell carcinoma (discussed in Chap. 2).

## Miscellaneous Lesions

### Renal-Adrenal Fusion

Renal-adrenal fusion is a developmental abnormality thought to arise from a failure to form a renal capsule that results in fusion of the adrenal gland with the renal parenchyma (Fig. 3.15) [72, 73]. Lesions are most often identified incidentally, usually in kidneys that are resected for another indication [73]. Renal-adrenal fusion may be radiographically mistaken for a renal mass due to the presence of adherent adrenal tissue to the kidney.

### Ectopic Adrenal Tissue

Ectopic adrenal tissue is most often located in the superior pole of the kidney. The adrenal tissue is composed of normal adrenal cortical parenchyma with no medullary tissue generally identified [73]. Although these lesions are not generally a pathological diagnostic dilemma, they may occasionally present a problem on frozen section analysis, where the clear cells of the adrenal cortex may be mistaken for a clear cell renal cell carcinoma.

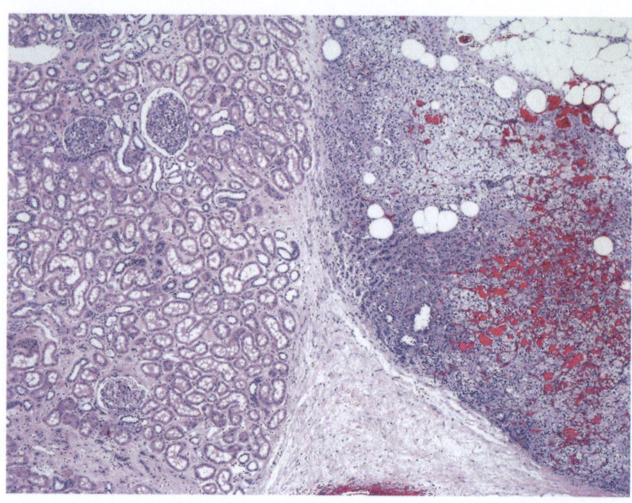

**Fig. 3.15** Renal-adrenal fusion. Example of renal-adrenal fusion, where the adrenal gland (*right*) is seen intermixed with the renal parenchyma (*left*). Grossly, the adrenal gland appears adherent to the renal parenchyma and is difficult to separate

## Splenorenal Fusion

Splenorenal fusion is a rare, benign abnormality typically involving the left kidney that can arise from a developmental anomaly resulting in fusion of splenic and renal tissues. It can also be acquired after trauma or splenectomy, where it is referred to as splenosis. This process may present as an asymptomatic solid-enhancing mass mimicking a renal neoplasm [74, 75]. It has also been known to present with anemia. A preoperative biopsy or a fine needle aspiration specimen will aid in the diagnosis of normal splenic tissue. Other diagnostic modalities include a 99mTc sulfur colloid scan, which will demonstrate uptake in splenic tissue or a ferumoxides-enhanced MRI [76]. Accurate diagnosis is invaluable to prevent unnecessary surgical intervention.

## Extramedullary Hematopoiesis (EMH)

Extramedullary hematopoiesis (EMH) is the development of hematopoietic tissue in a multitude of sites, most commonly involving the liver and the spleen. EMH has been rarely reported in the kidney [77–79]. Associations that have been reported for renal EMH include myelofibrosis, chronic myeloproliferative disorder, renal cell carcinoma, polycythemia vera, and other hematologic disorders [80, 81]. Renal involvement may be parenchymal, intrapelvic, or perirenal [82]. Imaging can reveal diffuse enlargement of the kidney, a single hypoattenuating mass, or multiple nodules surrounding or encasing the kidney [83]. Identification of a renal mass in patients with any of the previously mentioned hematologic disorders should alert the clinician to the possibility of EMH. Diagnosis rests on the identification of mature hematopoietic elements in association with the renal parenchyma. Lesions that are located in the perirenal tissue may mimic a renal mass and thus present a diagnostic challenge.

## Conclusions

A variety of nonneoplastic renal disease processes can present with signs, symptoms, imaging, and pathologic characteristics that can be easily confused with renal neoplasms. Knowledge of potential mimics and focused evaluation may prevent misdiagnosis and potentially avoid unnecessary interventions.

## References


1. Bhatt S, MacLennan G, Dogra V. Renal pseudotumors. AJR Am J Roentgenol. 2007;188(5):1380–7.
2. Conley SP, Frumkin K. Acute lobar nephronia: a case report and literature review. J Emerg Med. 2014; 46(5):624–6.

3. Huang JJ, Sung JM, Chen KW, Ruaan MK, Shu GH, Chuang YC. Acute bacterial nephritis: a clinicoradiologic correlation based on computed tomography. Am J Med. 1992;93(3):289–98.

4. Li Y, Zhang Y. Diagnosis and treatment of acute focal bacterial nephritis. Chin Med J (Engl). 1996;109(2):168–72.

5. Yang CC, Shao PL, Lu CY, Tsau YK, Tsai IJ, Lee PI, et al. Comparison of acute lobar nephronia and uncomplicated urinary tract infection in children. J Microbiol Immunol Infect. 2010;43(3):207–14.

6. Klar A, Hurvitz H, Berkun Y, Nadjari M, Blinder G, Israeli T, et al. Focal bacterial nephritis (lobar nephronia) in children. J Pediatr. 1996;128(6): 850–3.

7. Cheng CH, Tsau YK, Lin TY. Effective duration of antimicrobial therapy for the treatment of acute lobar nephronia. Pediatrics. 2006;117(1):e84–9.

8. Anderson KA, McAninch JW. Renal abscesses: classification and review of 40 cases. Urology. 1980;16(4):333–8.

9. Meng MV, Mario LA, McAninch JW. Current treatment and outcomes of perinephric abscesses. J Urol. 2002;168(4 Pt 1):1337–40.

10. Cancelinha C, Santos L, Ferreira C, Gomes C. Renal abscesses in childhood: report of two uncommon cases. BMJ Case Rep. 2014. doi:10.1136/bcr-2013-202408.

11. Doolittle KH, Taylor JN. Renal abscess in differential diagnosis of mass in kidney. J Urol. 1963;89(5):649.

12. Caplan LH, Siegelman SS, Bosniak MA. Angiography in inflammatory space-occupying lesions of the kidney. Radiology. 1967;88(1):14–23.

13. Merenich WM, Popky GL. Radiology of renal infection. Med Clin North Am. 1991;75(2):425–69.

14. Wang YT, Lin KY, Chen MJ, Chiou YY. Renal abscess in children: a clinical retrospective study. Acta Paediatr Taiwan. 2003;44(4):197–201.

15. Seguias L, Srinivasan K, Mehta A. Pediatric renal abscess: a 10-year single-center retrospective analysis. Hosp Pediatr. 2012;2(3):161–6.

16. Rabushka LS, Fishman EK, Goldman SM. Pictorial review: computed tomography of renal inflammatory disease. Urology. 1994;44(4):473–80.

17. Zia-ul-Miraj M, Cheema MA. Xanthogranulomatous pyelonephritis presenting as a pseudotumor in a 2-month-old boy. J Pediatr Surg. 2000;35(8):1256–8.

18. Dell'Aprovitola N, Guarino S, Del Vecchio W, Camera L, Chiancone F, Imbimbo C, et al. Xanthogranulomatous pyelonephritis mimicking a renal cell carcinoma: a unique and challenging case. Acta Radiol Short Rep. 2014;3(1):2047981613513763.

19. Dembry LM, Andriole VT. Renal and perirenal abscesses. Infect Dis Clin North Am. 1997;11(3): 663–80.

20. Eastham J, Ahlering T, Skinner E. Xanthogranulomatous pyelonephritis: clinical findings and surgical considerations. Urology. 1994;43(3):295–9.

21. Goodman M, Curry T, Russell T. Xanthogranulomatous pyelonephritis (XGP): a local disease with systemic manifestations. Report of 23 patients and review of the literature. Medicine. 1979;58(2):171–81.

22. Kim JC. US and CT findings of xanthogranulomatous pyelonephritis. Clin Imaging. 2001;25(2):118–21.

23. Loffroy R, Guiu B, Watfa J, Michel F, Cercueil JP, Krause D. Xanthogranulomatous pyelonephritis in adults: clinical and radiological findings in diffuse and focal forms. Clin Radiol. 2007;62(9):884–90.

24. Ganpule A, Jagtap J, Ganpule S, Bhattu A, Soni S, Sabnis R, et al. Xanthogranulomatous pyelonephritis (XGPN) mimicking a "renal cell carcinoma with renal vein thrombus and paracaval lymphadenopathy". F1000Research. 2013;2:263.

25. Gupta G, Singh R, Kotasthane DS, Kotasthane VD, Kumar S. Xanthogranulomatous pyelonephritis in a male child with renal vein thrombus extending into the inferior vena cava: a case report. BMC Pediatr. 2010;10:47.

26. Ozcan H, Akyar S, Atasoy C. An unusual manifestation of xanthogranulomatous pyelonephritis: bilateral focal solid renal masses. AJR Am J Roentgenol. 1995;165(6):1552–3.

27. Korkes F, Favoretto RL, Broglio M, Silva CA, Castro MG, Perez MD. Xanthogranulomatous pyelonephritis: clinical experience with 41 cases. Urology. 2008;71(2):178–80.

28. Tobias-Machado M, Lasmar MT, Batista LT, Forseto Jr PH, Juliano RV, Wroclawski ER. Laparoscopic nephrectomy in inflammatory renal disease: proposal for a staged approach. Int Braz J Urol. 2005;31(1):22–8.

29. Osca JM, Peiro MJ, Rodrigo M, Martinez-Jabaloyas JM, Jimenez-Cruz JF. Focal xanthogranulomatous pyelonephritis: partial nephrectomy as definitive treatment. Eur Urol. 1997;32(3):375–9.

30. Mollier S, Descotes JL, Pasquier D, Coquillat P, Michel A, Dalsoglio S, et al. Pseudoneoplastic xanthogranulomatous pyelonephritis. A typical clinical presentation but unusual diagnosis and treatment. Eur Urol. 1995;27(2):170–3.

31. Reul O, Waltregny D, Boverie J, de Leval J, Andrianne R. Pseudotumoral xanthogranulomatous pyelonephritis: diagnosis with percutaneous biopsy and success of conservative treatment. Prog Urol. 2001;11(6):1274–6.

32. Li L, Parwani AV. Xanthogranulomatous pyelonephritis. Arch Pathol Lab Med. 2011;135(5):671–4.

33. Sugie S, Tanaka T, Nishikawa A, Yoshimi N, Kato K, Mori H, et al. Fine-needle aspiration cytology of xanthogranulomatous pyelonephritis. Urology. 1991; 37(4):376–9.

34. Kumar N, Jain S. Aspiration cytology of focal xanthogranulomatous pyelonephritis: a diagnostic challenge. Diagn Cytopathol. 2004;30(2):111–4.

35. Diwakar R, Else J, Wong V, Carne A, Banerjee D, MacPhee I. Enlarged kidneys and acute renal failure--why is a renal biopsy necessary for diagnosis and treatment? Nephrol Dial Transplant. 2008;23(1):401–3.

36. Hammond NA, Nikolaidis P, Miller FH. Infectious and inflammatory diseases of the kidney. Radiol Clin North Am. 2012;50(2):259–70. vi.

37. Vourganti S, Agarwal PK, Bodner DR, Dogra VS. Ultrasonographic evaluation of renal infections. Radiol Clin North Am. 2006;44(6):763–75.
38. Abolhasani M, Jafari AM, Asgari M, Salimi H. Renal malakoplakia presenting as a renal mass in a 55-year-old man: a case report. J Med Case Reports. 2012;6:379.
39. Pickhardt PJ, Lonergan GJ, Davis Jr CJ, Kashitani N, Wagner BJ. From the archives of the AFIP. Infiltrative renal lesions: radiologic-pathologic correlation. Armed Forces Institute of Pathology. Radiographics. 2000;20(1):215–43.
40. Venkatesh SK, Mehrotra N, Gujral RB. Sonographic findings in renal parenchymal malacoplakia. J Clin Ultrasound. 2000;28(7):353–7.
41. Stanton MJ, Maxted W. Malacoplakia: a study of the literature and current concepts of pathogenesis, diagnosis and treatment. J Urol. 1981;125(2):139–46.
42. Tam VK, Kung WH, Li R, Chan KW. Renal parenchymal malacoplakia: a rare cause of ARF with a review of recent literature. Am J Kidney Dis. 2003;41(6):E13–7.
43. Mochizuki T, Tsuchiya K, Nitta K. Autosomal dominant polycystic kidney disease: recent advances in pathogenesis and potential therapies. Clin Exp Nephrol. 2013;17(3):317–26.
44. Collins AJ, Foley RN, Chavers B, Gilbertson D, Herzog C, Ishani A, et al. US renal data system 2013 annual data report. Am J Kidney Dis. 2014;63(1 Suppl):A7.
45. Torres VE, Harris PC. Autosomal dominant polycystic kidney disease: the last 3 years. Kidney Int. 2009;76(2):149–68.
46. Grantham JJ. Clinical practice. Autosomal dominant polycystic kidney disease. N Engl J Med. 2008;359(14):1477–85.
47. Srivastava A, Patel N. Autosomal dominant polycystic kidney disease. Am Fam Physician. 2014;90(5):303–7.
48. Pei Y, Obaji J, Dupuis A, Paterson AD, Magistroni R, Dicks E, et al. Unified criteria for ultrasonographic diagnosis of ADPKD. J Am Soc Nephrol. 2009;20(1):205–12.
49. Huang E, Samaniego-Picota M, McCune T, Melancon JK, Montgomery RA, Ugarte R, et al. DNA testing for live kidney donors at risk for autosomal dominant polycystic kidney disease. Transplantation. 2009;87(1):133–7.
50. Nascimento AB, Mitchell DG, Zhang XM, Kamishima T, Parker L, Holland GA. Rapid MR imaging detection of renal cysts: age-based standards. Radiology. 2001;221(3):628–32.
51. Lee DI, Andreoni CR, Rehman J, Landman J, Ragab M, Yan Y, et al. Laparoscopic cyst decortication in autosomal dominant polycystic kidney disease: impact on pain, hypertension, and renal function. J Endourol. 2003;17(6):345–54.
52. Dunn MD, Portis AJ, Elbahnasy AM, Shalhav AL, Rothstein M, McDougall EM, et al. Laparoscopic nephrectomy in patients with end-stage renal disease and autosomal dominant polycystic kidney disease. Am J Kidney Dis. 2000;35(4):720–5.
53. Wisenbaugh ES, Tyson 2nd MD, Castle EP, Humphreys MR, Andrews PE. Massive renal size is not a contraindication to a laparoscopic approach for bilateral native nephrectomies in autosomal dominant polycystic kidney disease (ADPKD). BJU Int. 2015;115(5):796–801.
54. Jilg CA, Drendel V, Bacher J, Pisarski P, Neeff H, Drognitz O, et al. Autosomal dominant polycystic kidney disease: prevalence of renal neoplasias in surgical kidney specimens. Nephron Clin Pract. 2013;123(1–2):13–21.
55. Gupta K, Vankalakunti M, Sachdeva MU. Glomerulocystic kidney disease and its rare associations: an autopsy report of two unrelated cases. Diagn Pathol. 2007;2:12.
56. Bissler JJ, Siroky BJ, Yin H. Glomerulocystic kidney disease. Pediatr Nephrol. 2010;25(10):2049–56. quiz 56–9.
57. Buscher R, Buscher AK, Weber S, Mohr J, Hegen B, Vester U, et al. Clinical manifestations of autosomal recessive polycystic kidney disease (ARPKD): kidney-related and non-kidney-related phenotypes. Pediatr Nephrol. 2014;29:1915–25.
58. Roy S, Dillon MJ, Trompeter RS, Barratt TM. Autosomal recessive polycystic kidney disease: long-term outcome of neonatal survivors. Pediatr Nephrol. 1997;11(3):302–6.
59. Adeva M, El-Youssef M, Rossetti S, Kamath PS, Kubly V, Consugar MB, et al. Clinical and molecular characterization defines a broadened spectrum of autosomal recessive polycystic kidney disease (ARPKD). Medicine. 2006;85(1):1–21.
60. Reuss A, Wladimiroff JW, Niermeyer MF. Sonographic, clinical and genetic aspects of prenatal diagnosis of cystic kidney disease. Ultrasound Med Biol. 1991;17(7):687–94.
61. Consugar MB, Anderson SA, Rossetti S, Pankratz VS, Ward CJ, Torra R, et al. Haplotype analysis improves molecular diagnostics of autosomal recessive polycystic kidney disease. Am J Kidney Dis. 2005;45(1):77–87.
62. Beaunoyer M, Snehal M, Li L, Concepcion W, Salvatierra Jr O, Sarwal M. Optimizing outcomes for neonatal ARPKD. Pediatr Transplant. 2007;11(3):267–71.
63. Bean SA, Bednarek FJ, Primack WA. Aggressive respiratory support and unilateral nephrectomy for infants with severe perinatal autosomal recessive polycystic kidney disease. J Pediatr. 1995;127(2):311–3.
64. Shukla AR, Kiddoo DA, Canning DA. Unilateral nephrectomy as palliative therapy in an infant with autosomal recessive polycystic kidney disease. J Urol. 2004;172(5 Pt 1):2000–1.
65. Martignoni G, Bonetti F, Pea M, Tardanico R, Brunelli M, Eble JN. Renal disease in adults with TSC2/PKD1 contiguous gene syndrome. Am J Surg Pathol. 2002;26(2):198–205.

66. Rajanna DK, Reddy A, Srinivas NS, Aneja A. Autosomal recessive polycystic kidney disease: antenatal diagnosis and histopathological correlation. J Clin Imaging Sci. 2013;3:13.
67. Dunnill MS, Millard PR, Oliver D. Acquired cystic disease of the kidneys: a hazard of long-term intermittent maintenance haemodialysis. J Clin Pathol. 1977;30(9):868–77.
68. Waterman J. Diagnosis and evaluation of renal cysts. Prim Care. 2014;41(4):823–35.
69. Grantham JJ. Acquired cystic kidney disease. Kidney Int. 1991;40(1):143–52.
70. Truong LD, Krishnan B, Cao JT, Barrios R, Suki WN. Renal neoplasm in acquired cystic kidney disease. Am J Kidney Dis. 1995;26(1):1–12.
71. Hosseini M, Antic T, Paner GP, Chang A. Pathologic spectrum of cysts in end-stage kidneys: possible precursors to renal neoplasia. Hum Pathol. 2014; 45(7):1406–13.
72. Honore LH, O'Hara KE. Combined adrenorenal fusion and adrenohepatic adhesion: a case report with review of the literature and discussion of pathogenesis. J Urol. 1976;115(3):323–5.
73. Ye H, Yoon GS, Epstein JI. Intrarenal ectopic adrenal tissue and renal-adrenal fusion: a report of nine cases. Mod Pathol. 2009;22(2):175–81.
74. Carneiro F, Sobreira Mde N, Dos Santos A, de Magalhaes A, Maurmo R. Splenorenal fusion mimicking renal neoplasm in a patient with von Hippel-Lindau disease. Intern Med. 2010;49(5):513–4.
75. Forino M, Davis GL, Zins JH. Renal splenic heterotopia, a rare mimic of renal neoplasia: case report of imaging and fine-needle aspiration biopsy. Diagn Cytopathol. 1993;9(5):565–9.
76. Karabulut N, Elmas N. Contrast agents used in MR imaging of the liver. Diagn Interv Radiol. 2006; 12(1):22–30.
77. Gibbins J, Pankhurst T, Murray J, McCafferty I, Baiden-Amissahk K, Shafeek S, et al. Extramedullary haematopoiesis in the kidney: a case report and review of literature. Clin Lab Haematol. 2005; 27(6):391–4.
78. Ricci D, Mandreoli M, Valentino M, Sabattini E, Santoro A. Extramedullary haematopoiesis in the kidney. Clin Kidney J. 2012;5:143.
79. Coyne JD. Extramedullary haemopoiesis. J Clin Pathol. 2005;58(4):448.
80. Saisorn I, Leewansangtong S, Sukpanichnant S, Ruchutrakool T, Leemanont P. Intrarenal extramedullary hematopoiesis as a renal mass in a patient with thalassemia. J Urol. 2001;165(2):507–8.
81. Talmon GA. Pure erythropoiesis in clear cell renal cell carcinoma. Int J Surg Pathol. 2010;18(6):544–6.
82. Choi H, David CL, Katz RL, Podoloff DA. Case 69: extramedullary hematopoiesis. Radiology. 2004; 231(1):52–6.
83. Rapezzi D, Racchi O, Ferraris AM. Perirenal extramedullary hematopoiesis in agnogenic myeloid metaplasia: MR imaging findings. AJR Am J Roentgenol. 1997;168(5):1388–9.

Gladell P. Paner

## Classification of Renal Neoplasms

The nosology of tumors of renal origin has tremendously evolved during the last three decades. Advancement in our knowledge of histology, immunohistochemistry, genetics, and molecular pathology of renal tumors brought the expansion in its types, particularly within the spectrum of renal cell carcinoma (RCC). The last World Health Organization (WHO) classification of renal tumors was published in 2004 that had evolved mainly from the prior Heidelberg 1996 and Rochester 1997 international consensus conferences. In 2010, the International Society of Urological Pathology (ISUP) conducted a consensus conference in Vancouver, Canada, to modify the 2004 WHO classification of renal tumors [1]. This latest classification scheme known as the *ISUP Vancouver classification of renal neoplasia* (Table 4.1) is the basis for the new WHO classification of renal tumors scheduled for release in 2016.

Several new subtypes of RCC are recognized in the ISUP Vancouver classification such as tubulocystic RCC, acquired cystic disease-associated RCC, clear cell (tubulo) papillary RCC, MiT family translocation RCC (including t(6;11) RCC), and hereditary leiomyomatosis RCC syndrome-associated RCC. Some newly described RCCs are also considered as provisional entities such as thyroid-like follicular RCC, succinic dehydrogenase B deficiency-associated RCC, and ALK-translocation RCC. Additional data are needed to help shed light on the biology of these rare unique tumors. Some innovations were also made on traditional tumor entities, such as renaming multicystic clear cell RCC as a neoplasm of low malignant potential, subtyping papillary RCC into type 1 or 2, accepting the hybrid oncocytic/chromophobe tumor as a discrete subtype of chromophobe RCC, and merging cystic nephroma with mixed epithelial stromal tumor into one tumor spectrum. Despite the inclusion of these novel entities, clear cell RCC, papillary RCC, and chromophobe RCC still comprise >90 % of the RCCs. The proportion of MiT family translocation RCC however is higher in pediatric and young adult patients.

## Staging of Renal Cancers

### Introduction

The tumor node metastasis (TNM) is the most widely accepted staging system for renal cancer [2]. This approach measures the extent of can-

G.P. Paner, M.D. (✉)
Department of Pathology and Surgery, Section of Urology, University of Chicago, MC MC6101, Room S-626, 5841 South Maryland Avenue, Chicago, IL 60637, USA
e-mail: Gladell.paner@uchospitals.edu

© Springer Science+Business Media New York 2016
D.E. Hansel et al. (eds.), *The Kidney*, DOI 10.1007/978-1-4939-3286-3_4

**Table 4.1** ISUP Vancouver modification of 2004 WHO classification of renal tumors

| |
|---|
| **Renal cell tumors** |
| Papillary adenoma |
| Oncocytoma |
| Clear cell renal cell carcinoma |
|    Multilocular cystic clear cell renal cell neoplasm of low malignant potential[a] |
| Papillary renal cell carcinoma |
| Chromophobe renal cell carcinoma |
|    Hybrid oncocytic/chromophobe tumor[a] |
| Carcinoma of the collecting ducts of Bellini |
| Renal medullary carcinoma |
| MiT family translocation renal cell carcinoma[a] |
|    Xp11 translocation renal cell carcinoma |
|    t(6;11) renal cell carcinoma |
| Carcinoma associated with neuroblastoma |
| Mucinous tubular and spindle cell carcinoma |
| Tubulocystic renal cell carcinoma[a] |
| Acquired cystic disease-associated renal cell carcinoma[a] |
| Clear cell (tubulo) papillary renal cell carcinoma[a] |
| Hereditary leiomyomatosis renal cell carcinoma syndrome-associated renal cell carcinoma[a] |
| Renal cell carcinoma, unclassified |
| **Metanephric tumors** |
| Metanephric adenoma |
| Metanephric adenofibroma |
| Metanephric stromal tumor |
| **Nephroblastic tumors** |
| Nephrogenic rests |
| Nephroblastoma |
|    Cystic partially differentiated nephroblastoma |
| **Mesenchymal tumors** |
| Occurring mainly in children |
|    Clear cell sarcoma |
|    Rhabdoid tumor |
|    Congenital mesoblastic nephroma |
|    Ossifying renal tumor of infants |
| Occurring mainly in adults |
|    Leiomyosarcoma (including renal vein) |
|    Angiosarcoma |
|    Rhabdomyosarcoma |
|    Malignant fibrous histiocytoma |
|    Hemangiopericytoma |
|    Osteosarcoma |
|    Synovial sarcoma[a] |
|    Angiomyolipoma |

(continued)

**Table 4.1** (continued)

| |
|---|
|    Epithelioid angiomyolipoma[a] |
|    Leiomyoma |
|    Hemangioma |
|    Juxtaglomerular cell tumor |
|    Renomedullary interstitial cell tumor |
|    Schwannoma |
|    Solitary fibrous tumor |
| **Mixed mesenchymal and epithelial tumors** |
|    Cystic nephroma/mixed epithelial stromal tumor |
| **Neuroendocrine tumors** |
|    Carcinoid (low-grade neuroendocrine tumor) |
|    Neuroendocrine carcinoma (high-grade neuroendocrine tumor) |
|    Primitive neuroectodermal tumor |
|    Neuroblastoma |
|    Pheochromocytoma |
| **Hematopoietic and lymphoid tumors** |
|    Lymphoma |
|    Leukemia |
|    Plasmacytoma |
| **Germ cell tumors** |
|    Teratoma |
|    Choriocarcinoma |
| **Metastatic tumors** |
| **Other tumors** |

[a]New additions or changes

cer spread at the primary organ site, regional lymph nodes, and distant sites (Table 4.2). The TNM system underwent considerable revisions over the past three decades with its latest edition (seventh) published in 2010, and a new version is being expected within the next 2 years as of 2015. Purely based on the tumor's anatomic extent, the different TNM stage categories are lumped into four main prognostic groups (Table 4.3). The clinical (c) stage is routinely used as a guide in determining the type of primary management, such as nephron sparing surgery (NSS) or ablative therapies for low stage renal tumors or systemic therapy for advanced stage tumors. The pathologic (p) stage mainly provides prognosis of outcome after surgical resection of renal cancer and is important on the decision for adjuvant therapy. TNM stage is often incorporated in the inclusion criteria and in stratifying

**Table 4.2** Definitions of the 2010 AJCC TNM staging for renal cancers

| *Primary tumor (T)* | |
|---|---|
| TX | Primary tumor cannot be assessed |
| T0 | No evidence of primary tumor |
| T1 | Tumor 7 cm or less in greatest dimension, limited to the kidney |
| T1a | Tumor 4 cm or less in greatest dimension, limited to the kidney |
| T1b | Tumor more than 4 cm but not more than 7 cm in greatest dimension, limited to the kidney |
| T2 | Tumor more than 7 cm in greatest dimension, limited to the kidney |
| T2a | Tumor more than 7 cm but less than or equal to 10 cm in greatest dimension, limited to the kidney |
| T2b | Tumor more than 10 cm, limited to the kidney |
| T3 | Tumor extends into major veins or perinephric tissues but not into the ipsilateral adrenal gland and not beyond Gerota's fascia |
| T3a | Tumor grossly extends into the renal vein or its segmental (muscle-containing) branches, or tumor invades perirenal and/or renal sinus fat but not beyond Gerota's fascia |
| T3b | Tumor grossly extends into the vena cava below the diaphragm |
| T3c | Tumor grossly extends into the vena cava above the diaphragm or invades the wall of the vena cava |
| T4 | Tumor invades beyond Gerota's fascia (including contiguous extension into the ipsilateral adrenal gland) |
| *Regional lymph nodes (N)* | |
| NX | Regional lymph nodes cannot be assessed |
| N0 | No regional lymph node metastasis |
| N1 | Metastasis in regional lymph node (s) |
| *Distant metastasis (M)* | |
| M0 | No distant metastasis |
| M1 | Distant metastasis |

**Table 4.3** 2010 AJCC TNM anatomic stage or prognostic groupings

| Stage I | T1 | N0 | M0 |
|---|---|---|---|
| Stage II | T2 | N0 | M0 |
| Stage III | T1 or T2 | N1 | M0 |
| | T3 | N0 or N1 | M0 |
| Stage IV | T4 | Any N | M0 |
| | Any T | Any N | M1 |

patients for clinical therapeutic trials. The accuracy of TNM stage in renal cancer can be further enhanced by its integration in the different prognostic and predictive models such as the MSKCC prognostic nomogram; the Mayo Clinic stage, size, grade, and necrosis (SSIGN) score; and the UCLA integrated staging system (UISS) [3–7].

## Historical Background

In 1958, Flocks and Kasdesky [8] introduced one of the first formal stagings for renal cancer based on the tumor's anatomic extent and patterns of spread. A year later, Petkovic [9] proposed a similar classification that subdivided intrarenal tumors into stages I and II (Flocks and Kasdesky's stage I). In the 1960s, Robson modified these systems, incorporated venous involvement, and subdivided localized extrarenal spread [10, 11]. However, Robson's system was hampered by inaccuracies in some of the stage definitions due to the lumping of prognostically different patterns of anatomic spread [11].

First developed in the 1940s by Pierre Denoix in France, the TNM system was adopted by the Union Internationale Contre le Cancer (UICC), while the American Joint Commission on Cancer (AJCC) used a slightly different classification. In 1987, the UICC and AJCC were unified, and the first major revision of the TNM staging was published that incorporated tumor size cutoffs derived from cross-sectional imaging studies. Since then, the TNM system underwent several major revisions published in 1993 (supplement), 1997, 2002, and the latest in 2010, building on experiences and evidences accumulated from each prior version in order to enhance its prognostic accuracies (Table 4.4). Revisions in the 2010 TNM system include T2 tumors divided into T2a (>7 cm but ≤10 cm) and T2b (>10 cm); ipsilateral adrenal gland contiguous invasion classified as T4 and, if not contiguous as M1, renal vein involvement reclassified as T3a; and nodal involvement simplified into N0 and N1 [2].

**Table 4.4** Evolution of renal cancer staging system

| Stage | Robson (1969)[a] | UICC/AJCC TNM, fourth edition (1987) | UICC/AJCC TNM, fifth edition (1997) | UICC/AJCC TNM, sixth edition (2002) | UICC/AJCC TNM, seventh edition (2010) |
|---|---|---|---|---|---|
| T1 | (I) Organ confined, any size | Organ confined, ≤2.5 cm | Organ confined, ≤7 cm | – | – |
| T1a | – | – | – | Organ confined, ≤4 cm | Organ confined, ≤4 cm |
| T1b | – | – | – | Organ confined, >4–7 cm | Organ confined, >4–7 cm |
| T2 | (II) Into perinephric tissue | Organ confined, >2.5 cm | Organ confined, >7 cm | Organ confined, >7 cm | – |
| T2a | – | – | – | – | Organ confined, >7–10 cm |
| T2b | – | – | – | – | Organ confined, >10 cm |
| T3a | (IIIa) Renal vein | Perinephric tissue or contiguous adrenal gland extension | Perinephric tissue or contiguous adrenal gland extension | Perinephric or sinus tissue or contiguous adrenal gland extension | Perinephric or sinus tissue or renal vein or its segmental branches |
| T3b | (IIIb) Node involvement | Renal vein | Renal vein or vena cava below diaphragm | Renal vein or vena cava below diaphragm | Vena cava below diaphragm |
| T3c | (IIIc) Both renal vein and node involvement | Vena cava below diaphragm | Vena cava above diaphragm | Vena cava above diaphragm | Vena cava above diaphragm or wall of vena cava at any level |
| T4 | – | – | Beyond Gerota's fascia | Beyond Gerota's fascia | Beyond Gerota's fascia or contiguous adrenal gland extension |
| T4a | (IVa) Invasion of adjacent structures | Beyond Gerota's fascia | – | – | – |
| T4b | (IVb) Distant metastasis | Vena cava above diaphragm | – | – | – |

[a]Staged as I, II, IIIa, IIIb, IIIc, IVa, IVb

## Components of the TNM Staging System for Renal Cancer

### Organ-Confined Tumors
### Tumors 7 cm or Smaller (T1)

Since the 2002 TNM version, T1 tumors are subdivided into T1a and T1b using 4 cm size cutoff (Figs. 4.1 and 4.2). This was mainly based on the study by Hafez et al. [12] wherein they reviewed 485 patients with localized renal cancer treated with NSS and showed a more favorable cancer-free survival in tumors $\leq 4$ cm compared to larger tumors. Since then, the prognostic impact of this subdivision has been validated in subsequent studies [13–17]. Despite of several studies suggesting a different optimal size cutoff for T1a and T1b and T1 versus T2, the 4 and 7 cm cutoffs are retained in the current 2010 TNM system [18–22]. By incidence, most renal cancers are diagnosed as T1 tumors (~55 to 70 %) and with greater T1a (35–45 %) than T1b cases (19–27 %) (Table 4.5) [23–25]. A practical usefulness of this T1 grouping is that most of the current guidelines recommend NSS for T1 renal cancer when technically feasible, and this recommendation is generally accepted for T1a tumors.

### Tumors Larger Than 7 cm (T2)

One of the revisions in the 2010 TNM system is the subdivision of T2 into T2a and T2b using 10 cm cutoff (Fig. 4.3). In an earlier study by Frank et al. [17] on 544 patients with organ confined >7 cm renal cancers treated with radical nephrectomies or NSS, tumors $\geq 10$ cm in size had a significantly better cancer-specific survival (CSS) than with <10 cm tumors even after adjusting for regional lymph node involvement and distant metastasis. The 10 cm cutoff outperformed the 9 cm cutoff [17]. The 10 cm cutoff for T2 tumors was supported by data obtained from the National Cancer Data Base (NCDB), wherein T2a and T2b showed 5 years observed survival of 57 % and 47.5 %, respectively [2].

## Locally Aggressive Tumors
### Perinephric or Sinus Fat, Renal Vein, and Vena Caval Extension (T3)

T3 tumors are subdivided into three categories: T3a defined by invasion of the perinephric or sinus tissues or of the renal vein and both T3b and T3c defined by extension into vena cava subdivided by the level of tumor thrombus relative to the diaphragm (Figs. 4.4, 4.5, 4.6, 4.7, and 4.8). Renal vein invasion includes involvement of its muscle-containing segmental branches. T3c also includes tumor invasion of the vena caval wall regardless if present at any level. The distribution of T3 tumors is disproportionate with most tumors falling under the T3a category (12–36 % overall). Only ~2 and ~0.5 % of renal cancers overall are staged as T3b and T3c, respectively. Contributory to the increase in T3a is the incorporation of sinus invasion into this category [26–28]. Renal sinus invasion is diagnosed pathologically by tumor involvement of any of structures of the renal sinus, including sinus fat, loose connective tissue, or any sinus-based endothelium-lined space [29]. In contrast, perinephric fat invasion is defined pathologically as either tumor touching the fat or extending as irregular tongues into the perinephric tissue, with or without the presence of desmoplasia [29]. Bonsib [28] showed that the frequency of renal sinus invasion is closely related to the tumor size, having a cutoff point of 4 cm, after which the frequency of sinus invasion increases sharply. He also showed that T2 (>7 cm) clear cell RCCs are uncommon if careful examination of the renal sinus for tumor invasion is performed [28]. Renal sinus invasion was shown to have a negative impact on CSS in renal cancers without nodal or distant metastasis [30]. With increasing tumor size, sinus invasion was also shown to be more frequent than perinephric fat invasion. It is possible that the uncommon T1 renal cancers with aggressive course may have unrecognized renal sinus fat invasion that was missed on sampling, particularly for small tumors close to the renal hilum [31, 32]. Since

**Fig. 4.1** Kidney with two synchronous organ-confined tumors. The smaller tumor (*top*) is T1a and the larger tumor (*bottom*) is T1b. Multiple tumors are staged according to the highest T stage, in this case as T1b

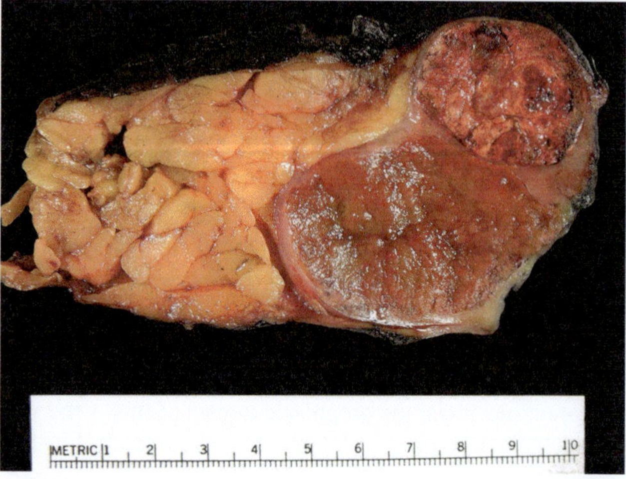

**Fig. 4.2** T1a clear cell RCC that is very close to the hilum. In this case, adequate sampling of the tumor-sinus interface is important to ascertain the absence of invasion (T3a)

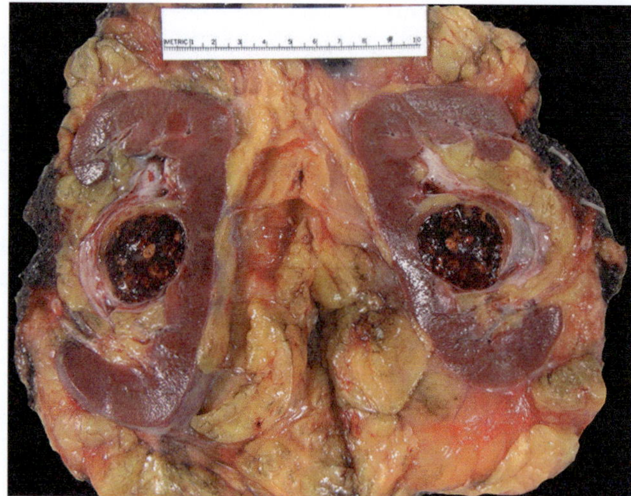

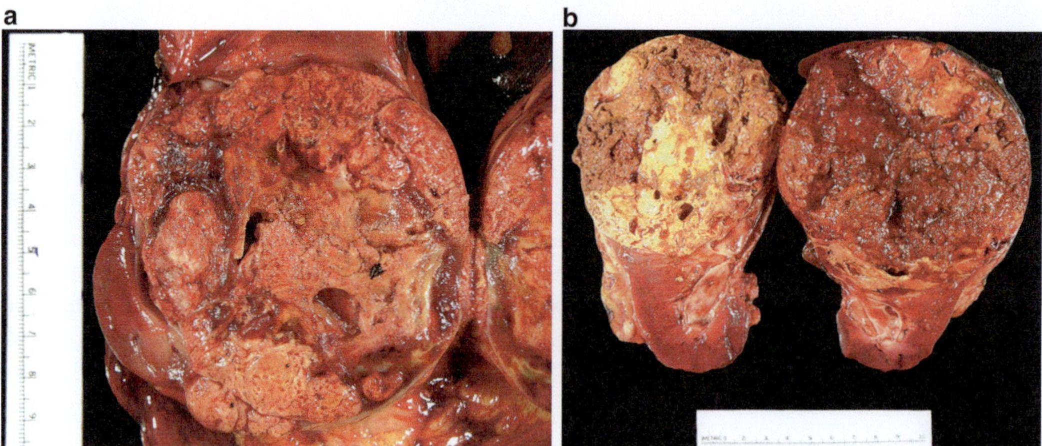

**Fig. 4.3** Large organ-confined tumors. (**a**) T2a clear cell RCC and (**b**) T2b papillary RCC

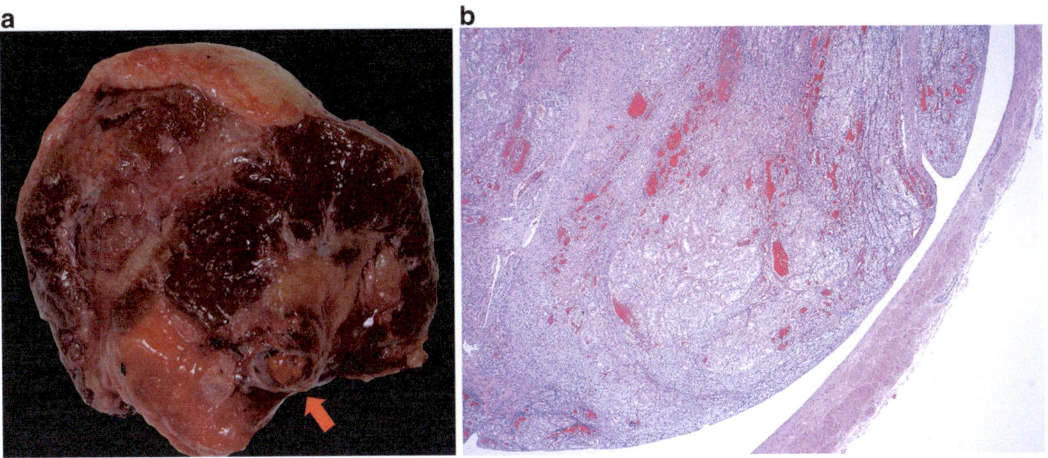

**Fig. 4.4** (**a**) T3a clear cell RCC with tumor thrombus in a segmental branch of renal vein (*arrow*) seen at the cut margin of a partial nephrectomy. (**b**) The tumor does not infiltrate into the vessel wall

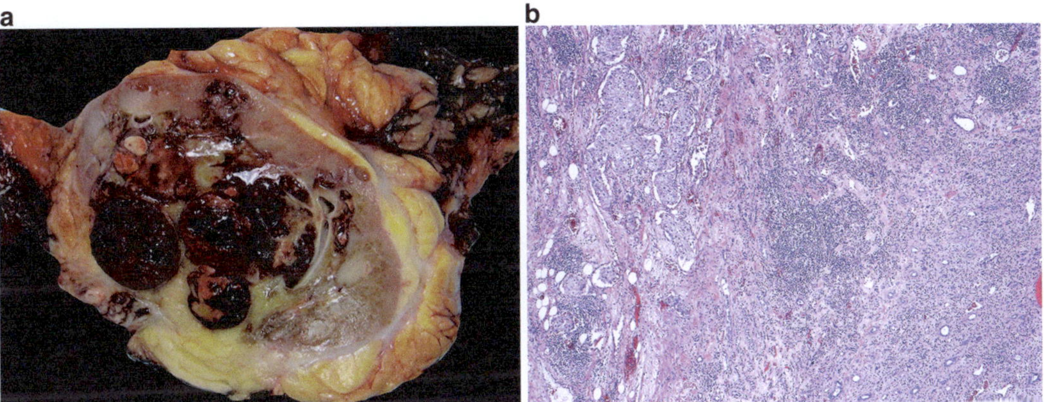

**Fig. 4.5** (**a**) T3a clear cell RCC with concomitant renal vein invasion and sinus fat invasion. (**b**) Infiltration of tumor into the renal sinus tissue

T3a has three different inclusion criteria (i.e., sinus invasion, perinephric invasion, and renal vein invasion) and has a relatively larger proportion of tumors among the different T categories (Table 4.5), this large group may also be prognostically heterogeneous. Thompson et al. [33], in a study of 205 T3a renal cancers treated with radical nephrectomy, showed that renal tumors invading the sinus are more aggressive than those invading into the perinephric fat. It is suggested that access by tumor to the lymphatic and vascular channels present at the sinus is responsible for the more aggressive course. Subsequent

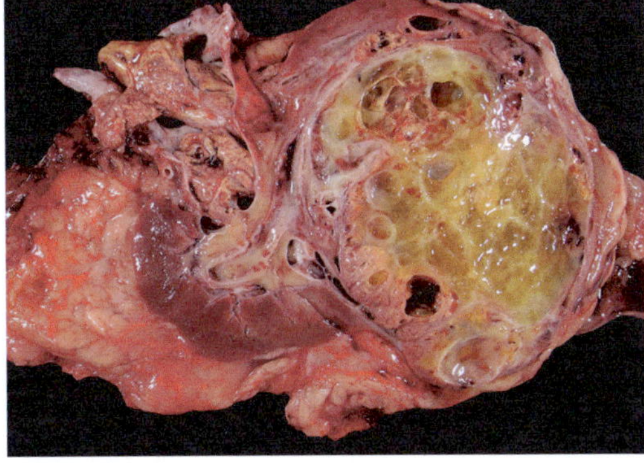

**Fig. 4.6** T3b Clear cell RCC with a tumor thrombus within the renal vein that extends into the vena cava

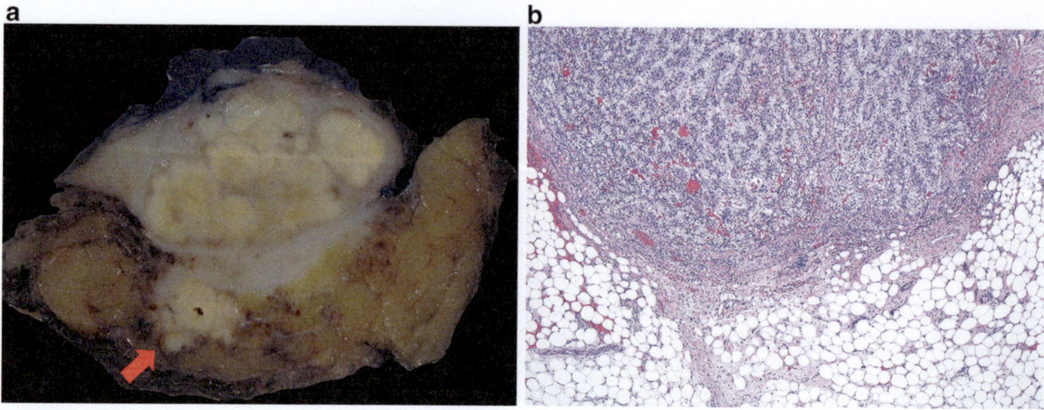

**Fig. 4.7** T3a clear cell RCC in a partial nephrectomy with invasion into the perinephric fat (**a**, *arrow*, and **b**)

**Table 4.5** Distribution of renal cancer patients by pathologic T stage

| pTstage | Novara et al. (2010) [23] | Lee et al. (2011) [24] | Pichler et al. (2013) [25] |
|---|---|---|---|
| N | 5339 | 1691 | 2739 |
| T1a (%) | 35.5 | 45.3 | 35.7 |
| T1b (%) | 27 | 24.8 | 19.2 |
| T2a (%) | 8 | 8.5 | 4.5 |
| T2b (%) | 3 | 4 | 1.6 |
| T3a (%) | 20 | 12.8 | 36.5 |
| T3b (%) | 2 | 2.2 | 1.6 |
| T3c (%) | 0.5 | 0.5 | 0.3 |
| T4 (%) | 4 | 1.8 | 0.7 |

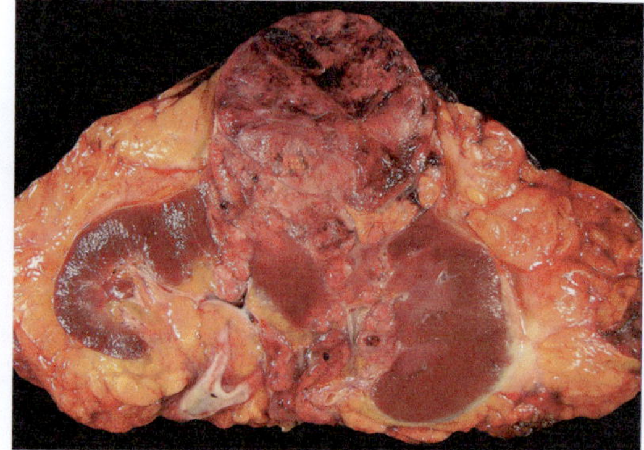

**Fig. 4.8** T3a clear cell RCC with concomitant perinephric fat and renal sinus invasion

studies also showed differences in outcome between sinus and perinephric fat invasion (see validation studies below).

In the 2010 TNM system, both T3b and T3c encompass extension of the tumor into the vena cava. Studies have shown that prognoses are different for tumors involving the renal vein (T3a) and sub- (T3b) and supradiaphragmatic (T3c) levels of the vena cava [34–36]. Kim et al. [36] showed that patients with tumor thrombus involving the vena cava above the diaphragm had a significantly worse survival than with renal vein involvement and vena

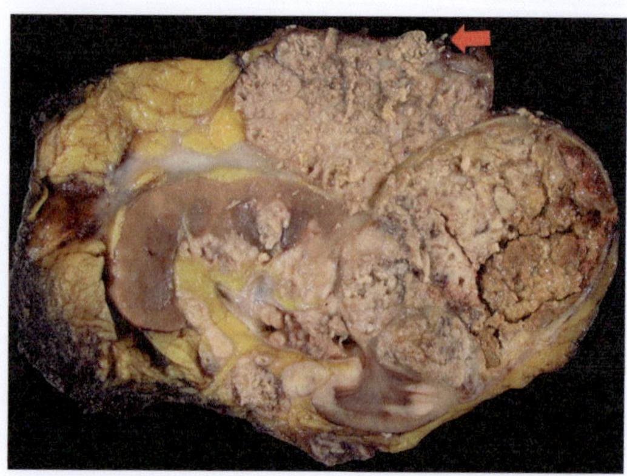

**Fig. 4.9** T4 renal cancer extending into Gerota's fascia (*arrow*)

cava involvement below the diaphragm. Leibovich et al. [35] showed that renal cancer with tumor thrombus in renal vein only has better prognosis than patients with T3 renal cancers with tumor thrombus extending 2 cm or less above the renal vein or beyond to the level above the diaphragm. Ficarra et al. [34] showed survival differences between renal cancers with tumor thrombus in renal vein (T3a) or vena cava below the diaphragm (T3b) versus vena caval thrombus above the diaphragm (T3b). These studies led to the reclassification of renal vein invasion into pT3a in the 2010 TNM system (vs. pT3b in 2002 TNM system).

### Invasion into Ipsilateral Adrenal Gland or Beyond Gerota's Fascia (T4)

Previous studies have shown that direct ipsilateral adrenal gland extension has poorer behavior than tumors involving the perinephric or sinus fat and is now lumped with tumor extending beyond Gerota's fascia (Fig. 4.9) [37–39]. Direct adrenal gland invasion is defined as contiguous spread of renal tumor through the peripheral perinephric fat into the ipsilateral adrenal gland [38]. Han et al. [37] showed a median survival of 12.5 months and 0 % 5-year CSS in renal cancer patients with adrenal gland involvement in contrast to a median survival of 36 months and a 36 % 5-year CSS for T3a renal cancer patients with perinephric or sinus fat invasion. The median survival of direct adrenal gland involvement is about similar to the median survival of tumors extending beyond Gerota's fascia (11 months) [37]. Thompson et al. [38] studied 424 renal cancer patients who underwent nephrectomy and adrenalectomy and showed that the CSS for tumors that directly invaded the adrenal gland (T4) was significantly worse compared with that of patients with perinephric, renal sinus, renal vein, or vena caval extension and without adrenal gland involvement (T3a–b). There was no difference in the 5-year CSS of patients with adrenal gland extension (20 %) and patients with extension beyond Gerota's fascia (14 %) [38]. Thus, ipsilateral adrenal gland extension was eventually designated as a T4 disease in the 2010 TNM system.

### Regional Lymph Nodes and Distant Metastasis

The regional lymph nodes for renal cancers include the hilar, caval (paracaval, precaval, and retrocaval), interaortocaval, and aortic (para-aortic, preaortic, and retroaortic) lymph nodes. The primary landing zone considered for right-sided renal tumors is the interaortocaval zone and for left-sided tumors is the aortic region; however, the patterns of tumor spread can be unpredictable. The 2010 TNM system lumps any positive lymph nodes altogether (N1 vs. N0), since most studies showed that any extent of lymph node involvement portends a poorer outcome.

Common distant metastatic sites for renal cancer are the bone, liver, lung, and brain. Involvement of distant or non-regional lymph nodes is staged as M1.

### Pathologist Handling of Kidney Resections for Staging Adequacy

Appropriate specimen handling is critical to the adequate pathologic staging of tumor nephrectomy specimens. In 2012, the ISUP held a consensus conference for the new classification of renal neoplasia [1]. Also covered in the consensus meeting is the pathological staging and specimen handling of renal tumors [29]. For specimen handling, it was agreed that kidneys with tumor should be sectioned along the long axis and perinephric fat extension should be determined by examining multiple perpendicular sections of the tumor/perinephric fat interface as well as areas that are suspicious for invasion. When measuring a renal tumor, the renal vein/vena caval thrombus, if present, is discounted from the measurement. Renal tumors should be sampled 1 block/cm with a minimum of 3 blocks per tumor. Recognizing the difficulty in identifying sinus invasion, the consensus recommended that at least 3 blocks of tumor-renal sinus interface should be submitted. If renal sinus invasion is grossly discernable, examination of one block of renal sinus tissue with tumor will suffice. When a caval thrombus is submitted by the surgeons for

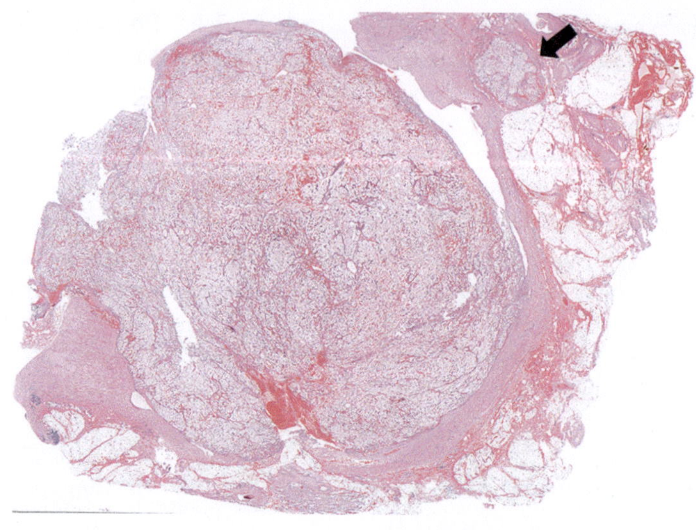

**Fig. 4.10** Section of the renal vein margin containing a tumor thrombus. This margin is considered positive because of tumor infiltration to the wall that is present at the margin (*arrow*)

**Table 4.6** Cancer-specific survival of renal cancer patients by pathologic T stage

| pT stage | 5-Year CSS | | 10-Year CSS |
|---|---|---|---|
| | Novara et al. (2010) [23] | Lee et al. (2011) [24] | Kim et al. (2011) [40] |
| T1a (%) | 94.9 | – | 96 |
| T1b (%) | 92.6 | – | 80 |
| T2a (%) | 85.4 | 83.2 | 66 |
| T2b (%) | 70 | 83.8 | 55 |
| T3a (%) | 64.7 | 62.6 | 36 |
| T3b (%) | 54.7 | 41.1 | 26 |
| T3c (%) | 17.9 | 50 | 25 |
| T4 (%) | 27.4 | 26.1 | 12 |

pathological examination, the recommendations is to submit at least two sections to look for wall invasion (classified as pT3c if present). Another recommendation is regarding the definition of a positive renal vein/caval margin in the presence of a tumor thrombus. It is not uncommon that a tumor thrombus when present may hang freely beyond the renal vein/caval resection margin, and such should not be automatically considered as a positive renal vein/caval margin. Renal vein/caval margin is considered positive only when there is adherent tumor visible microscopically at the actual cut margin (Fig. 4.10) [29].

## Validation Studies of the 2010 TNM Staging System

After its publication, several studies were conducted assessing the prognostic ability across all or select categories of the 2010 TNM system. The CSS of the different T categories in recent studies is presented in Table 4.6. While these studies were able to demonstrate the prognostic ability of the 2010 TNM system, its differences from the 2002 TNM system are only modest at best.

In a large multi-institutional study in Italy that included 5339 renal cancer patients, the 2010 TNM system was shown to be a strong predictor of CSS [23]. The substratification of T1 (T1a vs. T1b) tumors however was not retained as an independent prognostic variable. When only the non-metastatic tumors were considered, the survival differences between T1a and T1b, T2b and T3a, T3a and T3b, and T3c and T4 were not statistically significant. T3a was shown to be heterogeneous with renal vein invasion having a significantly higher CSS, followed by tumors with perirenal involvement and by those with both of these features present. The differences in the CSS of renal cancers with renal vein (T3a), infradiaphragmatic (T3b), and supradiaphragmatic vena caval thrombus (T3b) were statistically significant; however, these differences did not hold true in non-metastatic renal cancers.

In the study by Kim et al. [40] of 3996 renal cancer patients from a large tertiary institution, the 2010 TNM system likewise retained its robust predictive ability for CSS; however, it showed only modest improvement compared to the 2002 TNM system. The aggregation of nodal involvement to N0 or N1 did not contribute to any increase in the predictive ability than in the prior N subcategories. The T3a category was again shown to be heterogeneous where renal cancers with level 0 thrombus and no fat invasion had better CSS than patients with fat invasion only, while renal cancers with both level 0 thrombus and fat invasion had the poorest CSS.

In the study by Lee et al. [24] of 1691 renal cancer patients from Korea, the 2010 TNM system offered a good statistical power in predicting CSS; however, the findings suggested that the predictive ability of 2010 TNM system is not superior to that of the 2002 TNM system. The study also showed that the CSS of T2a and T2b renal cancers did not differ significantly. Pichler et al. [25] in another study of 2739 renal cancer patients from Austria showed the predictive ability of the 2010 TNM system for overall survival, CSS, and metastasis-free survival in renal cancers. However, the use of the 2010 TNM system was not associated with a net benefit in predicting these three clinical end points when compared with the 2002 TNM system [25]. In terms of metastasis-free survival, significant differences were observed for T1a versus T1b, T3a versus T3b, and T3b versus T3c [25]. The same authors showed similar lack of predictive advantage of the 2010 TNM system, specifically in clear cell RCC or in papillary RCC, regarding CSS compared to the 2002 TNM system [41].

Other studies focused only on some of the categories of the 2010 TNM system. Ingimarsson et al. [42] showed that the probability for synchronous metastases increased in a nonlinear fashion with increasing tumor size according to the 2010 TNM size cutoffs (T1a, T1b, T2a, and T2c) and that tumor size affected the probability of the disease-specific mortality. Bianchi et al. [43] showed the 10 cm cutoff for T2 tumors as an independent predictor of cancer-specific mortality; however, higher discrimination was achieved with either 9 or 11 cm cutoffs. In contrast, Waalkes et al. [44] in a study of 579 T2 renal cancer patients showed no significant difference in CSS between T2a and T2b.

Chevinsky et al. [45] in a study of 1809 T1–T3 renal cancer patients showed that T3a tumors had a greater risk of tumor recurrence than T1/T2 tumors. The risk of disease recurrence increased more rapidly as tumor size increased only with the presence of perinephric fat invasion. Veeratterapillay et al. [46] likewise showed that T3a and T3b were both significantly worse than T1 in the 2010 TNM system that were not demonstrated with the 2002 TNM stage. In a large multi-institutional study of 7384 T1a–T3a renal cancer patients pooled from 12 centers, the T3a tumors were grouped into those with perinephric fat invasion only (group 1) and those with renal vein invasion with or without perinephric fat invasion (group 2) [47]. The cancer-specific mortality was significantly higher for both group 1 and group 2 renal cancers compared to T1–T2 renal cancers. The cancer-specific mortality for group 1 and group 2 renal cancers did not differ, thus supporting the merging of perinephric fat invasion and renal vein invasion under a single stage category (pT3a) in the 2010 TNM system.

In a multi-institutional study that included 1215 renal cancer patients who underwent radical nephrectomy and tumor thrombectomy, the tumor thrombus level was shown to be an independent predictor of survival [48]. The 5-year survival of renal vein involvement (T3a), vena cava below diaphragm (T3b), and vena cava above diaphragm (T3c) were 43.2 %, 37 %, and 22 %, respectively. This finding supported the separation of these levels of vascular involvement in the 2010 TNM system.

# References


1. Srigley JR, Delahunt B, Eble JN, Egevad L, Epstein JI, Grignon D, et al. The International Society of Urological Pathology (ISUP) Vancouver classification of renal neoplasia. Am J Surg Pathol. 2013;37(10):1469–89.
2. Edge SB, Byrd DR, Compton CC, Fritz AG, Greene FL, Trotti III A. AJCC cancer staging manual. New York: Springer; 2010.
3. Kattan MW, Reuter V, Motzer RJ, Katz J, Russo P. A postoperative prognostic nomogram for renal cell carcinoma. J Urol. 2001;166(1):63–7.
4. Sorbellini M, Kattan MW, Snyder ME, Reuter V, Motzer R, Goetzl M, et al. A postoperative prognostic nomogram predicting recurrence for patients with conventional clear cell renal cell carcinoma. J Urol. 2005;173(1):48–51.
5. Frank I, Blute ML, Cheville JC, Lohse CM, Weaver AL, Zincke H. An outcome prediction model for patients with clear cell renal cell carcinoma treated with radical nephrectomy based on tumor stage, size, grade and necrosis: the SSIGN score. J Urol. 2002;168(6):2395–400.
6. Zisman A, Pantuck AJ, Dorey F, Said JW, Shvarts O, Quintana D, et al. Improved prognostication of renal cell carcinoma using an integrated staging system. J Clin Oncol. 2001;19(6):1649–57.
7. Sun M, Shariat SF, Cheng C, Ficarra V, Murai M, Oudard S, et al. Prognostic factors and predictive models in renal cell carcinoma: a contemporary review. Eur Urol. 2011;60(4):644–61.
8. Flocks RH, Kadesky MC. Malignant neoplasms of the kidney; an analysis of 353 patients followed five years or more. J Urol. 1958;79(2):196–201.
9. Petkovic SD. An anatomical classification of renal tumors in the adult as a basis for prognosis. J Urol. 1959;81(5):618–23.
10. Robson CJ. Radical nephrectomy for renal cell carcinoma. J Urol. 1963;89:37–42.
11. Robson CJ, Churchill BM, Anderson W. The results of radical nephrectomy for renal cell carcinoma. J Urol. 1969;101(3):297–301.
12. Hafez KS, Fergany AF, Novick AC. Nephron sparing surgery for localized renal cell carcinoma: impact of tumor size on patient survival, tumor recurrence and TNM staging. J Urol. 1999;162(6):1930–3.
13. Igarashi T, Tobe T, Nakatsu HO, Suzuki N, Murakami S, Hamano M, et al. The impact of a 4 cm. cutoff point for stratification of T1N0M0 renal cell carcinoma after radical nephrectomy. J Urol. 2001;165(4):1103–6.
14. Delahunt B, Kittelson JM, McCredie MR, Reeve AE, Stewart JH, Bilous AM. Prognostic importance of tumor size for localized conventional (clear cell) renal cell carcinoma: assessment of TNM T1 and T2 tumor categories and comparison with other prognostic parameters. Cancer. 2002;94(3):658–64.
15. Salama ME, Guru K, Stricker H, Peterson E, Peabody J, Menon M, et al. pT1 substaging in renal cell carcinoma: validation of the 2002 TNM staging modification of malignant renal epithelial tumors. J Urol. 2005;173(5):1492–5.
16. Ficarra V, Schips L, Guille F, Li G, De La Taille A, Prayer Galetti T, et al. Multiinstitutional European validation of the 2002 TNM staging system in conventional and papillary localized renal cell carcinoma. Cancer. 2005;104(5):968–74.
17. Frank I, Blute ML, Leibovich BC, Cheville JC, Lohse CM, Zincke H. Independent validation of the 2002 American Joint Committee on cancer primary tumor classification for renal cell carcinoma using a large, single institution cohort. J Urol. 2005;173(6):1889–92.
18. Zisman A, Pantuck AJ, Chao D, Dorey F, Said JW, Gitlitz BJ, et al. Reevaluation of the 1997 TNM classification for renal cell carcinoma: T1 and T2 cutoff point at 4.5 rather than 7 cm. better correlates with clinical outcome. J Urol. 2001;166(1):54–8.
19. Elmore JM, Kadesky KT, Koeneman KS, Sagalowsky AI. Reassessment of the 1997 TNM classification system for renal cell carcinoma. Cancer. 2003;98(11):2329–34.
20. Steiner T, Knels R, Schubert J. Prognostic significance of tumour size in patients after tumour nephrectomy for localised renal cell carcinoma. Eur Urol. 2004;46(3):327–30.
21. Kuczyk M, Wegener G, Merseburger AS, Anastasiadis A, Machtens S, Zumbragel A, et al. Impact of tumor size on the long-term survival of patients with early stage renal cell cancer. World J Urol. 2005;23(1):50–4.
22. Ficarra V, Guille F, Schips L, de la Taille A, Prayer Galetti T, Tostain J, et al. Proposal for revision of the TNM classification system for renal cell carcinoma. Cancer. 2005;104(10):2116–23.
23. Novara G, Ficarra V, Antonelli A, Artibani W, Bertini R, Carini M, et al. Validation of the 2009 TNM version in a large multi-institutional cohort of patients treated for renal cell carcinoma: are further improvements needed? Eur Urol. 2010;58(4):588–95.
24. Lee C, You D, Park J, Jeong IG, Song C, Hong JH, et al. Validation of the 2009 TNM classification for renal cell carcinoma: comparison with the 2002 TNM classification by concordance index. Korean J Urol. 2011;52(8):524–30.
25. Pichler M, Hutterer GC, Chromecki TF, Jesche J, Kampel-Kettner K, Groselj-Strele A, et al. Predictive ability of the 2002 and 2010 versions of the Tumour-Node-Metastasis classification system regarding metastasis-free, cancer-specific and overall survival in a European renal cell carcinoma single-centre series. BJU Int. 2013;111(4 Pt B):E191–5.
26. Grignon D, Paner GP. Renal cell carcinoma and the renal sinus. Adv Anat Pathol. 2007;14(2):63–8.
27. Bonsib SM, Gibson D, Mhoon M, Greene GF. Renal sinus involvement in renal cell carcinomas. Am J Surg Pathol. 2000;24(3):451–8.

28. Bonsib SM. T2 clear cell renal cell carcinoma is a rare entity: a study of 120 clear cell renal cell carcinomas. J Urol. 2005;174(4 Pt 1):1199–202.

29. Trpkov K, Grignon DJ, Bonsib SM, Amin MB, Billis A, Lopez-Beltran A, et al. Handling and staging of renal cell carcinoma: the International Society of Urological Pathology Consensus (ISUP) conference recommendations. Am J Surg Pathol. 2013;37(10):1505–17.

30. Bertini R, Roscigno M, Freschi M, Strada E, Petralia G, Pasta A, et al. Renal sinus fat invasion in pT3a clear cell renal cell carcinoma affects outcomes of patients without nodal involvement or distant metastases. J Urol. 2009;181(5):2027–32.

31. Thompson RH, Blute ML, Krambeck AE, Lohse CM, Magera JS, Leibovich BC, et al. Patients with pT1 renal cell carcinoma who die from disease after nephrectomy may have unrecognized renal sinus fat invasion. Am J Surg Pathol. 2007;31(7):1089–93.

32. Gorin MA, Ball MW, Pierorazio PM, Tanagho YS, Bhayani SB, Kaouk JH, et al. Outcomes and predictors of clinical T1 to pathological T3a tumor up-staging after robotic partial nephrectomy: a multi-institutional analysis. J Urol. 2013;190(5):1907–11.

33. Thompson RH, Leibovich BC, Cheville JC, Webster WS, Lohse CM, Kwon ED, et al. Is renal sinus fat invasion the same as perinephric fat invasion for pT3a renal cell carcinoma? J Urol. 2005;174(4 Pt 1):1218–21.

34. Ficarra V, Novara G, Iafrate M, Cappellaro L, Bratti E, Zattoni F, et al. Proposal for reclassification of the TNM staging system in patients with locally advanced (pT3-4) renal cell carcinoma according to the cancer-related outcome. Eur Urol. 2007;51(3):722–9.

35. Leibovich BC, Cheville JC, Lohse CM, Zincke H, Kwon ED, Frank I, et al. Cancer specific survival for patients with pT3 renal cell carcinoma-can the 2002 primary tumor classification be improved? J Urol. 2005;173(3):716–9.

36. Kim HL, Zisman A, Han KR, Figlin RA, Belldegrun AS. Prognostic significance of venous thrombus in renal cell carcinoma. Are renal vein and inferior vena cava involvement different? J Urol. 2004;171(2 Pt 1):588–91.

37. Han KR, Bui MH, Pantuck AJ, Freitas DG, Leibovich BC, Dorey FJ, et al. TNM T3a renal cell carcinoma: adrenal gland involvement is not the same as renal fat invasion. J Urol. 2003;169(3):899–903.

38. Thompson RH, Leibovich BC, Cheville JC, Lohse CM, Frank I, Kwon ED, et al. Should direct ipsilateral adrenal invasion from renal cell carcinoma be classified as pT3a? J Urol. 2005;173(3):918–21.

39. Thompson RH, Cheville JC, Lohse CM, Webster WS, Zincke H, Kwon ED, et al. Reclassification of patients with pT3 and pT4 renal cell carcinoma improves prognostic accuracy. Cancer. 2005;104(1):53–60.

40. Kim SP, Alt AL, Weight CJ, Costello BA, Cheville JC, Lohse C, et al. Independent validation of the 2010 American Joint Committee on Cancer TNM classification for renal cell carcinoma: results from a large, single institution cohort. J Urol. 2011;185(6):2035–9.

41. Pichler M, Hutterer GC, Chromecki TF, Jesche J, Kampel-Kettner K, Groselj-Strele A, et al. Comparison of the 2002 and 2010 TNM classification systems regarding outcome prediction in clear cell and papillary renal cell carcinoma. Histopathology. 2013;62(2):237–46.

42. Ingimarsson JP, Sigurdsson MI, Hardarson S, Petursdottir V, Jonsson E, Einarsson GV, et al. The impact of tumour size on the probability of synchronous metastasis and survival in renal cell carcinoma patients: a population-based study. BMC Urol. 2014; 14:72.

43. Bianchi M, Becker A, Trinh QD, Abdollah F, Tian Z, Shariat SF, et al. An analysis of patients with T2 renal cell carcinoma (RCC) according to tumour size: a population-based analysis. BJU Int. 2013;111(8): 1184–90.

44. Waalkes S, Becker F, Schrader AJ, Janssen M, Wegener G, Merseburger AS, et al. Is there a need to further subclassify pT2 renal cell cancers as implemented by the revised 7th TNM version? Eur Urol. 2011;59(2):258–63.

45. Chevinsky M, Imnadze M, Sankin A, Winer A, Mano R, Jakubowski C, et al. Pathological stage T3a significantly increases disease recurrence across all tumor sizes in renal cell carcinoma. J Urol. 2015;194:310–5.

46. Veeratterapillay R, Simren R, El-Sherif A, Johnson MI, Soomro N, Heer R. Accuracy of the revised 2010 TNM classification in predicting the prognosis of patients treated for renal cell cancer in the north east of England. J Clin Pathol. 2012;65(4):367–71.

47. Brookman-May SD, May M, Wolff I, Zigeuner R, Hutterer GC, Cindolo L, et al. Evaluation of the prognostic significance of perirenal fat invasion and tumor size in patients with pT1-pT3a localized renal cell carcinoma in a comprehensive multicenter study of the CORONA project. Can we improve prognostic discrimination for patients with stage pT3a tumors? Eur Urol. 2015;67(5):943–51.

48. Martinez-Salamanca JI, Huang WC, Millan I, Bertini R, Bianco FJ, Carballido JA, et al. Prognostic impact of the 2009 UICC/AJCC TNM staging system for renal cell carcinoma with venous extension. Eur Urol. 2011;59(1):120–7.

# Conventional Forms of Renal Neoplasia

**5**


Ithaar H. Derweesh, Omer A. Raheem, and Ahmed Shabaik


## Introduction

With approximately 65,000 cases and 15,000 deaths, renal cell carcinoma (RCC) is the third most common and deadliest urologic malignancy, accounting for 2 % of solid malignancies diagnosed in the United States (USA), making it the sixth most common malignancy in men and the seventh most common malignancy in women [1, 2]. Despite a robust downward stage migration due to increasing utilization of radiological imaging modalities and diagnoses in incidental settings, deaths from RCC continue to rise, raising the scepter of an even higher death rate in the absence of the impact of incidentally discovered disease. The underlying reasons for this are unclear, but are likely related to as of yet ill-defined complex interaction between environmental risk factors and metabolic drivers (obesity, hypertension) which give rise to RCC and continue to drive incidence up even as other prominent risk factors may be on the decline (smoking/tobacco use), lack of overarching successful systemic therapeutic strategy, and an aging population [3–7].

This chapter will review the major histopathological categorization and subtypes of RCC and major benign cortical tumors, staging classifications, as well as therapeutic strategies and options for different stages and ongoing controversies regarding management.

## Renal Tumor Pathology and Grading

Perhaps the earliest description of a renal tumor was that offered by Daniel Sennert in his textbook *Practicae Medicinae* in 1613. Under the term "Scirrhus renum," Sennert stated, "Sometimes the kidneys are attacked by hard growths and hard swellings, which often happen following poorly cared for inflammation. Moreover the hard swelling of bad kidneys which has the capacity to throw a person into cachexia and dropsy, is for the greater part incurable."

The first use of the word "Conventional" RCC was in the 1997 WHO classification of renal neoplasms, and it was used to denote the clear cell form of RCC. However, the editor's selection as a title for this chapter "Conventional Forms of Renal Neoplasia" intends to include more than just that. For this reason in this chapter, we will try to discuss the most common forms of renal neoplasms known to pathologists for some time before the plethora of the recently recognized special forms of renal neoplasms


I.H. Derweesh, M.D. (✉) • O.A. Raheem, M.D.
Department of Urology, University of California
San Diego, San Diego, CA, USA

A. Shabaik, M.D.
Department of Pathology, University of California,
San Diego Medical Center, 200 West Arbor Drive,
San Diego, CA 92103-8720, USA



© Springer Science+Business Media New York 2016
D.E. Hansel et al. (eds.), *The Kidney*, DOI 10.1007/978-1-4939-3286-3_5

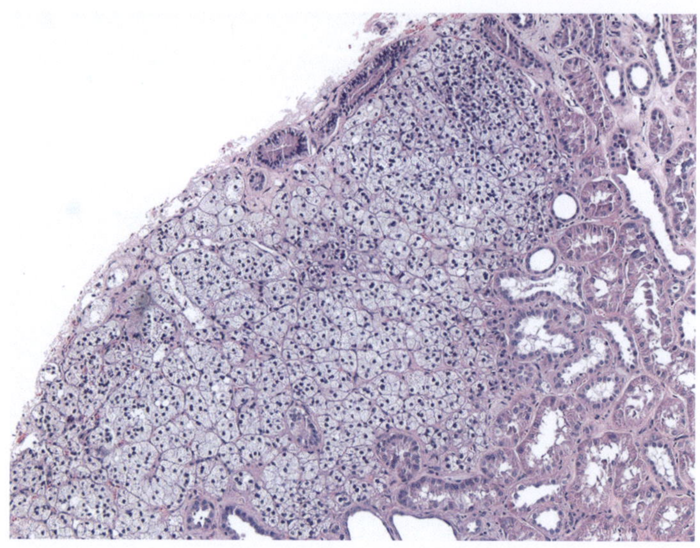

**Fig. 5.1** Adrenal rest in renal cortex. 100× magnification

that started around the mid-1980s with the introduction of chromophobe RCC by Theones and his colleagues. In this chapter, we will discuss clear cell RCC, multilocular cystic clear cell renal cell neoplasm of low malignant potential (multilocular cystic renal cell carcinoma), papillary RCC, papillary adenoma, chromophobe RCC, and oncocytoma.

## Clear Cell Renal Cell Carcinoma

Clear cell renal cell carcinoma (CCRCC) is the most common renal malignancy. It has been initially named the Grawitz tumor in reference to Grawitz who in 1883 recognized microscopically the presence of adrenal rests in the renal cortex, gave it the name "struma suprarenalis aberrata" (Fig. 5.1). He postulated that they are precursors of renal neoplasms [8]. However, in 1893 Sudeck published his observation of finding atypical tubules adjacent to renal tumors, postulated that these are the origin of renal tumors, and challenged Grawitz theory [8]. Such finding has been recently supported by one publication [9]. Despite Sudeck's challenge, in 1894 Lubarsch supported Grawitz theory and coined the term "hyperneph-roid tumor" which was later on modified to

"hypernephroma" by Birch-Hirschfeld [8]. This term remained in use until the late 1970s.

CCRCC occurs in sporadic and familial forms. Sporadic CCRCC is mostly found in the 6th decade with male to female ratio of 2–3:1 as solitary mass of the renal cortex commonly protruding on the renal surface as a globular or bosselated mass. Multiple or bilateral tumors or early age of onset should raise concern for the familial forms associated with von Hippel-Lindau (VHL) syndrome or constitutional chromosome 3 translocation. Familial cases comprise less than 5 % of all cases of CCRCC. A band of fibrosis of variable thickness (pseudocapsule) is present at the interface of the tumor with the nonneoplastic kidney. Generally, the cut surface is solid and golden yellow in color due to high fat content, but commonly displays foci of hemorrhage and necrosis and cyst formation. Calcification and even ossification may be encountered. The size is variable, but the majority of tumors nowadays are less than seven centimeters due to advances in the imaging and surgical techniques.

Microscopically as the name indicates, the tumor consists of cells with optically clear cytoplasm due to high content of lipid and glycogen, which dissolve during routine processing. A population of cells with eosinophilic cytoplasm can be found and

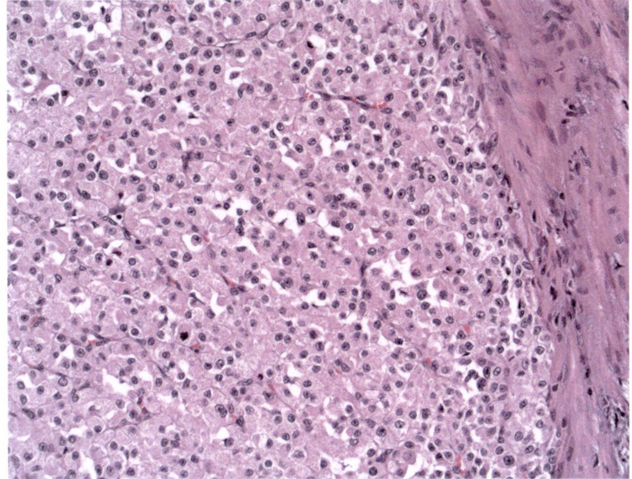

**Fig. 5.2** Clear cell renal cell carcinoma with predominantly eosinophilic cells. 200× magnification

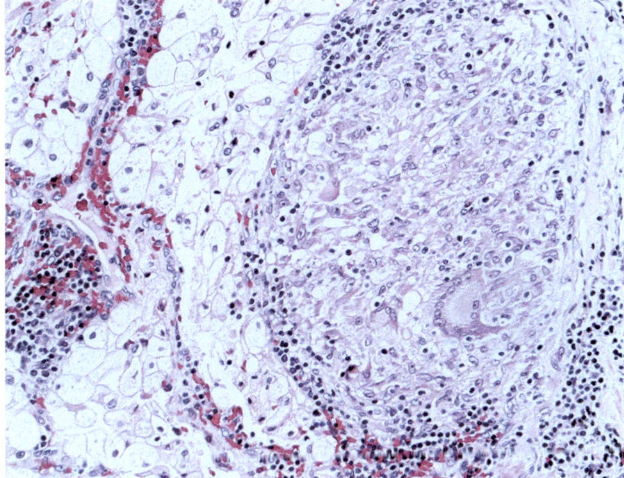

**Fig. 5.3** Granulomatous host response to clear cell renal cell carcinoma. 200× magnification

rarely may be the predominant cell type (Fig. 5.2). The cell border is distinct but not prominent. The cells are arranged in solid sheets and nests or alveoli and acini that may dilate to form microcystic or macrocystic spaces or combination of patterns. These spaces may be filled with serous fluid or blood ("blood lakes"). An elaborate network of thin-walled blood vessels invests these structures. The nuclei are usually round and uniform with evenly distributed chromatin. The size of the nucleus and the prominence of the nucleolus are the basis for the Fuhrman grading system. A host response of tumor infiltrating lymphocytes is usually present but can be very variable in intensity. Rarely a granulomatous response can be seen around tumor cells (Fig. 5.3). Host response and

tumor necrosis with subsequent organization may cause tumor regression and reduce the tumor to a small scar.

Immunohistochemistry can be helpful with the diagnosing CCRCC particularly in limited samples like core biopsies and fine needle aspiration. CCRCC is usually positive with the RCC marker, vimentin, PAX2, PAX8, CD10, carbonic anhydrase IX, and CK18 and usually negative with CK5, CK6, CK7, CK20, HMWKs, and CD117 [9]. AMACR and E-cadherin can be variable [10].

The tumor grade is second to the tumor stage in predicting prognosis. The most widely used grading system is the nuclear grading system published by Fuhrman et al. in 1982 [11]. It is a four-tier grading system based on the size of the nucleus and the prominence of the nucleolus at the 10× objective. Grade 1 tumors have nuclei that are less than 10 μm with dense chromatin and invisible nucleoli at the 100× magnification or higher. Grade 2 nuclei are less than 15 μm with finely granular chromatin and invisible nucleoli at 100× magnification but may be visible at 200×. Grade 3 nuclei are less than 20 μm and nucleoli are easily visible at 100× magnification. Grade 4 tumors display nuclei that are larger than 20 μm with noticeable hyperchromasia and pleomorphism and contain single or multiple macronucleoli. CCRCC can show areas with variable grades; however, the tumor grade is assigned based on the highest grade encountered. In 2013, ISUP proposed a modification of the Fuhrman grading system, which relies solely on the prominence of the nucleoli for grades 1–3. ISUP grade 4 tumors should encompass tumors with rhabdoid or sarcomatoid differentiation or those containing tumor giant cells or showing extreme nuclear pleomorphism with clumping of chromatin [12].

Staging of CCRCC is not discussed here extensively; however, CCRCC commonly spreads via blood stream. About 75 % of metastatic CCRCC are seen in the lungs. It is also known to metastasize to unusual sites like the eye, thyroid, parotid glands, pancreas, and cerebellum even after many years, which can reach up to 30 years. In such odd sites, the metastatic CCRCC may mimic primary tumors of these organs (e.g., clear cell myoepithelioma of parotid or hemangioblastoma of the central nervous system, which also shares the VHL mutation with CCRCC) [13]. In such situations, one may miss the diagnosis particularly if the history of prior RCC is not available due to long interval or due to patient changing hospitals. The clear cell morphology and the intricate delicate vascular network should stimulate the alert pathologist to think about possible metastatic CCRCC. The role of immunohistochemistry in directing the workup of such situations cannot be ignored.

Although most CCRCC are sporadic, cytogenetic studies have detected chromosomal abnormalities in the majority of them including 3p deletions involving the VHL locus at 3p25–26

[14, 15], the familial human RCC chromosomal translocation point at 3p13–14 [16], and 3p21–22 [17]. Chromosome 3p deletions were detected in very small CCRCC suggesting it to be an early event in its development [18]. Other chromosomal abnormalities like 9p loss [19] and 14q deletions [20] have been found in patients with higher grade and stage and they correlate with poor outcome.

## Multilocular Cystic Clear Cell Renal Cell Neoplasm of Low Malignant Potential (Multilocular Cystic Renal Cell Carcinoma)

A tumor closely related to CCRCC, these in its pure form have never been reported to have progressed, recurred, or metastasized and are seen in adults and more commonly in males. Previously regarded as a "carcinoma," in 2013 ISUP adopted a change in the nomenclature for these tumors to reflect its low malignant potential [21]. They are well-circumscribed masses with fibrous capsule and made up entirely of cysts. The cysts are lined by clear cells with grade 1 nuclei and the septa between the cysts may contain small nonexpansile groups of clear cells with grade 1 nuclei [22, 23].

## Papillary Renal Cell Carcinoma

Papillary renal cell carcinoma (PRCC) is the second most common malignant renal neoplasm and comprises about 10 % of RCC. Its age and sex distribution and clinical presentation are similar to that of CCRCC [24, 25]. Angiography studies suggest relative hypovascularity of PRCC [25]. Grossly PRCC is more prone to show multifocality and bilaterality particularly in cases of hereditary PRCC [26]. They frequently show areas of hemorrhage, necrosis, and cystic change. Well-circumscribed tumors have fibrous capsule. In the 1986 Mainz classification of renal tumors, PRCC was named chromophil RCC in contrast to the chromophobe RCC, and this was mainly due to its microscopic composition of either

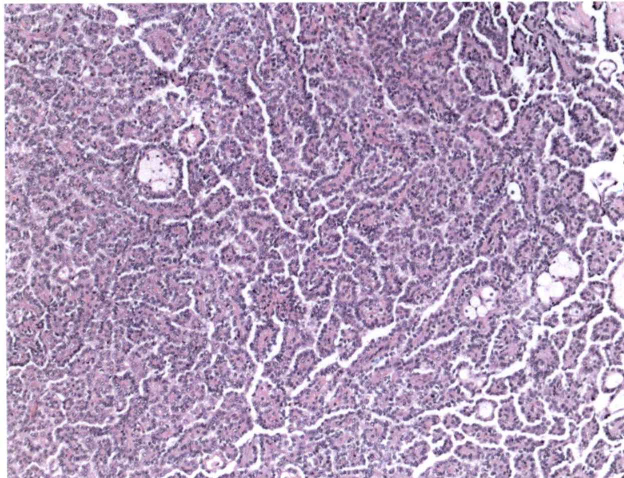

**Fig. 5.4** Type I papillary renal cell carcinoma. 100× magnification

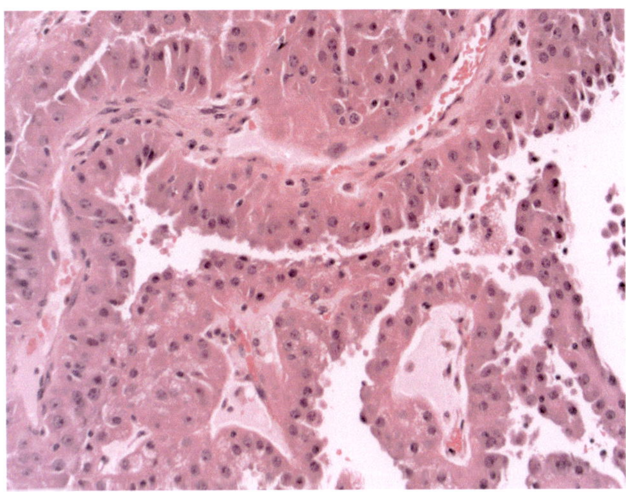

**Fig. 5.5** Type II papillary renal cell carcinoma. 400× magnification

basophilic or eosinophilic cells or combination. This chromophilic classification did not convey much prognostic significance. More recently Delahunt and Eble [27] proposed reclassifying PRCC into type 1 and type 2 based on that in type 1 the papillary fronds are lined by a single layer of small cells with scant cytoplasm (Fig. 5.4), while in type 2 tumor papillae are lined by larger cells with eosinophilic cytoplasm with pseudostratified nuclei of usually higher grade (Fig. 5.5). This classification proved to be of better prognostic significance [27, 28]. Type 1 is commonly multifocal, while type 2 is unifocal. PRCC is not always made entirely of papillary structures but can show variable proportions of papillae and tubules. Large cystic areas with

papillary fronds can also be found. Aggregates of foamy histiocytes and hemosiderin-laden macrophages can been seen mostly in the papillary cores. The lining epithelium may show hemosiderin granules decorating its luminal border. Calcifications and psammoma bodies can be found in PRCC. The so-called solid variant of PRCC is due to predominance of tubular and glomeruloid growths or to very compact papillae [29]. Sarcomatoid foci can be seen in up to 5 % of type 1 and type 2 PRCC, mainly as high-grade spindle cells [27].

By immunohistochemistry, PRCC is usually positive for RCC marker, CK7, vimentin, AMACR, PAX2, PAX8, and CD10 and usually negative for HMWK, E-cadherin, and CD117 and negative

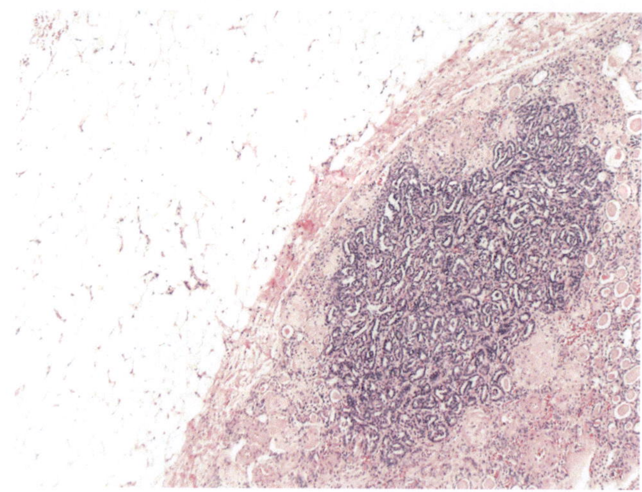

**Fig. 5.6** Papillary adenoma. 100× magnification

for uroplakin and p63, which help differentiate from papillary urothelial carcinoma if it is in the differential diagnosis of a papillary renal neoplasm. TFE3 is also negative in PRCC, which will be helpful in differentiating it from an Xp11 translocation carcinoma with papillary architecture [10, 30]. The non-sporadic (familial) PRCC are seen in patients with the hereditary PRCC syndrome and Birt–Hogg–Dube syndrome and these are usually type 1 [26, 31], while type 2 is usually seen in patients with the hereditary leiomyomatosis and RCC syndrome [32, 33].

The commonest cytogenetic abnormalities in PRCC are trisomy of chromosomes 7 and 17 and loss of chromosome Y [34]. These karyotypic abnormalities are diagnostic of PRCC even if the tumor lacks the papillary architecture. In their absence, a tumor cannot be classified as PRCC even if it displays papillary architecture. The type of PRCC, nuclear grade, and stage correlate with prognosis and survival [28]. However, in multivariate analysis, only the tumor stage seems to be the only significant variable [35].

## Papillary Adenoma

The term papillary adenoma is restricted to tumors that are 0.5 cm or less in diameter and composed of papillary or tubulo-papillary structures. With this definition they are the most common epithelial neoplasm of the kidney as suggested by autopsy studies which show exponential increase in their incidence from 10 % in patients younger than 40 years to 40 % in patients older than 70 years [36, 37]. They are also seen with higher frequency in kidneys of patients on long-term dialysis regardless of age [38, 39]. Grossly, they are frequently encountered as subcapsular yellow or greyish white nodules. Microscopically they are similar to type 1 PRCC (Fig. 5.6) but occasionally can look like type 2 also. Most tumors are not encapsulated, but if a capsule is present, it is usually thin. Foamy macrophages and psammoma bodies are frequently present. Papillary adenoma shares the same genetic abnormality like PRCC with loss of Y and trisomy 7 and 17.

## Chromophobe Renal Cell Carcinoma

Theones described chromophobe renal cell carcinoma (CRCC) in 1985 as renal carcinoma with large pale cells with prominent cell membrane [40]. It accounts for about 5 % of all renal tumors mostly encountered in the 6th decade with equal incidence in men and women [41]. Sporadic and hereditary forms exist.

Grossly they are usually solid circumscribed tumors with variegated light brown to tan cut surface. Microscopically they are characterized by large polygonal cells with clear to pale eosinophilic finely reticulated cytoplasm with prominent

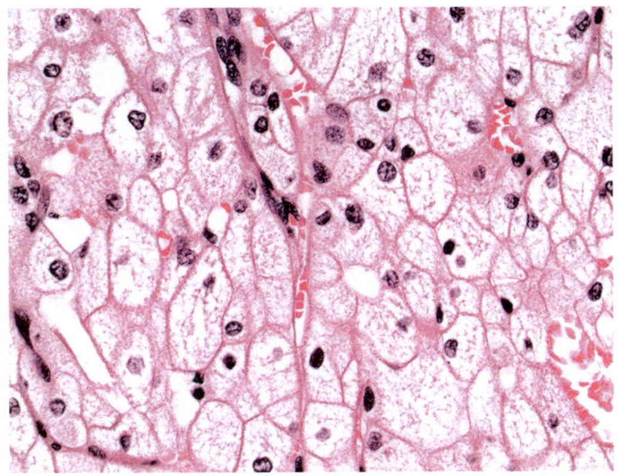

**Fig. 5.7** Chromophobe renal cell carcinoma, classic variant. 400× magnification

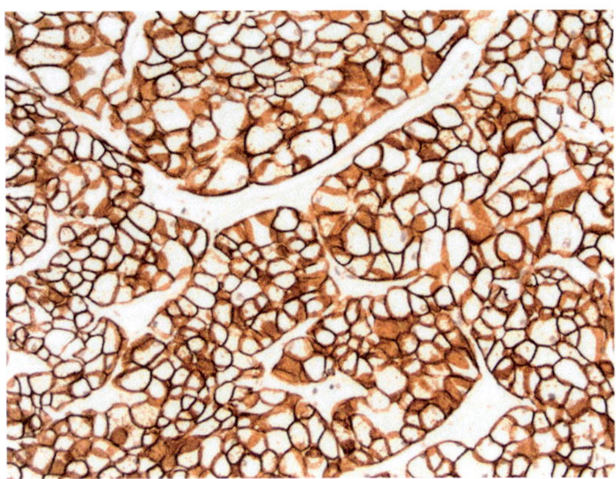

**Fig. 5.9** Cytokeratin 7 in chromophobe renal cell carcinoma. 200× magnification

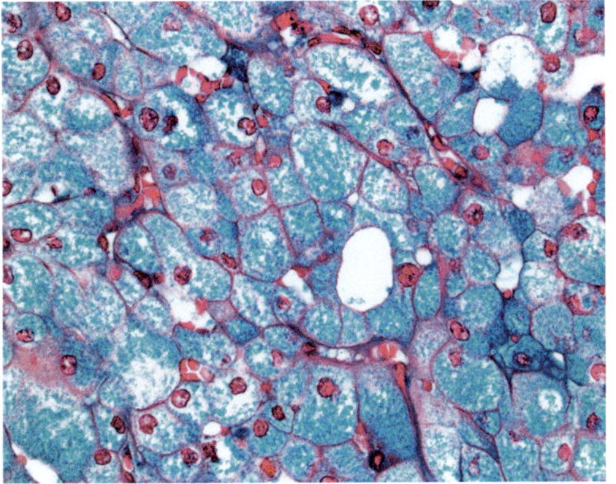

**Fig. 5.8** Positive colloidal iron stain in chromophobe renal cell carcinoma. 400× magnification

cell membrane. The nuclei are usually wrinkled with small nucleoli and a perinuclear halo (Fig. 5.7). Binucleation is common. An eosinophilic variant of CRCC has been described in which the cell cytoplasm is eosinophilic without reticulation [42]. Sarcomatoid areas can rarely be encountered in CRCC [43–46]. The cytoplasm of the CRCC cells stains positive with Hale's colloidal iron stain [40, 47] (Fig. 5.8). Ultrastructurally, CRCC shows abundant microvesicles and the eosinophilic type is rich in mitochondria. Grading of CRCC is controversial as many well-behaving and low-stage tumors show innate atypical nuclei [48]. The Fuhrman grading system was shown to be not applicable for CRCC [49, 50]. An alternative histologic grading system was proposed, but further validation is needed [50, 51].

The immunohistochemical profile of CRCC is positive for CK7 (Fig. 5.9), CK18, E-cadherin, kidney-specific cadherin, PAX8, and CD117 and negative for vimentin, AMACR, and variable with RCC marker and CD10, but mainly negative [10, 30, 47]. CRCC shows numerous chromosomal loss, which usually leads to hypodiploidy on DNA analysis [52, 53]. CRCC has good prognosis with no mortality at 5 years and 10 % mortality at 10 years [54]; however, sarcomatoid transformation is a poor prognostic indicator [45].

## Oncocytoma

A benign renal neoplasm made up of oncocytic cells with abundant granular eosinophilic cytoplasm rich in mitochondria. It was first described by Klein and Valensi in 1976 [55]. It constitutes about 5 % of all renal epithelial neoplasms and it is most frequent in the 7th decade with a male to female incidence ratio of 2:1. Most tumors are sporadic. It is believed that both oncocytoma and chromophobe RCC share origin from the intercalated cells of the cortical collecting ducts [47, 52, 55–59].

Grossly, oncocytomas are discrete well circumscribed but not encapsulated tumors. The cut surface is "mahogany brown" solid with a stellate scar in about 40 % of cases. Punctate hemorrhage may be encountered but no gross evidence of necrosis. Microscopically the tumor is composed of oncocytes that are round to polygonal with deeply eosinophilic granular cytoplasm with round regular centrally located nucleus with prominent nucleolus. The oncocytes are arranged in compact groups of small solid nests, acini, tubules, microcysts, or a combination of these structures embedded in loose edematous or hypocellular hyalinized stroma. Occasional clusters may display atypical degenerative nuclei, which does not affect the biologic behavior of the tumor. Mitoses are rare to absent and if present they are typical mitoses. Abundant clear cells or true papillary architecture is not a feature of oncocytoma and if encountered a diagnosis other than oncocytoma should be sought. Rarely oncocytoma may extend into perinephric fat or be seen within vessels [58–60]. Such features do not affect prognosis. Being a benign tumor, oncocytoma should not be graded or staged. Oncocytomas do not metastasize, although one report has claimed that two of seventy cases had metastasis. One case metastasized to the liver, which was histologically confirmed, and the second case metastasized to the liver and bone, but this was not histologically confirmed and could have been metastasized from other tumors [59].

Oncocytoma being related to CRCC should be differentiated from it. Oncocytomas have no fibrous capsule, show no prominent cell membranes, and do not show diffuse reticular positive reaction with Hale's colloidal iron stain, and nuclei are not wrinkled. Oncocytomas show overlapping immunophenotypic features with CRCC including the positivity for CD117. CK7 is usually negative in oncocytoma and if positive will be in the form of scattered positive cells (Fig. 5.10), in contrast to CRCC, which shows diffuse positive reaction. Few studies reported loss of chromosome Y and 1 in oncocytoma [61, 62].

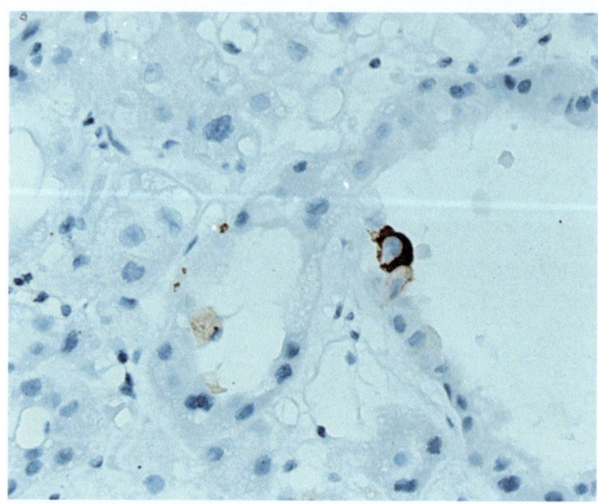

**Fig. 5.10** Cytokeratin 7 in oncocytoma

proposed erasure of the breakpoint between T1a and T1b at 4 cm was rejected, based on data suggesting that size appears to have continual prognostic significance, especially in the range of 2–6 cm [5, 6]. Nonetheless, the broad categories and breakdown of staging have remained unchanged and are as follows: stage I-T1N0M0, with T1 tumors being defined as <7 cm maximum dimension, and the breakpoint between T1a and T1b being 4 cm; stage II-T2N0M0, with T2 tumors being defined as >7 cm and the breakpoint between T2a and T2b being 10 cm; stage III-T3N0/1M0, with T3a being revised to include tumors breaking the renal capsule and tumor thrombus being confined to the renal vein, T3b including tumors with thrombus into the subdiaphragmatic inferior vena cava (IVC), and T3c comprising tumor thrombus into the supradiaphragmatic IVC; and stage IV comprising T4 (with extension into adjacent organs) with AnyN/AnyM or TAny/withN (>1 regional lymph node metastasis) or M1 [63].

## Staging of Renal Cell Carcinoma

Staging of RCC is based on the AJCC/TNM classification with its most recent iteration being in 2010, incorporating modifications based on increased understanding of tumor biology. The major change involved reclassification of T3a tumors with noncontiguous adrenal involvement (which had a worse prognosis to T4), while

## Evaluation and Workup of Cortical Renal Tumors

The cornerstone of evaluation is the history and physical. Careful attention should be paid to concurrent symptoms (e.g., hematuria or flank pain), as well as family history or symptomatic presentation which may guide further studies. Presence of physical exam findings may also indicate locally advanced (e.g., left-sided varicocele, lower extremity edema) or metastatic disease. The standard laboratory evaluation should include determination of renal function (BUN/creatinine and calculation of eGFR), liver function tests (including alkaline phosphatase), and a complete blood count. While several putative markers [nonspecific markers of systemic inflammation such as C-reactive protein (CRP), erythrocyte sedimentation rate (ESR), and platelet count] and tissue-based markers such as carbonic anhydrase IX have been demonstrated to have prognostic predictive utility, currently no single test or set of tests has gained widespread acceptance as an overarching tumor marker [3, 4].

Utilization of cross-sectional contrast-enhanced imaging studies (MRI or CT) remains as the confirmatory modalities of choice to assess local extent of disease and regional and abdominal metastases [64]. While data exist which demonstrate differential enhancement patterns between different tumor histologies, currently such data are of limited utility in clinical decision making [65, 66]. MRI may have added advantages in delineation of venous thrombus extent and allows utilization of contrast in patients with eGFR < 60; utilization of gadolinium contrast in patients with eGFR < 30 (severe CKD) is contraindicated given risk regarding progressive systemic fibrosis [67]. Chest imaging should be obtained as part of the workup, given the fact that the chest is the most common site of metastasis in RCC. Generally for lower-risk tumors, a chest X-ray is sufficient, with CT of the chest being preferred for higher-risk primary tumors or in patients with suggestive symptomatology. Current data do not support utilization of PET/CT for staging or follow-up of RCC, and utilization of adjunctive staging imaging (bone scintigraphy) or head CT should be limited to patients with elevated alkaline phosphatase (bone scintigraphy) or symptomatology (bone or neurological imaging) [6].

## Management

Treatment options are predicated by tumor stage, patient functional status, and whether or not indication exists to preserve nephron function.

Patients with a solitary kidney, bilateral synchronous masses, or preexisting chronic renal insufficiency (eGFR < 60) are considered to have imperative indication for nephron-sparing management approaches. Relative indications for nephron-sparing strategies include patients with significant medical drivers towards CKD (eGFR < 70, diabetes mellitus (DM) with sequelae, morbid and difficult to control hypertension, proteinuria) and a contralateral abnormal kidney even in the setting of a normal GFR [68, 69].

## Role of Percutaneous Biopsy of Renal Masses

Percutaneous renal mass biopsy is playing in increasingly important role in the management of RCC. With a greater understanding of the differential diagnosis and biological potential of RCC and improvements in biopsy technique and imaging technology, data suggest that risk for tumor seeding is minimal with diagnostic accuracy rates exceeding that of CT or MRI. While most localized renal masses in appropriate patients undergo definitive extirpative therapy without prior biopsy, given the overall diagnostic accuracy of contrast-enhanced CT and MRI which approaches that of biopsy, biopsy may be the preferred first-line approach in the diagnosis in the setting of metastatic disease (to confirm histology and guide systemic therapy), prior to ablative therapy (for risk stratification and to guide follow-up), and in select cases, prior to embarking on a strategy of active surveillance (and to rule out aggressive histology) [70].

## Management of Localized Renal Masses (Stage I/Stage II)

The main options for clinical stage I renal masses include nephrectomy (as the reference standard for cT1a masses and an alternate standard for cT1b masses), radical nephrectomy (an alternate standard for cT1a masses and the reference standard for cT1b masses), observation, and thermal ablation, in select patients, while for clinical stage II renal masses include radical nephrectomy as the standard and partial nephrectomy or observation in select patients [5, 6].

Data suggest that partial nephrectomy has equivalent oncological outcomes to radical nephrectomy for cT1a and cT2a, and emerging data suggest that equivalence may be extended to cT2 renal mass [68]. Furthermore, retrospective data suggest that partial nephrectomy may confer survival advantage by a reduction of cardiovascular events and metabolic sequelae compared to radical nephrectomy [5–7]. These data have been called into question by the recent publication of EORTC clinical trial 30904, while demonstrating equivalence in oncological outcomes between partial and radical nephrectomy for renal cell carcinomas of 1–5 cm, nonetheless did not demonstrate an improvement in overall survival [68]. While this clinical trial has been criticized for a number of valid reasons (including but not limited to early closure due to failure to accrue and resulting underpowering), the data nonetheless suggest that the impact of surgical nephron preservation may not be as great as previously thought and that retrospective data are heavily contaminated by selection bias [68].

Probe- or energy-based ablation is a valid option for patients with smaller renal masses (<3.5 cm). Long-term retrospective data has recently been published which demonstrate long-term satisfactory outcomes of cryoablation and radiofrequency ablation (RFA) for renal masses <3.5 cm in size. While overall and cancer-specific survival is similar to partial and radical nephrectomy, ablative treatment is nonetheless associated with a higher primary treatment failure rate, and concerns continue about the morbidity and efficacy of salvage treatment, as well as the need for more intensive ionizing radiation follow-up [71, 72].

Surveillance is an appropriate management option for patients with cT1a renal masses and who have limited life expectancy and/or whom immediate definitive management is not an immediate consideration because of intervening medical conditions. Recently published data also suggest that surveillance may be an appropriate option for larger (>cT1b) masses [73].

## Management of Locally Advanced and Metastatic Disease (Stage III/Stage IV)

Patients with clinical T3 renal masses are generally treated by radical nephrectomy with thrombectomy (renal vein or vena cava), with partial nephrectomy reserved as an option in select clinical scenarios. The role of targeted agents [tyrosine kinase inhibitors (TKI) and mTOR inhibitors] remains investigational in the adjuvant or neoadjuvant setting in stage II or stage III RCC, though it may facilitate resection of locally advanced and bulky disease or nephron-sparing surgery in imperative indications in bulky or metastatic disease. Several ongoing clinical trials have either been completed (ASSURE, PROTECT) or are currently accruing patients (EVEREST) to determine the utility of adjunctive targeted therapy in localized or locally advanced disease to reduce disease recurrence and improve survival [74].

The role of lymphadenectomy in T2 or T3 disease is not firmly established. While indication remains for regional lymphadenectomy in the presence of clinical lymphadenopathy (whether in preoperative imaging or intraoperative exam), the results of EORTC clinical trial were negative with respect to benefits of lymphadenectomy, though this clinical trial has also been criticized for its design which enrolled patients with lower-risk disease (i.e., cT1 tumors), whom were not likely to benefit from lymphadenectomy. Nonetheless, data suggest that lymphadenectomy may be of benefit in patients with >cT2b and in the presence of high-grade tumors (Fuhrman Grade III/IV in the event of a preoperative biopsy), or tumor necrosis [68].

Overall performance status (by ECOG score or Karnofsky score) and burden of metastatic disease/metastatic disease in the bone or brain continue to be most important prognostic factors associated with prognosis in metastatic renal cell carcinoma. The development of novel systemic targeted agents (TKI/mTOR inhibitors) has revolutionized the treatment of RCC with improvement of partial response and disease stabilization rates, complete response by pharmacologic means remains rare, and high-dose interleukin-2 (IL-2) therapy remains an option in patients with excellent performance status track record for achieving durable complete responses. While cytoreductive nephrectomy has remained a mainstay of therapy for metastatic disease in the targeted therapy era, based on Level I evidence from clinical trials in the immunotherapy era, the utility of cytoreductive nephrectomy and its timing have recently been questioned [75]. Nonetheless, retrospective data suggest that cytoreductive nephrectomy with or without metastasectomy is associated with improved outcomes in metastatic disease; clinical trials are underway to determine timing and utility of cytoreductive surgery [76]. The advent of programmed death (PD-1) inhibitor therapy as an immune modulator may further revolutionize the treatment of metastatic disease, and the results of clinical trials are eagerly awaited [77].

## Future Directions

While the last decade has witnessed numerous advances in therapy for localized and advanced RCC, much work remains to be done to improve outcomes in RCC. Tumor markers to assist in diagnosis and risk assessment of disease and risk stratification to guide surveillance or definitive surgical therapy are lacking. As our understanding improves of the molecular mechanisms underlying tumor aggressiveness and host response in different histological subtypes, the promise of an individualized integrative approach applying systemic therapy and surgery may yet be realized for localized and advanced disease.

## References


1. Siegel R, Ma J, Zou Z, Jemal A. Cancer statistics, 2014. CA Cancer J Clin. 2014;64:9–29.
2. National Cancer Institute. Surveillance, epidemiology, and end results program. SEER Stat Fact Sheets: Kidney and Renal Pelvis Cancer. http://seer.cancer.gov/statfacts/html/kidrp.html.
3. Malcolm JB, Bagrodia A, Derweesh IH, Mehrazin R, Diblasio CJ, Wake RW, et al. Comparison of rates and risk factors for developing chronic renal insufficiency, proteinuria and metabolic acidosis after radical or partial nephrectomy. BJU Int. 2009;104(4):476–81.
4. Bagrodia A, Kopp RP, Mehrazin R, Lee HJ, Liss MA, Jabaji R, et al. Impact of renal surgery for cortical neoplasms on lipid metabolism. BJU Int. 2014;114(6): 837–43.
5. Ljungberg B, Cowan NC, Hanbury DC, Hora M, Kuczyk MA, Merseburger AS, et al. EAU guidelines on renal cell carcinoma: the 2010 update. Eur Urol. 2010;58(3):398–406.
6. Campbell SC, Novick AC, Belldegrun A, Blute ML, Chow GK, Derweesh IH, et al. Guideline for management of the clinical T1 renal mass. J Urol. 2009;182(4):1271–9.
7. Van Poppel H, Da Pozzo L, Albrecht W, Matveev V, Bono A, Borkowski A, et al. A prospective, randomised EORTC intergroup phase 3 study comparing the oncologic outcome of elective nephron-sparing surgery and radical nephrectomy for low-stage renal cell carcinoma. Eur Urol. 2011;59(4):543–52.
8. Delahunt B, Thornton A. Renal cell carcinoma. A historical perspective. J Urol Pathol. 1996;4:31–49.
9. Mourad WA, Nestok BR, Saleh GY, Solez K, Power RF, Jewell LD. Dysplastic tubular epithelium in "normal" kidney associated with renal cell carcinoma. Am J Surg Pathol. 1994;18:1117–24.
10. Truong LD, Shen SS. Immunohistochemical diagnosis of renal neoplasms. Arch Pathol Lab Med. 2011; 135:92–109.
11. Fuhrman SA, Lasky LC, Limas C. Prognostic significance of morphologic parameters in renal cell carcinoma. Am J Surg Pathol. 1982;6:655–63.
12. Delahunt B, Cheville JC, Martignoni G, Humphrey PA, Magi-Galluzzi C, McKenney J, et al. The International Society of Urological Pathology (ISUP) grading system for renal cell carcinoma and other prognostic parameters. Am J Surg Pathol. 2013;37(10): 1490–504,
13. Kanno H, Kondo K, Ito S, Yamamoto I, Fujii S, Torigoe S, et al. Somatic mutations of the von Hippel-Lindau tumor suppressor gene in sporadic central nervous system hemangioblastomas. Cancer Res. 1994; 54:4845–7.
14. Gnarra JR, Tory K, Weng Y, Schmidt L, Wei MH, Li H, et al. Mutations of the VHL tumour suppressor gene in renal carcinoma. Nat Genet. 1994;7:85–90.
15. Shuin T, Kondo K, Torigoe S, Kishida T, Kubota Y, Hosaka M, et al. Frequent somatic mutations and loss of heterozygosity of the von Hippel-Lindau tumor suppressor gene in primary human renal cell carcinomas. Cancer Res. 1994;54:2852–5.
16. Velickovic M, Delahunt B, Grebe SK. Loss of heterozygosity at 3p14.2 in clear cell renal cell carcinoma is an early event and is highly localized to the FHIT gene locus. Cancer Res. 1999;59:1323–6.
17. van den Berg A, Hulsbeek MF, de Jong D, Kok K, Veldhuis PM, Roche J, et al. Major role for a 3p21 region and lack of involvement of the t(3;8) breakpoint region in the development of renal cell carcinoma

suggested by loss of heterozygosity analysis. Genes Chromosomes Cancer. 1996;15:64–72.

18. Zbar B, Brauch H, Talmadge C, Linehan M. Loss of alleles of loci on the short arm of chromosome 3 in renal cell carcinoma. Nature. 1987;327:721–4.

19. Moch H, Presti Jr JC, Sauter G, Buchholz N, Jordan P, Mihatsch MJ, et al. Genetic aberrations detected by comparative genomic hybridization are associated with clinical outcome in renal cell carcinoma. Cancer Res. 1996;56:27–30.

20. Beroud C, Fournet JC, Jeanpierre C, Droz D, Bouvier R, Froger D, et al. Correlations of allelic imbalance of chromosome 14 with adverse prognostic parameters in 148 renal cell carcinomas. Genes Chromosomes Cancer. 1996;17:215–24.

21. Srigley JR, Delahunt B, Eble JN, Egevad L, Epstein JI, Grignon D, et al. The International Society of Urological Pathology (ISUP) Vancouver classification of renal neoplasia. Am J Surg Pathol. 2013; 37(10):1469–89.

22. Takeuchi T, Tanaka T, Tokuyama H, Kuriyama M, Nishiura T. Multilocular cystic renal adenocarcinoma: a case report and review of the literature. J Surg Oncol. 1984;25:136–40.

23. Murad T, Komaiko W, Oyasu R, Bauer K. Multilocular cystic renal cell carcinoma. Am J Clin Pathol. 1991;95:633–7.

24. Mancilla-Jimenez R, Stanley RJ, Blath RA. Papillary renal cell carcinoma: a clinical, radiologic, and pathologic study of 34 cases. Cancer. 1976;38:2469–80.

25. Mydlo JH, Bard RH. Analysis of papillary renal adenocarcinoma. Urology. 1987;30:529–34.

26. Ornstein DK, Lubensky IA, Venzon D, Zbar B, Linehan WM, Walther MM. Prevalence of microscopic tumors in normal appearing renal parenchyma of patients with hereditary papillary renal cancer. J Urol. 2000;163:431–3.

27. Delahunt B, Eble JN. Papillary renal cell carcinoma: a clinicopathologic and immunohistochemical study of 105 tumors. Mod Pathol. 1997;10:537–44.

28. Allory Y, Ouazana D, Boucher E, Thiounn N, Vieillefond A. Papillary renal cell carcinoma. Prognostic value of morphological subtypes in a clinicopathologic study of 43 cases. Virchows Arch. 2003; 442:336–42.

29. Gobbo S, Eble JN, Maclennan GT, Grignon DJ, Shah RB, Zhang S, et al. Renal cell carcinomas with papillary architecture and clear cell components: the utility of immunohistochemical and cytogenetical analyses in differential diagnosis. Am J Surg Pathol. 2008; 32:1780–6.

30. Tan PH, Cheng L, Rioux-Leclercq N, Merino MJ, Netto G, Reuter VE, et al. Renal tumors: diagnostic and prognostic biomarkers. Am J Surg Pathol. 2013; 37:1518–31.

31. Schmidt L, Junker K, Weirich G, Glenn G, Choyke P, Lubensky I, et al. Two North American families with hereditary papillary renal carcinoma and identical novel mutations in the MET proto-oncogene. Cancer Res. 1998;58:1719–22.

32. Alam NA, Rowan AJ, Wortham NC, Pollard PJ, Mitchell M, Tyrer JP, et al. Genetic and functional analyses of FH mutations in multiple cutaneous and uterine leiomyomatosis, hereditary leiomyomatosis and renal cancer, and fumarate hydratase deficiency. Hum Mol Genet. 2003;12:1241–52.

33. Toro JR, Nickerson ML, Wei MH, Warren MB, Glenn GM, Turner ML, et al. Mutations in the fumarate hydratase gene cause hereditary leiomyomatosis and renal cell cancer in families in North America. Am J Hum Genet. 2003;73:95–106.

34. Kovacs G, Fuzesi L, Emanual A, Kung HF. Cytogenetics of papillary renal cell tumors. Genes Chromosomes Cancer. 1991;3:249–55.

35. Amin MB, Corless CL, Renshaw AA, Tickoo SK, Kubus J, Schultz DS. Papillary (chromophil) renal cell carcinoma: histomorphologic characteristics and evaluation of conventional pathologic prognostic parameters in 62 cases. Am J Surg Pathol. 1997; 21:621–35.

36. Xipell JM. The incidence of benign renal nodules (a clinicopathologic study). J Urol. 1971;106:503–6.

37. Reis M, Faria V, Lindoro J, Adolfo A. The small cystic and noncystic noninflammatory renal nodules: a postmortem study. J Urol. 1988;140:721–4.

38. Hughson MD, Buchwald D, Fox M. Renal neoplasia and acquired cystic kidney disease in patients receiving long-term dialysis. Arch Pathol Lab Med. 1986;110:592–601.

39. Tickoo SK, de Peralta-Venturina MN, Harik LR, Worcester HD, Salama ME, Young AN, et al. Spectrum of epithelial neoplasms in end-stage renal disease: an experience from 66 tumor-bearing kidneys with emphasis on histologic patterns distinct from those in sporadic adult renal neoplasia. Am J Surg Pathol. 2006;30:141–53.

40. Thoenes W, Störkel S, Rumpelt HJ. Human chromophobe cell renal carcinoma. Virchows Arch B Cell Pathol Incl Mol Pathol. 1985;48:207–17.

41. Crotty TB, Farrow GM, Lieber MM. Chromophobe cell renal carcinoma: clinicopathological features of 50 cases. J Urol. 1995;154:964–7.

42. Thoenes W, Storkel S, Rumpelt HJ, Moll R, Baum HP, Werner S. Chromophobe cell renal carcinoma and its variants—a report on 32 cases. J Pathol. 1988; 155:277–87.

43. Peralta-Venturina M, Moch H, Amin M, Tamboli P, Hailemariam S, Mihatsch M, et al. Sarcomatoid differentiation in renal cell carcinoma: a study of 101 cases. Am J Surg Pathol. 2001;25:275–84.

44. Tanaka Y, Koie T, Hatakeyama S, Hashimoto Y, Ohyama C. Chromophobe renal cell carcinoma with concomitant sarcomatoid transformation and osseous metaplasia: a case report. BMC Urol. 2013;13:72.

45. Lauer SR, Zhou M, Master VA, Osunkoya AO. Chromophobe renal cell carcinoma with sarcomatoid differentiation: a clinicopathologic study of 14 cases. Anal Quant Cytopathol Histpathol. 2013;35:77–84.

46. Daga D, Dana R, Kothari N. Chromophobe renal cell carcinoma with sarcomatoid changes: case report and

review of literature. Cent European J Urol. 2014; 67:31–4.

47. Cochand-Priollet B, Molinie V, Bougaran J, Bouvier R, Dauge-Geffroy MC, Deslignieres S, et al. Renal chromophobe cell carcinoma and oncocytoma. A comparative morphologic, histochemical, and immunohistochemical study of 124 cases. Arch Pathol Lab Med. 1997;121:1081–6.

48. Lohse CM, Blute ML, Zincke H, Weaver AL, Cheville JC. Comparison of standardized and nonstandardized nuclear grade of renal cell carcinoma to predict outcome among 2,042 patients. Am J Clin Pathol. 2002;118:877–86.

49. Delahunt B, Sika-Paotonu D, Bethwaite PB, McCredie MR, Martignoni G, Eble JN, et al. Fuhrman grading is not appropriate for chromophobe renal cell carcinoma. Am J Surg Pathol. 2007;31(6):957–60.

50. Paner GP, Amin MB, Alvarado-Cabrero I, Young AN, Stricker HJ, Moch H, et al. A novel tumor grading scheme for chromophobe renal cell carcinoma: prognostic utility and comparison with Fuhrman nuclear grade. Am J Surg Pathol. 2010;34(9):1233–40.

51. Finley DS, Shuch B, Said JW, Galliano G, Jeffries RA, Afifi AA, et al. The chromophobe tumor grading system is the preferred grading scheme for chromophobe renal cell carcinoma. J Urol. 2011;186(6): 2168–74.

52. Storkel S, Steart PV, Drenckhahn D, Thoenes W. The human chromophobe cell renal carcinoma: its probable relation to intercalated cells of the collecting duct. Virchows Arch B Cell Pathol Incl Mol Pathol. 1989;56:237–45.

53. Bugert P, Kovacs G. Molecular differential diagnosis of renal cell carcinomas by microsatellite analysis. Am J Pathol. 1996;149:2081–8.

54. Amin MB, Tamboli P, Javidan J, Stricker H, de Peralta-Venturina M, Deshpande A, et al. Prognostic impact of histologic subtyping of adult renal epithelial neoplasms: an experience of 405 cases. Am J Surg Pathol. 2002;26:281–91.

55. Klein MJ, Valensi QJ. Proximal tubular adenomas of kidney with so-called oncocytic features. A clinicopathologic study of 13 cases of a rarely reported neoplasm. Cancer. 1976;38:906–14.

56. Choi H, Almagro UA, McManus JT, Norback DH, Jacobs SC. Renal oncocytoma. A clinicopathologic study. Cancer. 1983;51:1887–96.

57. Davis Jr CJ, Mostofi FK, Sesterhenn IA, Ho CK. Renal oncocytoma. Clinicopathological study of 166 patients. J Urogen Pathol. 1991;1:41–52.

58. Amin MB, Crotty TB, Tickoo SK, Farrow GM. Renal oncocytoma: a reappraisal of morphologic features with clinicopathologic findings in 80 cases. Am J Surg Pathol. 1997;21:1–12.

59. Perez-Ordonez B, Hamed G, Campbell S, Erlandson RA, Russo P, Gaudin PB, et al. Renal oncocytoma: a clinicopathologic study of 70 cases. Am J Surg Pathol. 1997;21:871–83.

60. Trpkov K, Yilmaz A, Uzer D, Dishongh KM, Quick CM, Bismar TA, et al. Renal oncocytoma revisited: a clinicopathological study of 109 cases with emphasis on problematic diagnostic features. Histopathology. 2010;57:893–906.

61. Crotty TB, Lawrence KM, Moertel CA, Bartelt Jr DH, Batts KP, Dewald GW, et al. Cytogenetic analysis of six renal oncocytomas and a chromophobe cell renal carcinoma. Evidence that -y, -1 may be a characteristic anomaly in renal oncocytomas. Cancer Genet Cytogenet. 1992;61:61–6.

62. van den Berg E, van der Hout AH, Oosterhuis JW, Störkel S, Dijkhuizen T, Dam A, et al. Cytogenetic analysis of epithelial renal-cell tumors: relationship with a new histopathological classification. Int J Cancer. 1993;55:223–7.

63. Donat SM, Diaz M, Bishoff JT, Coleman JA, Dahm P, Derweesh IH, et al. Follow-up for clinically localized renal neoplasms: AUA guideline. J Urol. 2013;190(2): 407–16.

64. Kang SK, Huang WC, Pandharipande PV, Chandarana H. Solid renal masses: what the numbers tell us. AJR Am J Roentgenol. 2014;202(6):1196–206.

65. Millet I, Doyon FC, Pages E, Thuret R, Taourel P. Morphometric scores for renal tumors: what does the radiologist need to know? Eur J Radiol. 2014; 83(8):1303–10.

66. Kopp RP, Mehrazin R, Palazzi KL, Liss MA, Jabaji R, Mirheydar HS, et al. Survival outcomes after radical and partial nephrectomy for clinical T2 renal tumours categorised by R.E.N.A.L. nephrometry score. BJU Int. 2014;114(5):708–18.

67. Braunagel M, Radler E, Ingrisch M, Staehler M, Schmid-Tannwald C, Rist C, et al. Dynamic contrast-enhanced magnetic resonance imaging measurements in renal cell carcinoma: effect of region of interest size and positioning on interobserver and intraobserver variability. Invest Radiol. 2015;50(1): 57–66.

68. Scosyrev E, Messing EM, Sylvester R, Campbell S, Van Poppel H. Renal function after nephron-sparing surgery versus radical nephrectomy: results from EORTC randomized trial 30904. Eur Urol. 2014; 65(2):372–7.

69. Weight CJ, Miller DC, Campbell SC, Derweesh IH, Lane BR, Messing EM. The management of a clinical t1b renal tumor in the presence of a normal contralateral kidney. J Urol. 2013;189(4):1198–202.

70. Halverson SJ, Kunju LP, Bhalla R, Gadzinski AJ, Alderman M, Miller DC, et al. Accuracy of determining small renal mass management with risk stratified biopsies: confirmation by final pathology. J Urol. 2013;189(2):441–6.

71. Thompson RH, Atwell T, Schmit G, Lohse CM, Kurup AN, Weisbrod A, et al. Comparison of partial nephrectomy and percutaneous ablation for cT1 renal masses. Eur Urol. 2014;67(2):252–9. doi:10.1016/j.eururo.2014.07.021.

72. Chang X, Zhang F, Liu T, Ji C, Zhao X, Yang R, et al. Radiofrequency ablation versus partial nephrectomy for clinical T1b renal cell carcinoma: long-term clinical and oncologic outcomes. J Urol. 2015;29(5): 518–25.

73. Smaldone MC, Kutikov A, Egleston BL, Canter DJ, Viterbo R, Chen DY, et al. Small renal masses progressing to metastases under active surveillance: a systematic review and pooled analysis. Cancer. 2012; 118(4):997–1006.

74. Pal SK, Haas NB. Adjuvant therapy for renal cell carcinoma: past, present, and future. Oncologist. 2014; 19(8):851–9.

75. Stroup SP, Raheem OA, Palazzi KL, Liss MA, Mehrazin R, Kopp RP, et al. Does timing of cytoreductive nephrectomy impact patient survival with metastatic renal cell carcinoma in the tyrosine kinase inhibitor era? A multi-institutional study. Urology. 2013;81(4):805–11.

76. Kroeger N, Choueiri TK, Lee JL, Bjarnason GA, Knox JJ, MacKenzie MJ, et al. Survival outcome and treatment response of patients with late relapse from renal cell carcinoma in the era of targeted therapy. Eur Urol. 2014;65(6):1086–92.

77. Choueiri TK, Fay AP, Gray KP, Callea M, Ho TH, Albiges L, et al. PD-L1 expression in nonclear-cell renal cell carcinoma. Ann Oncol. 2014;25(11):2178–84.

# Familial Forms of Renal Cell Carcinoma and Associated Syndromes

Charles C. Guo, Armine K. Smith, and Christian P. Pavlovich

## Chapter

Familial renal cell carcinoma (FRCC) is a hereditary renal neoplasm presenting within more than one member of a family. FRCC is uncommon and accounts for approximately 1–4 % of renal cancers [1]. In contrast to sporadic renal cell carcinomas (RCCs), FRCCs usually occur at a relatively young age and present as multiple tumors in both kidneys. In addition, patients may develop neoplastic disease in other nonrenal organs, such as the skin, lungs, uterus,

C.C. Guo, M.D. (✉)
Department of Pathology Unit 085, MD Anderson Cancer Center, University of Texas,
1515 Holcombe Blvd., Houston, TX, USA
e-mail: ccguo@mdanderson.org

A.K. Smith, M.D.
Department of Urology, Johns Hopkins University School of Medicine, Sibley Memorial Hospital, Ste 300, 5215 Loughboro Road, NW, Washington, DC 20016, USA
e-mail: asmit165@jhmi.edu

C.P. Pavlovich, M.D.
Department of Urology, Johns Hopkins University School of Medicine, Johns Hopkins Bayview Medical Center, Ste 3200, Bldg 301, 4940 Eastern Avenue, Baltimore, MD 21218, USA
e-mail: cpavlov2@jhmi.edu

and central nervous system. The majority of FRCCs are autosomal dominant diseases with variable penetrance [2]. Specific genetic alterations have been identified in most FRCCs, and the majority of these alterations are known to be involved in metabolic pathways that regulate oxygen, iron, glucose, and energy levels. Environmental or lifestyle factors may also play a role in the oncogenesis in FRCC [3]. It is important to identify these diseases, as this can help assess the cancer risk and extrarenal manifestation risk of individual family members and plan for cancer screening and prevention. In addition, appropriate psychosocial support and counseling may be provided to affected family members.

FRCC is a heterogeneous disease comprised of a number of syndromes. Each syndrome/subtype exhibits distinct genetic alterations, pathologic characteristics, and clinical features. In this chapter, we will primarily discuss five major hereditary syndromes that are associated with FRCCs: von Hippel-Lindau syndrome, hereditary papillary RCC, hereditary leiomyomatosis and RCC, Birt-Hogg-Dubé syndrome, and tuberous sclerosis syndrome (Table 6.1). A number of other heritable syndromes may also be associated with FRCC and are briefly discussed here, including the hyperparathyroidism-jaw tumor syndrome, PTEN hamartoma, and constitutional chromosome 3 translocations [4–6].

© Springer Science+Business Media New York 2016
D.E. Hansel et al. (eds.), *The Kidney*, DOI 10.1007/978-1-4939-3286-3_6

**Table 6.1** Major hereditary syndromes associated with renal cell neoplasms

| Syndrome (abbreviation) | Gene (protein) | Chromosome location | Renal pathology | Other clinical manifestations |
|---|---|---|---|---|
| Von Hippel-Lindau (VHL) syndrome | *VHL* (pVHL) | 3p25 | Clear cell RCC, cystic renal cell carcinoma, renal cysts | Central nervous system hemangioblastomas, pheochromocytomas, pancreatic cysts, neuroendocrine tumors; endolymphatic sac tumors; epididymal and broad ligament cystadenomas |
| Hereditary papillary RCC (HPRCC) | *MET* (HGFR) | 7q31 | Papillary type 1 RCC | None |
| Hereditary leiomyomatosis and RCC (HLRCC) | *FH* (pFH) | 1q42-43 | Papillary type 2 RCC; often solitary | Uterine leiomyomas and leiomyosarcoma, cutaneous leiomyomas |
| Birt-Hogg-Dubé (BHD) syndrome | *FLCN* (Folliculin) | 17p11.2 | Hybrid oncocytic RCC, chromophobe RCC, clear cell RCC, oncocytoma, oncocytosis | Cutaneous papules, lung cysts, spontaneous pneumothoraces |
| Tuberous sclerosis (TS) syndrome | *TSC1* (hamartin) | 9q34 | Angiomyolipoma, papillary RCC, hybrid oncocytic RCC | Facial angiofibromas, periungual fibromas, shagreen patches, cardiac rhabdomyomas, lung and kidney cysts, cortical tubers |
| | *TSC2* (tuberin) | 16p13 | | |
| Succinate dehydrogenase mutation | *SDHB* (pSDHB) | 1p36 | B – solid and cystic tumors, variable pathology, oncocytic and clear cell RCC | Paragangliomas/pheochromocytomas, GIST, pituitary adenomas, pulmonary chondromas |
| | *SHDC* (pSDHC) | 1q23 | C – solid tumors, clear cell RCC, low grade | |
| | *SDHD* (pSDHD) | 11q23 | D – solid tumors, clear cell RCC | |
| Cowden/PTEN hamartoma tumor syndrome | *PTEN* (pPTEN) | 10q23 | Variable pathology, including clear cell, chromophobe, and papillary RCC | Breast, thyroid, and endometrial cancer, mucocutaneous lesions, acral keratoses, facial trichilemmomas, papillomatous papules, macrocephaly, Lhermitte-Duclos disease, benign thyroid conditions, mental retardation, GI hamartomas, lipomas, fibromas, breast fibrocystic disease |
| Microphthalmia transcription (MiT) family translocations | Fusion chimeric proteins with TFE3 or TFEB | Xp11.2 | Solid or cystic tumors, variable architecture RCC | None |
| | | t(6;11) | | |
| Microphthalmia-associated factor mutation | *MITF* (pE318K) | 3p14 | Solid or cystic tumors, clear cell and papillary RCC | Melanoma |
| Chromosome 3 translocation | Fusion chimeric protein | t(3;8) | Clear cell RCC | None |
| BRCA1-associated protein-1 (BAP1) mutation | *BAP1* (pBAP1) | 3p21 | Solid and cystic tumors, high-grade clear cell RCC | Uveal/cutaneous melanoma, mesothelioma |

## Von Hippel-Lindau

### Introduction

Von Hippel-Lindau (VHL) syndrome is a hereditary disease with an autosomal dominant pattern. The VHL incidence is estimated to about 1:36,000 [7]. Patients usually develop characteristic neoplasms in multiple organs, including clear cell RCC, capillary hemangioblastomas of the central nervous system and retina, pheochromocytoma, pancreatic tumors, and inner ear tumors [7]. The mean age of RCC onset in patients with VHL syndrome is 37 years, which is much earlier than that for sporadic RCC (61 years).

VHL disease is caused by germline mutations of the *VHL* gene, which is located on the short arm of chromosome 3 (3p26-25) [8]. The *VHL* gene is a relatively small tumor suppressor gene with a coding sequence of 639 nucleotides on three exons [9]. The VHL protein is responsible for proteomic degradation of hypoxia-inducible factors (HIFs) [10]. HIF-1α and HIF-2α regulate a number of downstream genes, including vascular endothelial and platelet-derived growth factors (VEGF and PDGF), transforming growth factor-α (TGF-α), erythropoietin, glucose transporter protein-1, carbonic anhydrase IX, and C-mesenchymal-epithelial transition factor (c-MET) [2]. These downstream genes are involved in the cell cycle, angiogenesis, and tumorigenesis. Mutations of the *VHL* gene, which may occur in any exon, are most commonly missense mutations, but nonsense mutations such as deletions, insertions, and translocations may also occur. The germline mutation is found in nearly all VHL families [11]. The type of mutation is associated with the clinical presentation of VHL disease. Somatic VHL alterations are also common in sporadic clear cell RCCs, but they are usually absent in papillary, chromophobe, or collecting duct RCCs.

### Clinical Presentation

The earliest manifestations of VHL are usually not related to renal pathology. Central nervous system (CNS) hemangioblastomas, including retinal hemangioblastomas, can present as vision loss or neurologic symptoms as early as age 1 [7]. Other early manifestations in specific families include pheochromocytoma and pancreatic cysts, with ages of onset as young as 5 having been reported. Renal tumors have been noted as early as the teenage years, but generally present in the 4th decade of life on routine screening exams or with gross or microscopic hematuria. Overall some 25–60 % of VHL patients develop renal tumors, renal cysts, or cystic renal cell carcinomas; these are often bilateral and multifocal, as with most all forms of FRCC. Therefore, screening efforts for renal tumors in individuals affected by VHL generally start at age 18, when annual axial imaging (CT or MRI) is recommended.

### Pathology

Grossly, the tumors often present as multiple, well-circumscribed, bright yellow masses in both kidneys. There are often numerous cysts containing clear fluid in the kidneys. Some patients may develop up to 600 microscopic tumors and over 1000 cysts in each kidney [12]. Microscopically, the tumors are typically composed of clear cell RCC, which is characterized by nests or sheets of tumor cells with clear cytoplasm separated by a delicate vascular network (Fig. 6.1a). The tumor may show focal papillary, tubular, or cystic features (Fig. 6.1b). The renal cysts are usually lined by a single layer of tumor cells with clear cytoplasm, sometimes forming small tufts and papillary structures (Fig. 6.1c). In addition, multiple, small, incipient tumors (under 0.5 cm in the largest dimension), which are also composed of clear cell RCC, are often scattered in the renal parenchyma (Fig. 6.1d).

The immunohistochemical profile of VHL-associated RCC is similar to that of sporadic clear cell RCC. They usually show strong positive immunoreactivity for carbonic anhydrase IX (CAIX) and CD10 and are negative or focally positive for cytokeratin 7 (CK7). The reactivity for alpha-methylacyl-CoA racemase (AMACR) is variable. Deletion of chromosome 3p is also

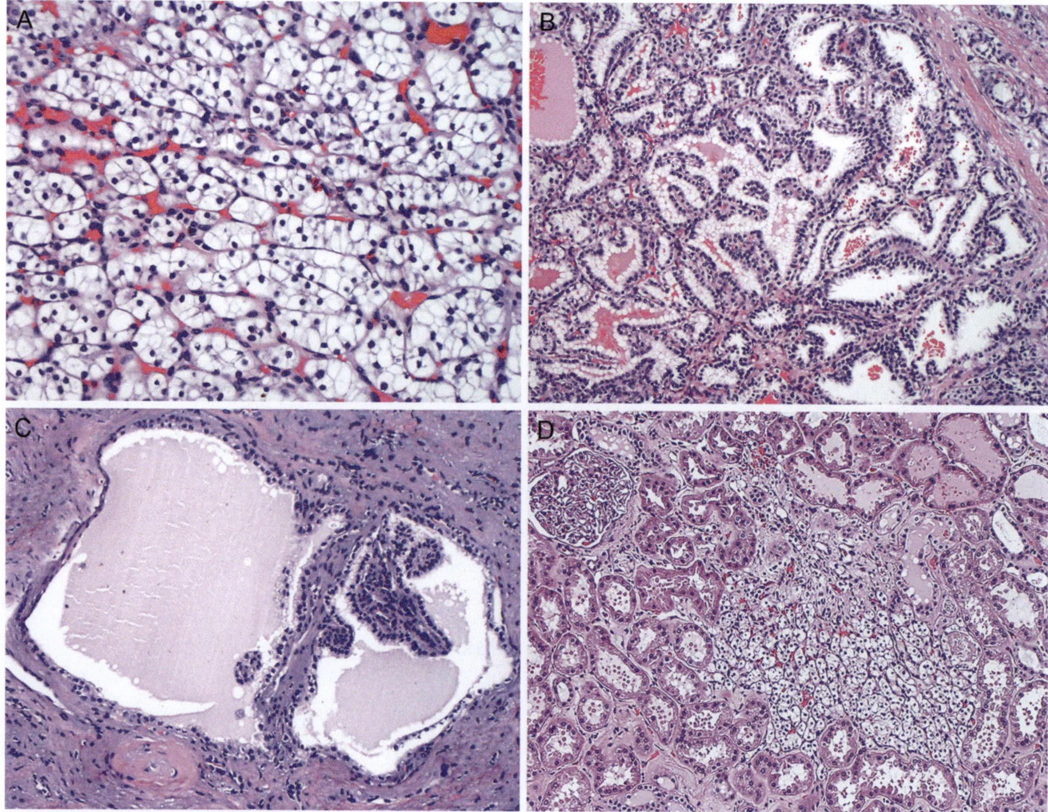

**Fig. 6.1** Renal cell carcinoma in von Hippel-Lindau syndrome. The tumor is typically the clear cell type, which is characterized by small nests of tumor cells with clear cytoplasm separated by a delicate vascular network (**a**). Tumor cells may form papillae and tubules (**b**). Renal cysts are lined by a single layer of clear tumor cells, forming small tufts and papillae (**c**). Small tumors (less than 0.5 cm) of clear cell RCCs are common (**d**)

common in VHL-associated RCC (82 %), at a level similar to that observed in sporadic clear cell RCC (80 %) [13].

VHL-associated RCC may have focal areas of tubular, papillary, and cystic structures lined by tumor cells with clear cytoplasm, which mimics clear cell papillary RCC (CCPRCC). CCPRCC is a new entity that has not been included in the current WHO classification [14]. However, unlike VHL-associated RCC, CCPRCC is characterized by positive immunoreactivity for CK7 and negative reactivity for AMACR and CD10. Furthermore, while VHL-associated RCC frequently exhibits 3p deletion, CCPRCC lacks 3p deletion but may exhibit chromosome 7 or 17 abnormalities in a subset of cases [13].

## Treatment

Historically many patients with VHL underwent radical nephrectomy, but renal parenchymal-sparing treatments are generally preferred in this and most other FRCC syndromes. Given the proclivity of most patients with VHL to form multiple and bilateral clear cell renal cell carcinomas over their lifetime, nephron-sparing should be entertained whenever oncologically feasible. Partial nephrectomy is now the standard extirpative approach to all but the largest renal tumors, and percutaneous ablation (with radiofrequency or cryotherapy) can also be offered to patients in lieu of radical nephrectomy unless the solid tumors have grown too large for such modalities [15]. A 3 cm size threshold prior to intervention for solid renal masses has been studied in order to limit the number of interventions in patients with some forms of FRCC such as VHL [16]. Data to date suggest that the metastatic potential of lesions less than 3 cm in diameter in VHL is close to zero, so solid renal masses in VHL, invariably clear cell RCC, are routinely observed until they grow. At that point, partial nephrectomy is performed if feasible, as well as enucleation of all smaller tumors and cysts that can be handled safely. If percutaneous ablation is chosen, only the 3 cm+ tumor is ablated and the smaller lesions are followed.

## Hereditary Papillary Renal Cell Carcinoma (HPRCC)

### Introduction

HPRCC is an inherited renal tumor syndrome characterized by an autosomal dominant trait with a high penetrance [17]. Affected individuals are at a high risk of developing a large number of tumors in both kidneys. This syndrome chiefly affects the kidney, and no extrarenal involvement has been reported to be associated with HPRCC. The tumors are invariably composed of papillary type 1 RCC. The onset of HPRCC is usually late in most patients, in the 6th to 8th decades of life, but a few cases of early onset have been reported [18].

HPRCC is commonly associated with germline mutations in the proto-oncogene MET, which is located at chromosome 7q31 [19]. MET encodes a transmembranous protein kinase, hepatocyte growth factor receptor [20]. Normally, hepatocyte growth factor receptor binds and activates MET tyrosine kinase, which in turn phosphorylates a number of signal transduction proteins. The MET tyrosine kinase plays an important role in cell proliferation and differentiation. Missense mutations in the MET tyrosine kinase domain lead to ligand-independent constitutive activation of the MET protein [21]. The aberrant activation of the MET protein leads to phosphorylation of signal transducers and adaptors, resulting in cancer develop-ment. *MET* somatic mutations have also been reported in some patients with sporadic papillary type 1 RCC [22].

## Clinical Presentation

Solid papillary renal tumors are the only clinical manifestation of this form of FRCC, and therefore these tumors are picked up incidentally, by screening of families known to be affected or on workup for gross or microscopic hematuria. These tumors are invariably solid (though some cysts have been noted in affected individuals) and enhance only minimally compared to other solid renal tumors: +10–30 Hounsfield units on contrast CT or +15 % on contrast MRI [23]. No mature routine screening recommendations for mutation carriers exist, though abdominal imaging by CT or MR is generally recommended every 2 years.

## Pathology

Typically, there are numerous tumors in bilateral kidneys, which may number in the hundreds to thousands on gross examination. Histologically, the renal tumors are composed of papillary type 1 RCC, which is characterized by papillae lined with a single layer of small tumor cells with scant amphophilic cytoplasm and low nuclear grade (Fig. 6.2a). Papillae may coalesce to impart solid growth patterns with glomeruloid structures (Fig. 6.2b). There is a variable amount of foamy histiocytes and psammomatous calcification in the papillary cores (Fig. 6.2c). Necrosis and hemosiderin deposits may be found. Clear cell changes may be present, especially in areas adjacent to necrosis. A large number of small papillary renal neoplasia that are identical to sporadic renal papillary adenomas are frequently seen in the renal parenchyma (Fig. 6.2d).

It is difficult, if not impossible, to distinguish HPRCCs from sporadic papillary type 1 RCCs based on pathologic analysis, as they share similar histologic and immunohistochemical features

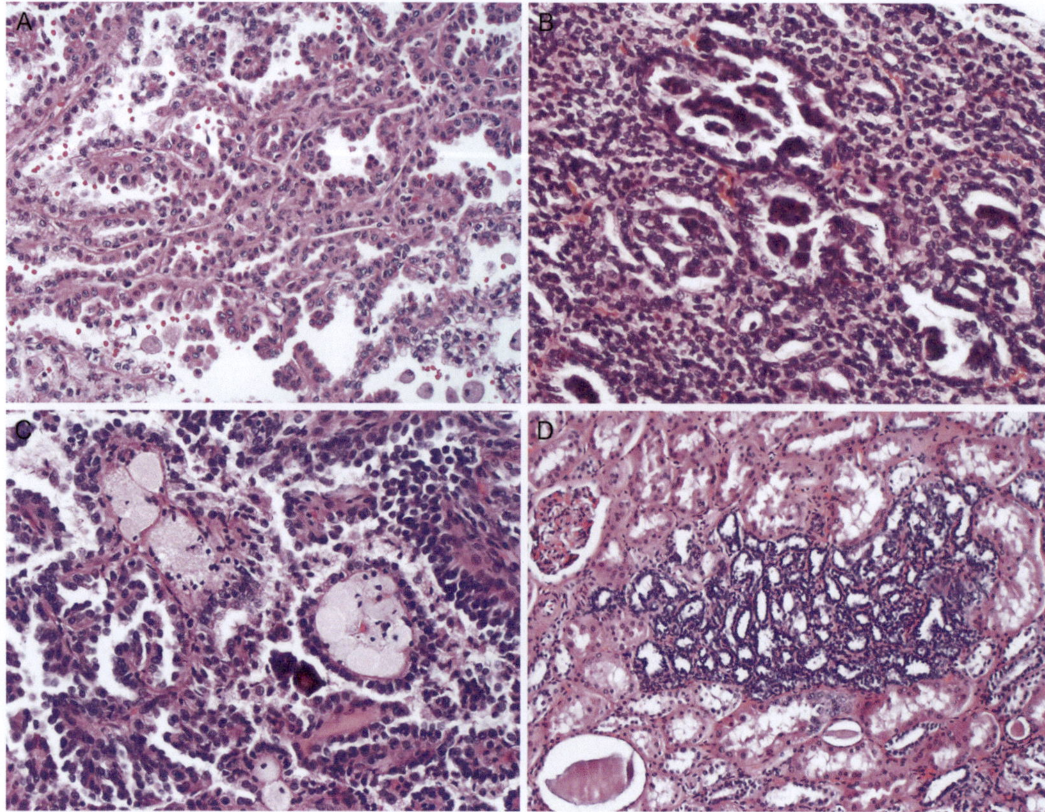

**Fig. 6.2** Hereditary papillary renal cell carcinoma. The tumor is invariably a papillary type 1 RCC, which is characterized by papillae lined with a single layer of tumor cells with low nuclear grade (**a**). Papillae may coalesce a solid growth pattern with glomeruloid structures (**b**). Foamy histiocytes and psammomatous calcification are observed in the papillary cores (**c**). A large number of renal papillary adenomas are frequently seen in the grossly normal renal parenchyma (**d**)

[24]. A diagnosis of HPRCC may be entertained when a patient presents with a large number of papillary type 1 RCC and a family history of renal tumor. The diagnosis of HPRCC can be further supported by identifying the germline MET mutations on DNA sequencing.

## Treatment

Type I papillary RCCs typically grow slowly and have low metastatic potential. They are therefore generally managed observationally until the 3 cm threshold for intervention is reached, as for many other forms of FRCC. The options of radical nephrectomy, partial nephrectomy, and percutaneous ablation are similarly offered for these tumors.

# Hereditary Leiomyomatosis and Renal Cell Carcinoma (HLRCC)

## Introduction

HLRCC is an autosomal dominant cancer syndrome with a high penetrance [25]. These patients are at risk of developing papillary type 2 RCC, cutaneous and uterine leiomyomas. In affected patients, the penetrance of RCC is approximately 20–30 %, whereas the penetrance of cutaneous and uterine leiomyomas is much higher: 76 % of individuals and 100 % of women at a mean age of 25 years or 30 years [25–27]. Occasionally patients may develop leiomyosarcoma in the uterus. The median age of patients at onset of RCC is 36–44 years, which is much earlier than when sporadic kidney cancer manifests. The onset of leiomyomas occurs at a relatively young age: at 10–47 years for cutaneous leiomyomas and 18–52 years for uterine leiomyomas.

The gene responsible for HLRCC is fumarate hydratase (*FH*), a tumor suppressor which is located on chromosome 1 (1q42.3-q43) [25–27]. Germline mutations in *FH* gene have been found in 85 % of the HLRCC patients. The majority of germline mutations are missense mutations, although truncation and whole-gene deletion may occur. A "second hit" or somatic inactivation of the remaining *FH* allele is usually required to cause functional loss of FH protein. Because the FH protein regulates the conversion of fumarate to malate in the citric acid (Krebs) cycle, the inactivation of this protein increases the level of fumarate, which competitively inhibits the HIF prolyl hydroxylase [28]. Subsequently, the HIF level increases, influencing the expression of the downstream genes. There is no evidence to support a relationship between the *FH* gene mutation and sporadic RCC.

## Clinical Presentation

This is a disorder with cutaneous, uterine, and renal manifestations, only the latter being cancerous. Patients generally develop cutaneous leiomyomata (trunk and extremity) in their 20s, and these can be painful. Females almost always develop multiple, large uterine leiomyomata during their young adulthood, which typically become quite symptomatic though rarely cancerous. In addition, some 10–16 % of affected patients also develop papillary RCC type 2 renal tumor [29]. These cancers are very aggressive, highly malignant, and quite different in behavior from most other papillary RCC and even from many clear cell RCC. Unlike other forms of FRCC, these tumors grow so rapidly that a patient will often present with just one large (and symptomatic) tumor despite their hereditary predisposition to multiple and bilateral tumors.

## Pathology

### Renal Cancer

On gross examination, HLRCC tumors are typically solitary and unilateral, unlike tumors of other hereditary RCC syndromes, which are characterized by bilateral distribution of multiple renal tumors. HLRCC tumors are usually large, tan, and firm with necrosis. Microscopically, HLRCC usually exhibits a large number of papillae covered by large tumor cells with abundant eosinophilic cytoplasm (Fig. 6.3a), as is seen in papillary type 2 RCC. The most characteristic feature of HLRCC is the presence of a large nucleus with a very prominent inclusion-like nucleolus that is surrounded by a clear halo, resembling cytomegalovirus nuclear inclusions (Fig. 6.3b). The tumor may also have solid, tubular, or tubulopapillary growth patterns (Fig. 6.3c). The tumor is often associated with desmoplastic and cystic changes, mimicking collecting duct carcinoma (CDC), but CDC lacks the characteristic nucleolar features of HLRCC. Furthermore, CDC is positive for CK7 and ULEX on immunostaining, while HLRCC is often negative or only focally positive for CK7 and negative for ULEX-1. Occasionally, the tumor may develop sarcomatoid dedifferentiation (Fig. 6.3d). The tumors often present at an advanced stage with invasion into renal vein, renal sinus, and perinephric soft tissue [30]. Recent studies have shown that the presence of *S*-(2-succino)-cysteine (2SC) positivity by immunohistochemical analysis predicts genetic alterations of the *FH* gene in patients and that this immunoreactivity is generally absent in non-HLRCC-related tumors [31, 32].

### Leiomyomas of the Skin and Uterus

Cutaneous leiomyomas often appear as multiple, firm nodules ranging from 0.2 to 2.0 cm in the largest dimension. Microscopically, cutaneous leiomyomas are composed of anastomosing bundles of smooth muscle cells with inconspicuous nuclei. Uterine leiomyomas often present as

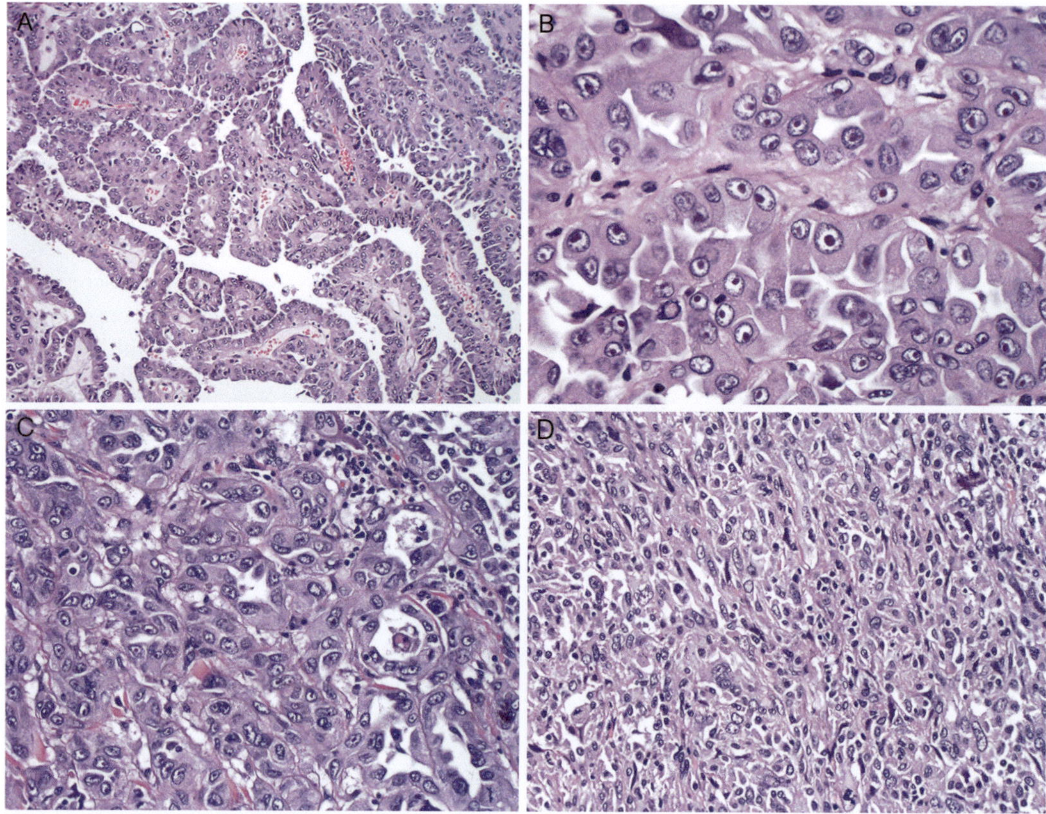

**Fig. 6.3** Hereditary leiomyomatosis and renal cell carcinoma. The tumor typically appears like papillary type 2 RCC, which is composed of papillae covered by large tumor cells with a high nuclear grade and abundant eosinophilic cytoplasm (**a**). The most characteristic feature is the presence of a large nucleus with a prominent inclusion that is surrounded by a clear halo (**b**). The tumor may have solid, tubular, or tubulopapillary growth patterns (**c**). The RCC may develop focal sarcomatoid dedifferentiation (**d**)

numerous, well-circumscribed, and firm masses. Histologically, most leiomyomas are composed of whorled, interlacing fascicles of uniform, fusiform smooth muscle cells. A small number of patients develop uterine leiomyosarcomas [33], which are usually large and fleshy with poorly defined margins. The leiomyosarcomas are usually hypercellular with conspicuous nuclear atypia and increased mitotic activity.

## Treatment

Prompt surgical management is recommended for HLRCC patients with a renal mass of any size. Unlike other forms of FRCC, where it is generally prudent to wait until a renal tumor grows to 3 cm prior to intervening, HLRCC renal tumors are treated on diagnosis. While there are not enough data to recommend nephron-sparing vs. radical nephrectomy for these tumors, prompt and aggressive treatment is warranted for these patients. Unfortunately, given that this syndrome has only recently been characterized, more than half of patients already had locally advanced or metastatic disease at presentation in the initial series [34].

## Birt-Hogg-Dubé (BHD) Syndrome

## Introduction

BHD syndrome is a rare autosomal dominant cancer syndrome with incomplete penetrance [35]. Renal tumors occur in 14–34 % of affected individuals with an onset commonly in the 6th decade of life (ranging 31–73 years). The majority of the renal tumors that develop are hybrid oncocytic tumors (50 %), chromophobe RCCs (33 %), or oncocytomas (5 %), but clear cell and papillary RCCs have occasionally been seen as well [36]. More than half of patients with BHD syndrome also have multifocal oncocytosis in the surrounding renal parenchyma [36].

BHD syndrome is caused by germline mutations in the folliculin gene (*FLCN*) [37], which is located at chromosome 17p11.2 [38]. These mutations can be insertions, deletions, or nonsense mutations. The *FLCN* gene, which functions as a tumor suppressor gene, requires mutations in both alleles to be inactivated. Usually, one allele has a germline mutation and the other allele has a somatic mutation. FLCN protein forms a complex with interacting proteins, which regulates the mammalian target of rapamycin (mTOR) signaling pathway via AMP-activated protein kinase (AMPK) [39]. Mutations in the *FLCN* gene may also be involved in the development of a number of sporadic RCCs [40].

## Clinical Presentation

BHD is a hereditary disorder predisposing patients to benign skin lesions, lung cysts and spontaneous pneumothorax, and renal tumors. BHD patients develop asymptomatic cutaneous fibrofolliculomas and other benign skin lesions during their young adulthood—skin-colored papules typically distributed over the nose, face, neck shoulders, and back. Benign lung cysts develop in the lung bases most typically, and these lead to spontaneous pneumothorax in many patients over time (~50× compared to the general population). BHD patients also have a 7× incidence of renal tumor compared to unaffected relatives and tend to present in their 5th decade of life [41]. As for any renal tumor, they may be found incidentally, on screening exams, or may present with hematuria or flank symptomatology. Screening for renal tumor is recommended every 2 years at least given that some patients with BHD have indeed died from metastatic RCC.

## Pathology

Patients with BHD syndrome often have multiple, well-circumscribed, tan or brown tumors in both kidneys (Fig. 6.4a). The average size of the largest tumor at presentation was 5.7 cm (ranging 1.2–15 cm), and the average number of tumors was 5.3 per kidney (ranging 1–28 cm) in the initial series [36]. Various histologic characteristics have been reported for patients with this syndrome. Half of the renal tumors are hybrid oncocytic tumors, which usually demonstrate features of both oncocytomas and chromophobe RCCs (Fig. 6.4b). Oncocytic hybrid renal tumors are usually positive for CD117 and focally positive for CK7 (Fig. 6.4c). Another common feature of hybrid renal oncocytic tumors is a mixture of oncocytic cells with abundant eosinophilic cytoplasm and clear cells with no prominent irregularity of the nuclear membrane (Fig. 6.4d). Other tumors may include chromophobe RCC (34 %), clear cell RCC (9 %), oncocytoma (7 %), or papillary RCC (2 %). Most patients (56 %) also exhibit renal oncocytosis in the grossly normal renal parenchyma. Metastatic disease is rare and occurs only occasionally in patients with renal tumors larger than 3 cm.

## Skin and Other Lesions

Several skin lesions are associated with the BHD syndrome [41]. The most characteristic is fibrofolliculoma, a benign tumor associated with the hair follicle. Fibrofolliculomas usually appear as skin papules on the neck, upper chest, upper back, and face. Histologically, these tumors show a proliferation of follicular epithelium surrounded by a perifollicular fibrous sheath. The stroma surrounding the epithelium may be densely fibrous or loose. Alcian blue may demonstrate the presence of abundant mucin. Trichodiscomas and acrochordons are also frequently associated with BHD syndrome. Pulmonary cystic lesions are present in 24 % of patients with BHD syndrome; these lesions may rupture, leading to spontaneous pneumothorax

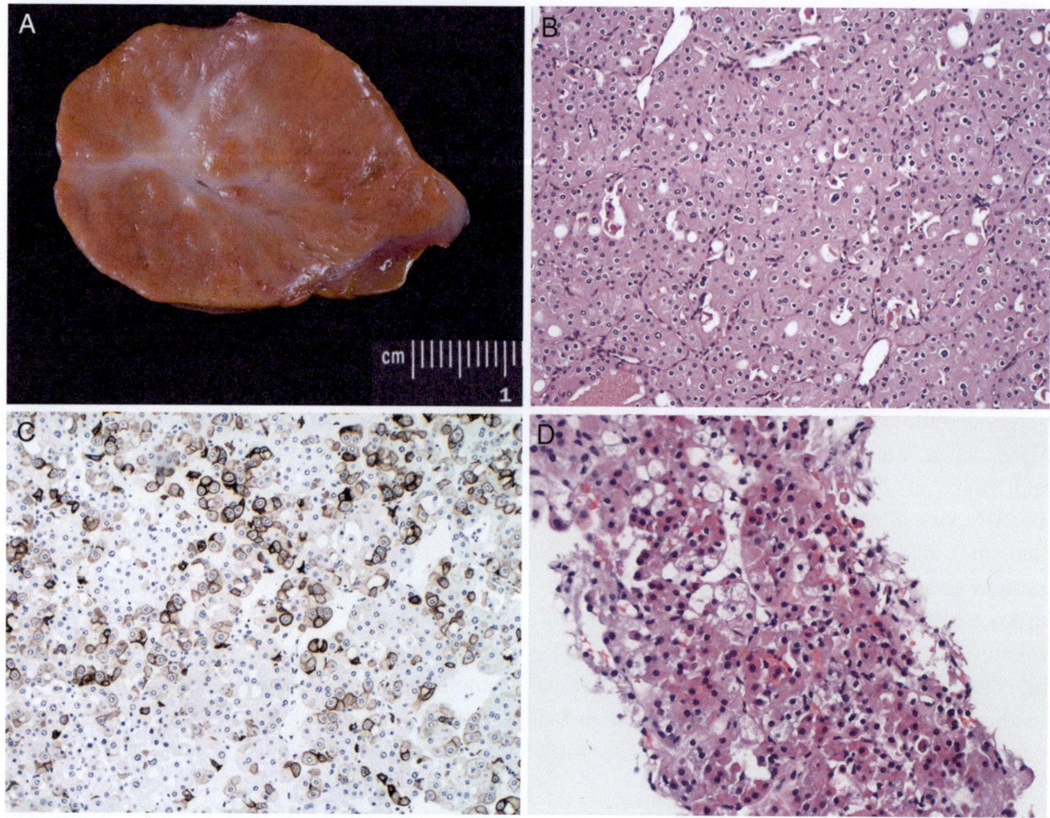

**Fig. 6.4** Renal cell carcinoma in Birt-Hogg-Dubé syndrome. The tumor is usually well circumscribed and tan or brown in color (**a**). The most common histologic feature is a hybrid oncocytic tumor, which shows features of both oncocytomas and chromophobe RCCs (**b**) and focal immunoreactivity for CK7 (**c**). Another hybrid renal tumor is composed of oncocytic cells with abundant eosinophilic cytoplasm and clear cells with no prominent nuclear membrane irregularity (**d**)

[42]. Multiple lipomas and mucosa papules have also been described for patients with BHD syndrome. A large number of other tumors may also occur in these patients, but a causal relationship between the syndrome and these tumors has not been proven [42].

ney. Given that there is an increased incidence of clear cell RCC in BHD, no renal mass in a BHD patient can be considered completely benign, and partial nephrectomy, percutaneous ablation, or radical nephrectomy are all considered on individual bases in these patients [43].

## Treatment

BHD renal tumors are treated and followed per 3 cm FRCC guideline. As most of these tumors are indolent (oncocytic hybrid tumors, oncocytoma) or of low malignant potential (chromophobe RCC), they may be followed until they reach 3 cm in diameter or become symptomatic in order to minimize repeated procedures on an affected kid-

## Tuberous Sclerosis (TS) Syndrome

### Introduction

Affecting 1 in 6000 live births in the United States, TS syndrome is a relatively common genetic disease [44]. The syndrome encompasses neoplastic diseases that can affect virtually any organ in the body but particularly the brain, kidney, lungs, eyes, and skin [45]. TS syndrome is transmitted in an autosomal dominant fashion and has variable penetrance. The characteristic renal tumor is angiomyolipoma (AML), which is present in 60–80 % of individuals with TS syndrome and represents the most common cause of TSC-related mortality in adults [46].

TS syndrome is associated with the mutations of two tumor suppressor genes, tuberous sclerosis complex 1 and 2 (*TSC1* and *TSC2*) [47, 48]. *TSC1* is located at chromosome 9q34 and encodes the protein hamartin, and *TSC2* is located at chromosome 16p13.3 and encodes the protein tuberin. Hamartin and tuberin bind and form a complex that downregulates the mTOR signaling pathway [49]. Mutations of *TSC1* or *TSC2* inactivate hamartin and tuberin, respectively, leading to upregulation of the mTOR signaling pathway. The majority of genetic mutations in TSC are sporadic and not inherited.

## Clinical Presentation

TS patients develop multiple, bilateral AML in their kidneys at an early age and have a slightly higher incidence of RCC over their lifetime as well (see below). Unlike in sporadic cases where AML are more commonly found in women, a majority of TS patients whether male or female develop renal AML by age 30. These are found incidentally, or on imaging for symptoms, which are generally related to bleeding from these very vascular tumors. Bleeding complications related to AML typically occur once a lesion grows to over 4 cm in diameter [50] and present either as gross hematuria or perinephric hematoma that may lead to hemodynamic instability. Infiltration by AML may also result in mass effect and hypertension and contribute to eventual renal failure.

## Pathology

Unlike sporadic AMLs, AMLs of the TS syndrome are characterized by multiple, well-circumscribed, small tumors in bilateral kidneys. Most AMLs present in the renal parenchyma, but some may be located on the renal capsule. Sometimes AMLs may involve other organs. The gross appearance depends on the relative proportion of tumor components. Microscopically, AMLs are composed of three typical components in various proportions: blood vessel, spindle cells, and adipose tissue (Fig. 6.5). Vessels typically have an eccentrically thickened wall with spindle cells spun off the wall. Epithelioid AMLs are reported to be more frequent in TS than in sporadic settings. Approximately 20–30 % of patients with TS develop renal cortical cysts. Renal cell carcinoma may occur in 2–4 % of patients. The most common RCC in TSC exhibits

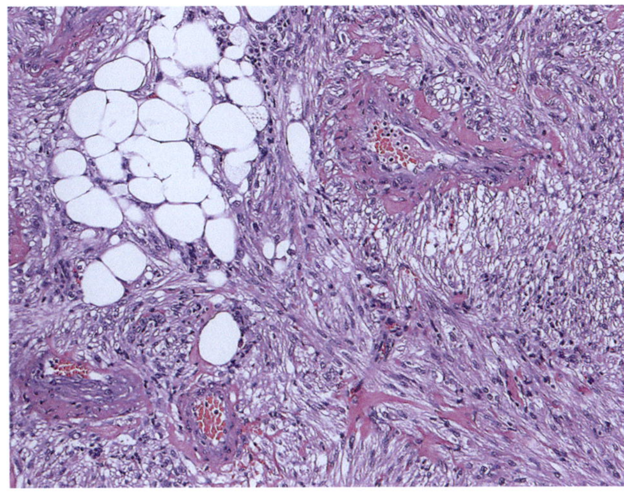

**Fig. 6.5** Angiomyolipoma in tuberous sclerosis syndrome. The tumor is typically composed of blood vessels, smooth muscle spindle cells, and adipose tissue

papillary features and uniformly lacks succinate dehydrogenase subunit B expression, prompting the novel term "TSC-associated papillary RCC" [51]. Another RCC associated with TSC is featured by hybrid oncocytic tumor and chromophobe RCC.

Patients with TS syndrome often develop neoplastic disease in multiple organs [52]. The typical skin lesions include facial angiofibromas, periungual fibromas, shagreen patches, and hypopigmented macules. Central nervous system lesions include subependymomas and giant cell astrocytomas. Patients may develop cardiac rhabdomyomas, pulmonary lymphangioleiomyomatosis, and retinal hamartomas.

## Treatment

The management of renal AML in TS is usually noninvasive, with selective angioembolization used for most bleeding or preemptively for significantly enlarging lesions. Partial nephrectomy has been performed for larger lesions, while nephrectomy has been performed for severely affected renal units. More recently, molecular exploration of the TSC pathways described above has led to trials of mTOR inhibitors in patients with TS. Everolimus is being used successfully to shrink AML in TS patients over a 1-year interval, with promising results of 30–80 % shrinkage of renal lesions in an ongoing study [53, 54].

## Succinate Dehydrogenase Mutation

Similar to FH in HLRCC, succinate dehydrogenase (SDH) is a critical enzyme in the Krebs cycle and electron transport chain, and its mutation shifts the cells towards aerobic glycolysis, resulting in rapid growth and proliferation. The enzyme is made of four subunits, SDHA, SDHB, SDHC, and SCHD, and mutations in the latter three predispose to aggressive RCC. These patients also present with paragangliomas (PGL) and pheochromocytomas (PCC), gastrointestinal stromal tumors (GIST), pituitary adenomas, and

pulmonary chondromas. The kidney tumors can be cystic or solid and may present with variable pathology, including oncocytic features in SDHB-associated tumors. The low grade of clear cell tumors on histopathology may be deceptive, for they behave aggressively, metastasizing early. Given the potential for multifocality and lifelong risk for metachronous tumor development, the recommendation for these patients, when feasible, is nephron-sparing surgery with lifelong surveillance [55].

## Cowden/PTEN Hamartoma Tumor Syndrome

A number of syndromes with differing phenotypical manifestations have been associated with mutations in *PTEN* gene, and of these, more than 300 mutations are associated with Cowden syndrome [56]. PTEN is a tumor suppressor, and its mutated form allows dysregulated activation of PI3K/AKT pathway and resultant activation of mTOR pathway. Besides increased risk for development of RCC, Cowden syndrome is associated with increased risk for breast, endometrial, and thyroid malignancy. Pathognomonic phenotypic features include mucocutaneous lesions such as acral keratosis, facial trichilemmomas, and papillomatous papules. Other nonmalignant conditions associated with this syndrome include macrocephaly, Lhermitte-Duclos disease, benign thyroid conditions, mental retardation, GI hamartomas, lipomas, fibromas, and breast fibrocystic disease. Due to its low penetrance, patients may not have a convincing history of familial RCC; however, the phenotype of the associated dermatologic features and macrocephaly, along with the presence of other cancers, should raise the suspicion for *PTEN* mutation. Histopathology of the kidney tumors associated with this syndrome is variable, and papillary, chromophobe, and clear cell variants of RCC have been described. The biologic behavior of these tumors is not different than their sporadic histopathologically matched counterparts; however, obtaining genetic diagnosis may allow selection of targeted therapy, should surgery not be an option.

## Microphthalmia Transcription (MiT) Family Translocations

This includes a variety of chromosomal translocations which result in fusion proteins activating the MET receptor with uncontrolled proliferation and downstream mTOR pathway activation [57–59]. The largest family is the Xp11.2 translocations/*TFE3* fusions with several genes including *ASPL*, *PRCC*, *PSF*, *NonO*, and *CLTC*. Another less common subtype involves t(6;11)(p21;q12)/*alpha-TFEB* gene fusion. The Xp11.2 is the most common etiology for RCC in pediatric population, comprising about 50 % of total neoplasms. Although rare in adult population, these translocations account for 15 % of RCC in patients younger than 45 years of age. There is speculation that these cancers are associated with exposure to chemotherapy. Interestingly, whereas in children these tumors may have indolent course, in adults they are very aggressive and tend to metastasize early, showing propensity for retroperitoneal lymph node involvement. There is no consensus about architectural uniformity in these tumors, but they tend to be diagnosed by TFE3 and TFEB staining and fluorescent in situ histochemistry (FISH). Grossly they may be cystic or solid and may resemble clear cell or papillary morphology with psammoma bodies and hyaline nodules. The treatment recommendation is partial or radical nephrectomy with regional lymphadenectomy and lifelong surveillance.

## Microphthalmia-Associated Factor (MITF) Mutation

Most recently a germline mutation in MITF, which is another member of the family of MiT transcription factors, was identified in families which have RCC and melanoma. This missense mutation at the Mi-318K locus of MITF gene stimulates transcription of genes affecting multiple oncogenic pathways, including *MET* and *HIF1A*. These tumors are of variable architecture, and the prognosis remains under investigation [60].

## BAP1 Mutation

BAP1 (BRCA1-associated protein-1) is an enzyme that functions as both an effector and regulator of breast cancer gene 1 (*BRCA1*). Its function is implicated in multiple pathways, including cell cycle regulation, protein trafficking, chromatin modulation, and DNA repair. Individuals with *BAP1* mutation have increased susceptibility for early onset clear cell RCC, along with cutaneous and uveal melanomas and mesothelioma. This is a new member of familial RCC attributable to genetic mutation, and more studies are needed to ascertain the prognosis of BAP1-associated renal tumors [61].

## Chromosome 3 Translocation

This is a balanced germline translocation between chromosome 3 and 8, which includes multiple genes important for renal cell cancer development, including *VHL*, *BAP1*, *PBRM1*, and *SETD2*. These patients can present with multifocal cystic and solid clear cell RCC, similar to VHL; however, the age of onset is later, usually in 4th or 5th decade of life [60]. The later age of onset can be explained by the 3-step tumorigenesis model, which includes inheritance of the constitutional translocation, loss of the derivative chromosome carrying the 3p segment as a result of chromatid separation, and, finally, a somatic mutation that renders the tumor suppressor gene inactive. There are no other malignancies associated with this genotype.

## References


1. Pavlovich CP, Schmidt LS. Searching for the hereditary causes of renal-cell carcinoma. Nat Rev Cancer. 2004;4:381–93.
2. Barrisford GW, Singer EA, Rosner IL, et al. Familial renal cancer: molecular genetics and surgical management. Int J Surg Oncol. 2011;2011:658767.
3. Lipworth L, Tarone RE, Lund L, et al. Epidemiologic characteristics and risk factors for renal cell cancer. Clin Epidemiol. 2009;1:33–43.

4. Tan MH, Teh BT. Renal neoplasia in the hyperparathyroidism-jaw tumor syndrome. Curr Mol Med. 2004;4:895–7.

5. Mester JL, Zhou M, Prescott N, et al. Papillary renal cell carcinoma is associated with PTEN hamartoma tumor syndrome. Urology. 2012;79:e1–7.

6. Bonne AC, Bodmer D, Schoenmakers EF, et al. Chromosome 3 translocations and familial renal cell cancer. Curr Mol Med. 2004;4:849–54.

7. Lonser RR, Glenn GM, Walther M, et al. von Hippel-Lindau disease. Lancet. 2003;361:2059–67.

8. Clark PE, Cookson MS. The von Hippel-Lindau gene: turning discovery into therapy. Cancer. 2008;113(7 Suppl):1768–78.

9. Latif F, Tory K, Gnarra J, et al. Identification of the von Hippel-Lindau disease tumor suppressor gene. Science. 1993;260:1317–20.

10. Iliopoulos O, Levy AP, Jiang C, et al. Negative regulation of hypoxia-inducible genes by the von Hippel-Lindau protein. Proc Natl Acad Sci U S A. 1996;93:10595–9.

11. Stolle C, Glenn G, Zbar B, et al. Improved detection of germline mutations in the von Hippel-Lindau disease tumor suppressor gene. Hum Mutat. 1998;12:417–23.

12. Walther MM, Lubensky IA, Venzon D, et al. Prevalence of microscopic lesions in grossly normal renal parenchyma from patients with Von Hippel-Lindau disease, sporadic renal cell carcinoma and no renal disease: clinical implications. J Urol. 1995;154:2010–5.

13. Williamson SR, Zhang S, Eble JN, et al. Clear cell papillary renal cell carcinoma-like tumors in patients with von Hippel-Lindau disease are unrelated to sporadic clear cell papillary renal cell carcinoma. Am J Surg Pathol. 2013;37:1131–9.

14. Gobbo S, Eble JN, Grignon DJ, et al. Clear cell papillary renal cell carcinoma: a distinct histopathologic and molecular genetic entity. Am J Surg Pathol. 2008;32:1239–45.

15. Herring JC, Enquist EG, Chernoff A, et al. Parenchymal sparing surgery in patients with hereditary renal cell carcinoma:10 year experience. J Urol. 2001;165:177.

16. Duffey BG, Choyke PL, Glenn G, et al. The relationship between renal tumor size and metastases in patients with von Hippel-Lindau disease. J Urol. 2004;172:63–5.

17. Zbar B, Tory K, Merino M, et al. Hereditary papillary renal cell carcinoma. J Urol. 1994;151:561–6.

18. Schmidt LS, Nickerson ML, Angeloni D, et al. Early onset hereditary papillary renal carcinoma: germline missense mutations in the tyrosine kinase domain of the MET proto-oncogene. J Urol. 2004;172:1256–61.

19. Schmidt L, Duh FM, Chen F, et al. Germline and somatic mutations in the tyrosine kinase domain of the MET proto-oncogene in papillary renal carcinomas. Nat Genet. 1997;16:68–73.

20. Bottaro DP, Rubin JS, Faletto DL, et al. Identification of the hepatocyte growth factor receptor as the c-met proto-oncogene product. Science. 1991;251:802–4.

21. Schmidt L, Junker K, Nakaigawa N, et al. Novel mutations of the MET proto-oncogene in papillary renal carcinomas. Oncogene. 1999;18:2343–50.

22. Choi JS, Kim MK, Seo JW, et al. MET expression in sporadic renal cell carcinomas. J Korean Med Sci. 2006;21:672–7.

23. Choyke PL, Glenn GM, Walther MM, et al. Hereditary renal cancers. Radiology. 2003;226(1):33–46.

24. Lubensky IA, Schmidt L, Zhuang Z, et al. Hereditary and sporadic papillary renal carcinomas with c-met mutations share a distinct morphological phenotype. Am J Pathol. 1999;155:517–26.

25. Launonen V, Vierimaa O, Kiuru M, et al. Inherited susceptibility to uterine leiomyomas and renal cell cancer. Proc Natl Acad Sci U S A. 2001;98:3387–92.

26. Tomlinson IP, Alam NA, Rowan AJ, et al. Germline mutations in FH predispose to dominantly inherited uterine fibroids, skin leiomyomata and papillary renal cell cancer. Nat Genet. 2002;30:406–10.

27. Toro JR, Nickerson ML, Wei MH, et al. Mutations in the fumarate hydratase gene cause hereditary leiomyomatosis and renal cell cancer in families in North America. Am J Hum Genet. 2003;73:95–106.

28. Isaacs JS, Jung YJ, Mole DR, et al. HIF overexpression correlates with biallelic loss of fumarate hydratase in renal cancer: novel role of fumarate in regulation of HIF stability. Cancer Cell. 2005;8:143–53.

29. Pithukpakorn M, Toro JR. Hereditary leiomyomatosis and renal cell cancer. In: Pagon RA, Adam MP, Ardinger HH, Bird TD, Dolan CR, Fong CT, Smith RJH, Stephens K, editors. GeneReviews® [Internet]. Seattle: University of Washington; 2006. 1993–2014. 2006 Jul 31 [updated 2010 Nov 02].

30. Merino MJ, Torres-Cabala C, Pinto P, et al. The morphologic spectrum of kidney tumors in hereditary leiomyomatosis and renal cell carcinoma (HLRCC) syndrome. Am J Surg Pathol. 2007;31:1578–85.

31. Bardella C, El-Bahrawy M, Frizzell N, et al. Aberrant succination of proteins in fumarate hydratase-deficient mice and HLRCC patients is a robust biomarker of mutation status. J Pathol. 2011;225:4–11.

32. Chen YB, Brannon AR, Toubaji A, et al. Hereditary leiomyomatosis and renal cell carcinoma syndrome-associated renal cancer: recognition of the syndrome by pathologic features and the utility of detecting aberrant succination by immunohistochemistry. Am J Surg Pathol. 2014;38:627–37.

33. Lehtonen R, Kiuru M, Vanharanta S, et al. Biallelic inactivation of fumarate hydratase (FH) occurs in nonsyndromic uterine leiomyomas but is rare in other tumors. Am J Pathol. 2004;164:17–22.

34. Grubb 3rd RL, Franks ME, Toro J, et al. Hereditary leiomyomatosis and renal cell cancer: a syndrome associated with an aggressive form of inherited renal cancer. J Urol. 2007;177(6):2074–9. discussion 2079–80.

35. Birt AR, Hogg GR, Dube WJ. Hereditary multiple fibrofolliculomas with trichodiscomas and acrochordons. Arch Dermatol. 1977;113:1674–7.

36. Pavlovich CP, Walther MM, Eyler RA, Hewitt SM, Zbar B, Linehan WM, Merino MJ. Renal tumors in the Birt-Hogg-Dubé syndrome. Am J Surg Pathol. 2002;26:1542–52.

37. Nickerson ML, Warren MB, Toro JR, et al. Mutations in a novel gene lead to kidney tumors, lung wall defects, and benign tumors of the hair follicle in patients with the Birt-Hogg-Dubé syndrome. Cancer Cell. 2002;2:157–64.

38. Schmidt LS, Warren MB, Nickerson ML, et al. Birt-Hogg-Dubé syndrome, a genodermatosis associated with spontaneous pneumothorax and kidney neoplasia, maps to chromosome 17p11.2. Am J Hum Genet. 2001;69:876–82.

39. Baba M, Hong SB, Sharma N, et al. Folliculin encoded by the BHD gene interacts with a binding protein, FNIP1, and AMPK, and is involved in AMPK and mTOR signaling. Proc Natl Acad Sci U S A. 2006;103:15552–7.

40. Nahorski MS, Lim DH, Martin L, et al. Investigation of the Birt-Hogg-Dubé tumour suppressor gene (FLCN) in familial and sporadic colorectal cancer. J Med Genet. 2010;47:385–90.

41. Menko FH, van Steensel MA, Giraud S, et al. Birt-Hogg-Dubé syndrome: diagnosis and management. Lancet Oncol. 2009;10:1199–206.

42. Toro JR, Pautler SE, Stewart L, et al. Lung cysts, spontaneous pneumothorax, and genetic associations in 89 families with Birt-Hogg-Dubé syndrome. Am J Respir Crit Care Med. 2007;175:1044–53.

43. Pavlovich CP, Grubb RL 3rd, Hurley K et al. Evaluation and management of renal tumors in the Birt-Hogg-Dubé syndrome. J Urol. 2005;173(5):1482–6; Erratum in: J Urol. 2005;174(2):796

44. Osborne JP, Fryer A, Webb D. Epidemiology of tuberous sclerosis. Ann N Y Acad Sci. 1991;615:125–7.

45. Crino PB, Nathanson KL, Henske EP. The tuberous sclerosis complex. N Engl J Med. 2006;355:1345–56.

46. Rakowski SK, Winterkorn EB, Paul E, et al. Renal manifestations of tuberous sclerosis complex: incidence, prognosis, and predictive factors. Kidney Int. 2006;70:1777–82.

47. van Slegtenhorst M, de Hoogt R, Hermans C, et al. Identification of the tuberous sclerosis gene TSC1 on chromosome 9q34. Science. 1997;277:805–8.

48. European Chromosome 16 Tuberous Sclerosis Consortium. Identification and characterization of the tuberous sclerosis gene on chromosome 16. Cell. 1993;75:1305–15.

49. Kwiatkowski DJ. Tuberous sclerosis: from tubers to mTOR. Ann Hum Genet. 2003;67:87–96.

50. Ouzaid I, Autorino R, Fatica R, et al. Active surveillance for renal angiomyolipoma: outcomes and factors predictive of delayed intervention. BJU Int. 2014;114(3):412–7. PMID:24325283 Epub 2014 Apr 16.

51. Yang P, Cornejo KM, Sadow PM, et al. Renal cell carcinoma in tuberous sclerosis complex. Am J Surg Pathol. 2014;38:895–909.

52. Northrup H, Krueger DA, International Tuberous Sclerosis Complex Consensus Group. Tuberous sclerosis complex diagnostic criteria update: recommendations of the 2012 International Tuberous Sclerosis Complex Consensus Conference. Pediatr Neurol. 2013;49:243–54.

53. Budde K, Gaedeke J. Tuberous sclerosis complex-associated angiomyolipomas: focus on mTOR inhibition. Am J Kidney Dis. 2012;59(2):276–83.

54. Kingswood JC, Jozwiak S, Belousova ED, et al. The effect of everolimus on renal angiomyolipoma in patients with tuberous sclerosis complex being treated for subependymal giant cell astrocytoma: subgroup results from the randomized, placebo-controlled, Phase 3 trial EXIST-1. Nephrol Dial Transplant. 2014;29(6):1203–10. Epub 2014 Apr 11.

55. Ricketts CJ, Shuch B, Vocke CD, et al. Succinate dehydrogenase kidney cancer: an aggressive example of Warburg effect in cancer. J Urol. 2012;188(6):2063–71.

56. Shuch B, Ricketts CJ, Vocke CD, et al. Germline PTEN mutation cowden syndrome: an underappreciated form of hereditary kidney cancer. J Urol. 2013;190(6):1990–8.

57. Delahunt B, Srigley JR, Montironi R, et al. Advances in renal neoplasia: recommendations from the 2012 International Society of Urological Pathology Consensus Conference. Urology. 2014;83(5):969–74.

58. Klaassen Z, Tatem A, Burnette JO, et al. Adult Xp11 translocation associated renal cell carcinoma: time to recognize. Urology. 2012;80(5):965–8.

59. Kuroda N, Mikami S, Pan CC, et al. Review of renal carcinoma associated with Xp11.2 translocations/TFE3 gene fusions with focus on pathobiological aspect. Histol Histopathol. 2012;27(2):133–40.

60. Linehan WM, Srinivasan R, Garcia JA. Non-clear cell renal cancer: disease-based management and opportunities for targeted therapeutic approaches. Semin Oncol. 2013;40(4):511–20.

61. Battaglia A. The importance of multidisciplinary approach in early detection of BAP1 tumor predisposition syndrome: clinical management and risk assessment. Clin Med Insights Oncol. 2014;8:37–47.

# Translocation-Associated Carcinoma


Zachary Klaassen, John M. DiBianco, and Martha K. Terris


## Abbreviations

RCC    Renal cell carcinoma
tRCC    Translocation renal cell carcinoma
IHC    Immunohistochemical
H&E    Hematoxylin and eosin

## Introduction

Although mortality rates for renal cell carcinoma (RCC) in the United States remain stable, the incidence of RCC continues to rise [1, 2]. In 2014, there will be an estimated 63,920 new cases of RCC and an estimated 13,860 estimated RCC-related deaths [2]. Generally accepted risk factors for RCC include cigarette smoking, obesity, hypertension, occupational exposure, and certain genetic mutations. However, the implication of genetic factors and their effect on pathological and clinical outcomes remains to be completely elucidated [1]. Since the mapping of the human genome, advanced genetic diagnostic tests have been used to facilitate diagnosis and treatment of rare genetic malignancies. Particularly for RCC, an emerging family of genetic mutations, translocation-associated RCC (tRCC), was recognized in 2004 as a subtype of RCC by the World Health Organization (WHO) [3, 4]. A number of genetic subtypes of tRCCs have been described, the most common of which is Xp11.2 and to a lesser extent t(6;11) and tRCCs involving chromosome 3.

## History and Epidemiology

tRCC was originally considered to be a pediatric disease. Since RCC in children is less likely to be secondary to environmental factors, these tumors were investigated more thoroughly for genetic variation compared to adult RCC [5]. tRCC accounts for up to 33 % of all pediatric RCCs, up to 15 % of RCC's diagnosed in patients less than 45 years of age [6, 7], and more recent data demonstrates a female predominance [8]. The diagnosis of tRCC has become a recognized entity, and it is now estimated that tRCC makes up approximately 5 % of all RCC diagnoses [6, 7] and may comprise >1.5 % of all clear cell RCC [3].

Xp11 tRCC is currently the most common subtype of tRCC. Xp11 tRCC involves the splice site Xp11.2 and was first found by karyotype of


Z. Klaassen, M.D. • J.M. DiBianco (✉)
M.K. Terris, M.D.
Department of Surgery, Section of Urology,
Medical College of Georgia – Georgia Regents
University, 1120 15th Street, Augusta,
GA 30912, USA
e-mail: zklaassen@gru.edu;
jmdibi32@gmail.com; meterris@gru.edu



© Springer Science+Business Media New York 2016
D.E. Hansel et al. (eds.), *The Kidney*, DOI 10.1007/978-1-4939-3286-3_7

two apical renal masses presenting in infant males [9, 10]. After further study using TFE3 immunoassays, Xp11 tRCC was found to constitute approximately 40 % of pediatric RCC cases [11–14]. In these cases, Xp11 tRCC was discovered in the setting of children having undergone chemotherapy with DNA ligating agents for non-RCC malignancies. Argani et al. speculated that early exposure to DNA-altering agents, such as DNA topoisomerase II inhibitors or cyclophosphamide, could potentially serve as a precipitating factor for developing Xp11 tRCC [15]. These tumors typically presented at an advanced stage and with characteristics similar to other RCC; however, the prognosis remained relatively uncertain with occasional indolent progression. While the natural history and pathophysiology of the disease remained poorly defined, the accumulation of these studies led most investigators to believe that tRCC was an anomalous malignancy unique to the pediatric population [11].

The belief that Xp11 tRCC may have been a pediatric specific disease has since been refuted. Since 2007, studies have emerged identifying Xp11 tRCC in adult populations with an incidence of 1–5 % [14, 16–18]. Similar to the pediatric population, these patients typically present at an advanced stage, with metastases and similar histological features to traditional histologic subtypes of RCC [16–18]. Despite aggressive surgical intervention, these patients universally have a poor prognosis with a rapid terminal course. These outcomes have prompted increased interest, time, and resources dedicated to investigating, understanding, and describing Xp11 tRCC.

Rare subtypes of tRCC include t(6;11), also known as TFEB-RCC, and tRCCs involving chromosome 3. The relatively low incidence is likely due to a combination of lack of recognition and histologic similarity with traditional RCC [19]. Most of the early studies describing t(6;11) tRCC, similar to Xp11 tRCC, demonstrated a pediatric age predilection; however, more recent studies have highlighted cases of adults with this unique disease [19, 20]. Hora et al. examined ten cases of tRCC, including six Xp11 and four

t(6;11), and found that tRCCs were more common in females (seven of ten patients) [8]. They also reported that Xp11 was diagnosed at an older age than t(6;11) (51 vs. 32 years of age), and while both entities have the potential to be an aggressive malignancy, t(6;11) tRCC had a better prognosis than Xp11.

Although the most common genetic mutation involving chromosome 3 is 3p25 (von Hippel-Lindau (VHL) disease), much less is known about tRCCs involving chromosome 3. t(3;6) tRCC has an estimated incidence of <2 % in patients diagnosed with bilateral RCC [21]. Cohen et al. in 1979 were the first to describe t(3;8) tRCC in association with familial RCC [22]. Due to the rarity of this tRCC subtype, few cases have been reported, and little is known about its clinical course; however, these patients typically have bilateral, multifocal disease in the fourth or fifth decade of life [23].

## Genetics

Xp11 tRCC was initially described based on a chromosomal translocation t(X;1)(p11.2;q21.2) resulting in the fusion of a novel gene designated PRCC at 1q21.2 to the TFE3 gene at Xp11.2 [24]. Mutations of Xp11 result in gene fusion products between the helix-loop-helix leucine zipper transcription factor (TFE3) and the alveolar soft part sarcoma locus (ASPL), along with several other genes (*PRCC*, *NonO* (*p54^{nrb}*), *PSF*, and *CLTC*) [25]. TFE3, a member of the microphthalmia transcription factor family, is believed to mediate transcription factor upregulation of the MET tyrosine kinase receptor [26], the activation of which triggers downstream signaling pathways. One of the downstream pathways activated is the mammalian rapamycin pathway target, which subsequently leads to unregulated cell proliferation seen in Xp11 tRCC and believed to play a significant role in the poor prognosis of the disease [27]. Xp11 tRCC has a unique and unparalleled upregulation of TFE3, and testing for TFE3 is done by immunohistochemical (IHC) assay. This process has a high degree of sensitivity (97.5 %) and specificity

(99.6 %) compared with standard cytogenetics [28] and can be further improved using dual-color break-apart fluorescence in situ hybridization (FISH) assay as a confirmatory test to potentially eliminating false-positive outcomes that result from over staining [29].

While there are many gene products formed as a result of Xp11 mutations, the most commonly observed is the *ASPL-TFE3* gene fusion product. This product contains breakpoints identical to those found in alveolar soft part sarcoma (ASPS), which is an exceedingly rare soft tissue tumor. While Xp11 tRCC can share similar gross and histopathologic appearance on hematoxylin and eosin (H&E) stain with clear cell and papillary RCC [6], it most likely has a different pathologic and tumorigenesis process owing to its more aggressive disease processes and outcomes.

t(6,11) tRCC involves a genetic fusion of the 11q12, 5′ alpha portion, with TEFB at chromosome 6p21 [19]. Originally, alpha fusion points and breakpoints were seen upstream of the TFEB exon 3; however, more recent studies examining t(6,11) tRCC have shown these points occur within the breakpoint cluster region [19]. The consequence of this finding is a more diverse transcription product than previously identified [19]. Both TFE3 and TFEB genes are considered microphthalmia transcription factors (MiTs). Secondary to their TFE3 and TFEB gene fusions, t(6;11) and Xp11 tRCC were classified in a new subgroup of renal carcinoma by the International Society of Urological Pathology (ISUP) known as the MiT family tRCC [8].

In 1993, Boldog et al. conducted an extensive genetic analysis of t(3;8) translocation in relation to familial RCCs, identifying the gene HRCA1 (hereditary renal cancer associated 1) mapped immediately adjacent to the 3;8 breakpoint [30]. More recent laboratory and case series analyses of familial RCCs have identified many chromosome 3 translocations: t(1;3)(q32; q13), t(2;3)(q33;q21), t(2;3)(q35;q21), t(3;4)(p13; p16), t(3;6)(q12;q15), t(3;8)(p13;q24), and t(3;8) (p14.1; q24.23), t(3;6) (p13;q25.1), t(3;6)(q23; q16.2) [5]. tRCC genomic profiling and the first full genome-wide RNA and exome sequence by Malouf et al. have revealed new markers for better understanding of the disease and for possible diagnosis tRCC [3]. The genomic sequencing was done on seven different confirmed tRCC samples, so it is still unknown if these results are truly universal for all tRCCs. Regardless, this information has the potential to expand the understanding of tRCC and provide insight into more accurate and timely diagnosis in the future [3].

## Diagnosis and Pathologic Analysis

Xp11 tRCC is most commonly seen in patients <45 years of age and has no unique CT or MRI findings that would differentiate it from clear cell RCC (Fig. 7.1) [8, 31–33]. Diagnosis of tRCC is primarily made by a combination of histology, immunohistochemistry, and genetic testing [4, 6, 16, 18, 25, 34]. The H&E staining of the Xp11 tRCC can be confounding due to the overlap with papillary and clear cell RCC. Typical gross pathology includes a well-circumscribed tumor without areas of necrosis, and histologically a polygonal neoplastic cell possessing cytoplasm ranging from predominantly clear to eosinophilic [16] (Fig. 7.2a, b). There are subsets of Xp11 tRCC that exhibit a unique histological appearance [16, 17]. *ASPL-TFE3* gene fusion variant demonstrates a distinct characteristic of mixed clear cell papillary tumors containing tumor cells with voluminous cytoplasm and psammomatous calcifications (Fig. 7.2c). The *ASPL-TFE3* gene fusion variant is the most common subtype of Xp11 tRCC and one of the most aggressive, associated with metastases at presentation and poor outcomes [16, 17]. In order to sufficiently diagnose Xp11 tRCC, TFE3 IHC and genetic analysis are imperative. Klatte et al. demonstrated that 23 % of tumors suspected of being Xp11.2 tRCC demonstrated TFE3 immunoreactivity (Fig. 7.3) and concluded that strong TFE3 expression was associated with metastatic spread and poor prognosis [35]. If histological analysis shows clear cell RCC or mixed clear cell and papillary features, particularly in a child or young adult, this should prompt further histological and molecular characterization of the tumor to rule out tRCC [36].

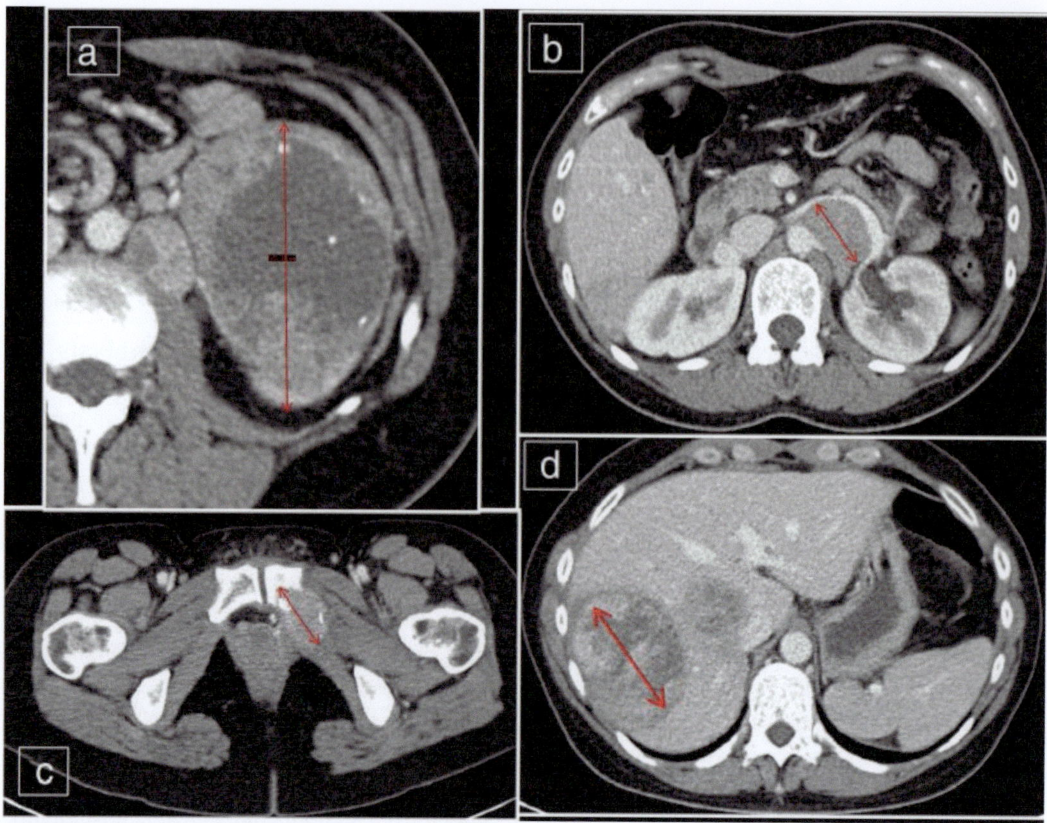



**Fig. 7.1** Computed tomography scan from a 34-year-old woman with (**a**) a tumor of the left kidney (T3aN2M1), (**b**) metastases to the paraaortal lymph nodes, (**c**) left pubic bone, and (**d**) liver. Biopsy confirmed Xp11.2 tRCC (*red arrows* depicting tumor involvement) (Reprinted with open access permission from Hora M, Urge T, Travnicek I, Ferda J, Chudacek Z, Vanecek T, Michal M, Petersson F, Kuroda N, Hes O. MiT Translocation renal cell carcinomas: two subgroups of tumors with translocations involving 6p21 [t(6;11)] and Xp11.2 [t(X;1 or X or 17)]. SpringerPlus. 2014; 3:245)

Recent technologic and genetic analysis advances, including polymerase chain reaction (PCR) and FISH, have further improved the diagnosis of Xp11 tRCC (Fig. 7.4). The goal is to more accurately identify tRCC by testing for specific biomarkers, gene mutations, polymorphisms, and gene split products [14]. Pfleuger et al. performed whole transcriptome sequencing in order to identify diagnostic molecular markers [14]. They identified two novel gene signatures within chimeric RNA molecules: eukaryotic translocation elongation factor 1 alpha 2 (EEF1A2) and Contactin 3 (CNTN3), both of which the clinical significance remains to be determined. Newer and more advanced technologies may allow for more accurate tRCC diagnoses, allowing for improved clinical correlation.

In general, tRCC, t(6,11) has similar histopathologic features of other tRCCs, as well as clear cell RCC and epithelioid angiomyolipoma (Fig. 7.5) [19, 20]. Grossly, these tumors are not easily discernable from other RCCs, as they may appear gray, tan, circumscribed, or uncircumscribed, with and without necrosis [19, 20]. The histopathological characteristics of t(6,11) include a biphasic epithelial cell morphology of large clear cells surrounding a second population of smaller cells with focal basement membrane material deposition, pseudorosette formation, and HMB-45 IHC reactivity [17, 20, 37, 38]. In a case series of three patients with t(6,11) tRCC, Inamura et al. reported that the most efficacious way to identify t(6,11) tRCC was with histopathological nuclear staining for the TFEB protein

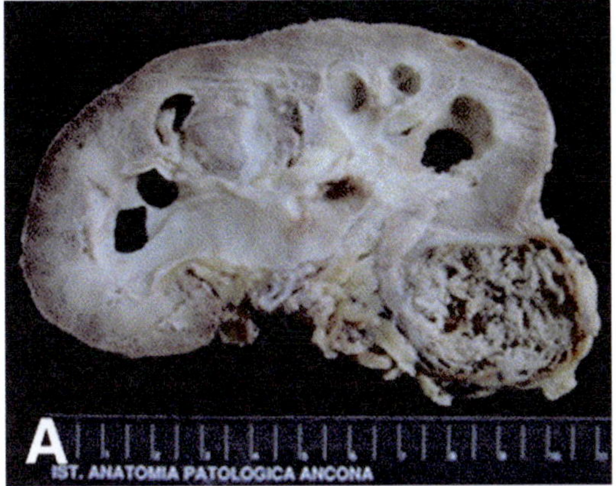


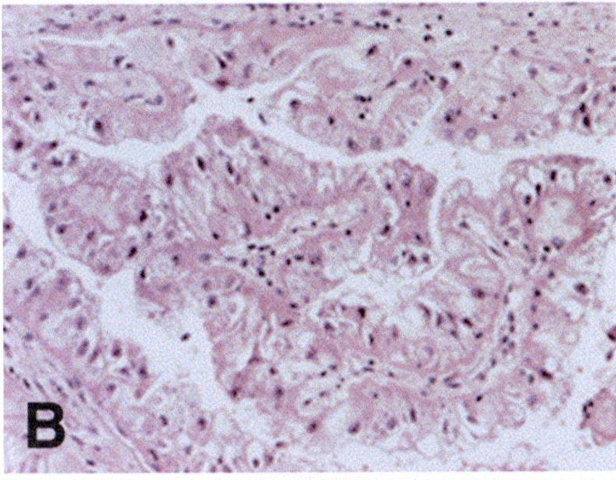


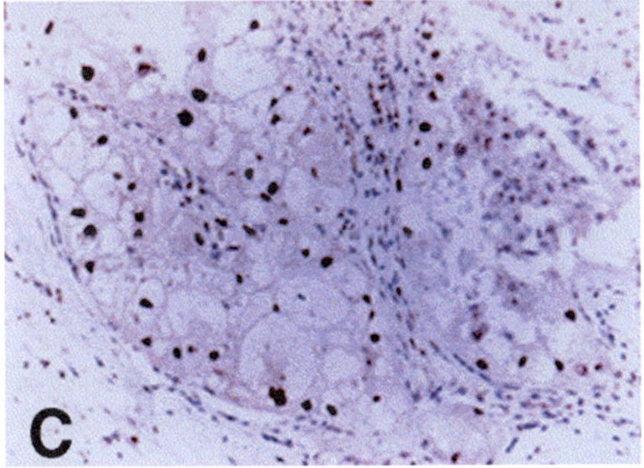


**Fig. 7.2** Xp11 tRCC showing (**a**) gross and (**b**) histological features with papillary architecture. (**c**) Nuclear immunoreactivity for TFE-3 protein is characteristic (Reprinted with permission from Lopez-Beltran A, Scarpelli M, Montironi R, Kirkali Z. 2004 WHO classification of the renal tumors of the adults. Eur Urol. 2006; 49(5):798–805)

[19]. This finding was corroborated by Rao et al. in their seven-patient case series; they found that all tumors displayed 100 % reactivity to TFEBS1 and TFEBS2 [38]. Petersson et al. described a case series of four patients with t(6;11) tRCC and concluded that HMB-45 and cathepsin K are the

most consistent IHC reactivity finding. In contrast to Xp11, none of the t(6;11) tumors displayed reactivity to TFE3 [20]. These varying degrees of reactivity illustrate the variation within this disease process. Based on the available literature, a combination of HMB-45 reactivity and TFEB staining may be the IHC profile with the highest positive predictive value.

To date there is no consensus for identifying and diagnosing t(3;6) tRCC. Due to the paucity of available literature, most studies describe laboratory genetic identification through microarray and FISH as the most feasible means of diagnosis [5]. This is not dissimilar to VHL disease, which is diagnosed by DNA sequencing and/or Southern blot testing [39]. Sporadic clear cell RCC is caused by VHL inactivation in 60 % of patients, and Foster et al. hypothesize that there may be a non-VHL-dependent sporadic clear cell RCC pathway that is caused by chromosome 3 translocations [5, 40, 41]. It seems reasonable to test for t(3;6) tRCC and other tRCC subtypes when an absence of VHL inactivation has been confirmed.

## Treatment

To date, there is no reliable and effective treatment protocol for tRCC. Currently, the principal treatment for RCC in the pediatric population is tumor resection either with partial or radical nephrectomy [42]. Although tRCCs have been more commonly associated with the pediatric population, there is no consensus on whether the treatment regimen and surveillance protocol should be altered. Children with RCC and regional lymph node involvement demonstrate improved cancer-specific and all-cause mortality as well as higher cancer-free survival than adults diagnosed at the same stage [42].

Even with more common RCC subtypes, there is still debate and controversy regarding usefulness and reliability of renal biopsy and radiographic criteria for concerning renal lesions (Fig. 7.6) [43]. This lack of consensus and histological criteria leads to misdiagnosis of tRCC as well as creating confusion as to treatment response. The best treatment outcomes involve protocols that recommend radical nephrectomy

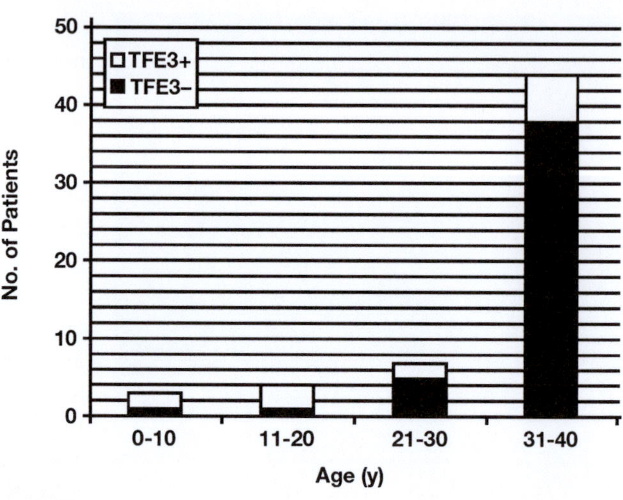



**Fig. 7.3** Incidence of positive TFE3 immunostaining in renal cell carcinoma in age ranges of 0–10, 11–20, 21–30, and 31–40 years (Reprinted with permission from Klatte T, Streubel B, Wrba F, Remzi M, Krammer B, de Martino M, Waldert M, Marberger M, Susani M, Haitel A. Renal cell carcinoma associated with transcription factor E3 expression and Xp11.2 translocation. Am J Clin Pathol. 2012; 137(5):761–8)

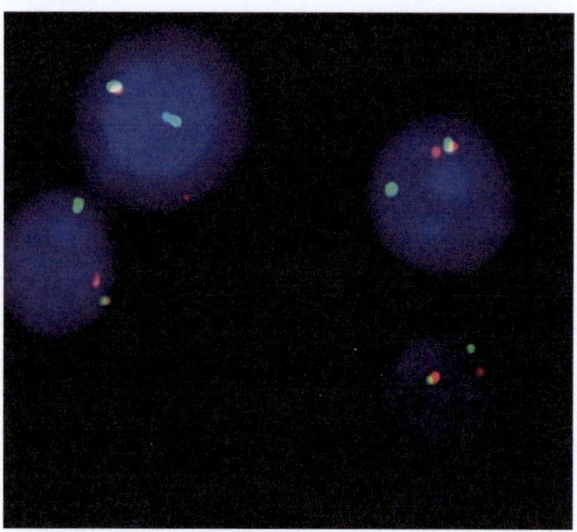

**Fig. 7.4** Fluorescence in situ hybridization with probes flanking TFE3 shows *red-green fusion signal* representing the normal *TFE3* gene and *separate red and green signals* demonstrating a *TFE3* rearrangement in all tumor cells (Reprinted with permission from Klatte T, Streubel B, Wrba F, Remzi M, Krammer B, de Martino M, Waldert M, Marberger M, Susani M, Haitel A. Renal cell carcinoma associated with transcription factor E3 expression and Xp11.2 translocation. Am J Clin Pathol. 2012; 137(5):761–8)

and lymph node dissection prior to distant metastases [44, 45]. Hung et al. reviewed eight cases of Xp11 tRCC treated at their institution from 2007 to 2010 [45]. They concluded that the factor that directly effects patient survival is the presence of distant metastases at the time of diagnosis or at the time of surgery. Of the four patients who presented with stage I or II disease at the time of nephrectomy, three were disease-free at 24, 16, and 2 months postoperatively. With such a limited number of cohorts, any conclusive recommendation is difficult in regard to advantage of radical versus partial nephrectomy and/or the impact of an extended lymph node dissection.

In general, tRCC response to standard immunotherapy or chemotherapy is poor, and patients have a relatively short overall survival [27]. Modest results have been reported with the receptor tyrosine kinase inhibitor sunitinib [46, 47]. In a 2010 study, Malouf et al. examined 21 adult patients with Xp11 tRCC and metastatic disease that had received targeted anti-VEGF or mTOR inhibitors [47]. They observed an 8.2-month

**Fig. 7.5** t(6,11) tRCC. (**a**) The tumor consists of large and epithelioid cells arranged in a nested alveolar or acinar pattern and separated by thin capillaries. (**b**) The small cells have narrow eosinophilic cytoplasm, and dark nuclei are characteristically clustered around hyaline basement membrane material with large acini. (**c, d**) Tumor cells are diffusely positive for vimentin and Melan-A and widely stained with AE1/AE3, CK8, and Cam5.2 anticytokeratin antibodies. (**e**) Nuclear staining with TFEB antibody is present in the majority of tumor cells (Reprinted with permission from Zhan HQ, Wang CF, Zhu XZ, Xu XL. Renal cell carcinoma with t(6;11) translocation: a patient case with a novel alpha-TFEB fusion point. J Clin Oncol. 2010; 28(34):e709–13)

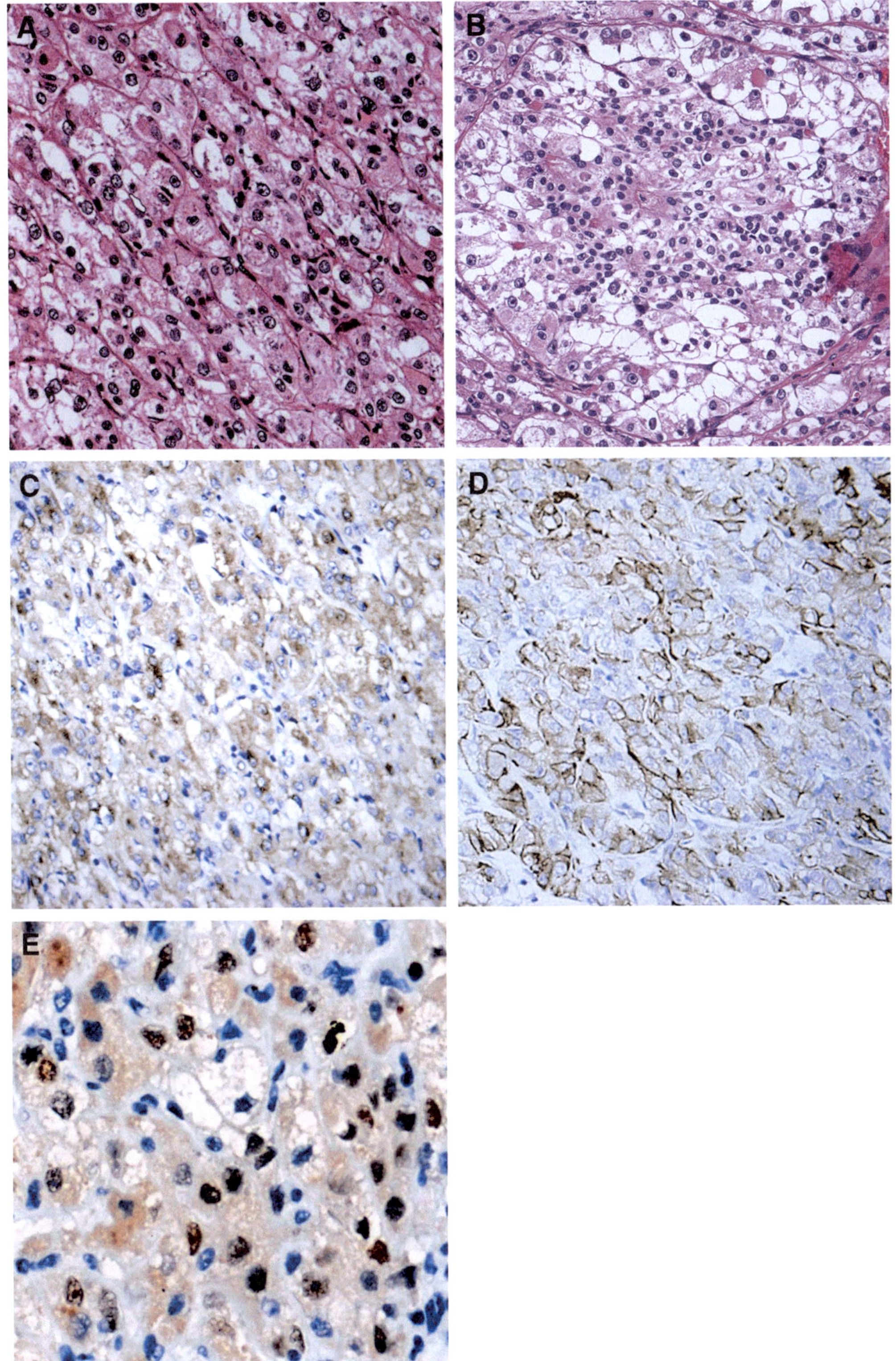

**Fig. 7.5** (continued)

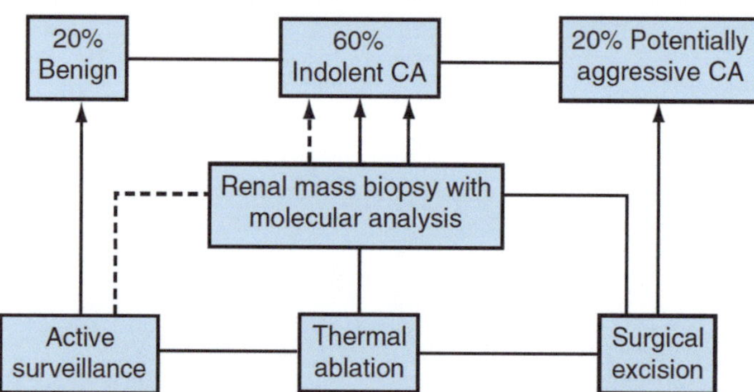


**Fig. 7.6** The AUA guideline panel for the management of the clinical T1 renal mass strongly advocates research priority for renal mass biopsy with molecular profiling to facilitate more rational management (Reprinted with permission from Campbell SC, Lane BR. Malignant Renal Tumors. In: Wein AJ, Kavoussi LR, Novick AC, Partin AW, Peters CA, editors. Campbell-Walsh Urology. 10th ed. Philadelphia. Elsevier Saunders; 2012)

progression-free survival in the sunitinib group compared with 2-month progression-free survival observed in the group receiving cytokine therapy. A retrospective review of 15 adult patients (12 females; median age 40 years) with tRCC who were treated with targeted therapy at four centers in the United States showed an overall response rate of 20 %, with median progression-free survival of 7.1 months and median overall survival of 14.3 months [36, 48]. A Children's Oncology Group (COG) clinical trial is currently testing the effectiveness of antiangiogenesis agents comparing Xp11 tRCC with adult RCC [49]. A second current trial with tivantinib (agent ARQ 197) for the treatment of tRCCs showed limited effectiveness [50]; however, this is an area of continued clinical research. Although ultimately fatal, targeted therapy with both temsirolimus and sunitinib appears to be the optimal management of metastatic Xp11 tRCC [27, 46, 47].

t(6;11) tRCC has been described as having an indolent pathologic course [37]. Among the patients with t(6;11) tRCC who have documented outcomes, the majority are treated with radical nephrectomy and present with localized disease [19, 20, 37, 51–57]. However, until long-term clinical outcomes are available, a potential aggressive clinical course for patients with t(3;6) tRCC should not be underestimated as they may require assertive treatment and follow-up.

Due to the aggressive nature and advanced-stage presentation of Xp11 tumors, the effectiveness of metastasectomy has been brought into question. Although the usefulness and feasibility of metastasectomy in advanced Xp11 tRCC has not been established, studies have reported successful results performing metastasectomy for patients with limited metastatic disease and with histopathologic variants similar to prototypical RCC [58–60]. In general, as with typical RCC, isolated pulmonary metastases are lesions most amenable to metastasectomy, with median 5-year survival rates of 35–50 % [58–60]. Kavolius et al. reported a series of 278 patients with recurrent RCC, of whom 141 (50.7 %) underwent curative metastasectomy and 70 (25.2 %) underwent non-curative metastasectomy [59]. Multivariate analysis identified a solitary metastatic lesion, age <60 years, and disease-free survival of >12 months as favorable prognostic factors [59]. These findings, along with tRCC's relative lack of sensitivity to current chemotherapeutic and radiotherapeutic agents, add evidence albeit weak, to the prospect of utilizing metastasectomy in the treatment protocol of patients with metastatic Xp11 tRCC.

## Surveillance

As with diagnosis and treatment, there is currently no proven, reliable, or effective surveillance algorithm for tRCC for patients after radical nephrectomy. However, in 2006, Chin et al. developed and proposed a novel staging system for RCC that incorporated the 1997 TNM classification with the Eastern Cooperative Oncology Group performance status and Fuhrman grade (UCLA Integrated Staging System) into a single prognostic algorithm [61]. They recommended treatment follow-up according to stratification into low-, intermediate-, or high-risk categories. Because Xp11 tRCC has an unpredictable and aggressive disease course, it is reasonable to stratify patients with Xp11 tRCC as high risk and place them into the proposed post-nephrectomy surveillance algorithm developed by Chin et al. Their protocol recommends (a) history, physical examinations, and laboratory tests every 6 months for 3 years and then yearly until 10 years; (b) chest computed tomography every 6 months for 3 years and then yearly until 10 years (chest computed tomography alternating with chest radiography after 3 years); and (c) abdominal computed tomography every 6 months for 2 years, yearly until 5 years, and then every 2 years until 10 years [61]. In addition to their recommendations, because Xp11 tRCC is often diagnosed in young adults, it may be reasonable to suggest lifelong surveillance with yearly history, physical examination, and laboratory tests and chest and/or abdominal imaging, as deemed clinically necessary, after completing the previously described 10-year surveillance regimen (Table 7.1) [62]. The rarity of t(6;11) tRCC and chromosomal 3 tRCCs does not enable definitive recommendations regarding a surveillance protocol after treatment. At this point, it seems reasonable to recommend the same surveillance protocol as with Xp11 tRCC until further clinical outcomes are reported.

There is currently no difference between the surveillance protocol for adults and children treated for RCC. Furthermore, the National Comprehensive Cancer Network (NCCN) guidelines do not distinguish these age-specific populations [63]. A similar surveillance protocol for adults and children with tRCC appears reasonable; however, ultrasound surveillance for children may be more appropriate given the more indolent course of tRCC and risk of radiation exposure from multiple CT scans in the pediatric population.

## Conclusion

Translocation-associated RCC is a recently recognized genetic variant subtype of RCC; Xp11 tRCC is the most common variant, historically associated with the pediatric population. Secondary to an increasing number of incidental

**Table 7.1** Surveillance protocol after radical nephrectomy for Xp11 tRCC

| |
| --- |
| At 6, 12, 18, and 24 months—history/physical/lab tests, chest CT, abdominal CT |
| At 2.5 years—history/physical/lab tests, chest CT |
| At 3, 4, and 5 years—history/physical/lab tests, chest CTa, abdominal CT |
| At 6 years—history/physical/labs tests, chest CT[a] |
| At 7 years—history/physical/labs tests, chest CT[a], abdominal CT |
| At 8 years—history/physical/labs tests, chest CT[a] |
| At 9 years—history/physical/labs tests, chest CT[a], abdominal CT |
| At 10 years—history/physical/labs tests, chest CT[a] |
| Yearly thereafter—history/physical/labs tests, imaging as deemed clinically relevant |

Copyright © MedReviews®, LLC. Reprinted with permission of MedReviews®, LLC. Chin AI et al. Surveillance strategies for renal cell carcinoma patients following nephrectomy. Rev Urol. 2006;8(1):1–7
Reviews in Urology is a copyrighted publication of MedReviews®, LLC. All rights reserved
[a]Chest radiography can alternate with chest computed tomography (Adapted from Chin et al. [61])

renal masses detected, particularly for young adults, knowledge regarding the potentially aggressive and fatal nature of tRCC is important for the urologist and general clinician. Similar to traditional RCC, curative surgery with close postoperative surveillance remains the best treatment option for these patients. Systemic regimens for distant disease remain largely ineffective and have been demonstrated to marginally extend life expectancy. With continually improving histopathologic and genetic analysis, the incidence of tRCC will continue to increase, requiring longterm follow-up data to further develop the optimal treatment algorithm for these patients.

# References


1. Chow WH, Dong LM, Devesa SS. Epidemiology and risk factors for kidney cancer. Nat Rev Urol. 2010;7(5):245–57.
2. Siegel R, Ma J, Zou Z, Jemal A. Cancer statistics, 2014. CA Cancer J Clin. 2014;64(1):9–29.
3. Malouf GG, Monzon FA, Couturier J, Molinie V, Escudier B, Camparo P, Su X, Yao H, Tamboli P, Lopez-Terrada D, Picken M, Garcia M, Multani AS, Pathak S, Wood CG, Tannir NM. Genomic heterogeneity of translocation renal cell carcinoma. Clin Cancer Res. 2013;19(17):4673–84.
4. Lopez-Beltran A, Scarpelli M, Montironi R, Kirkali Z. 2004 WHO classification of the renal tumors of the adults. Eur Urol. 2006;49(5):798–805.
5. Foster RE, Abdulrahman M, Morris MR, Prigmore E, Gribble S, Ng B, Gentle D, Ready S, Weston PM, Wisener MS, Kishida T, Yao M, Davison V, Barbero JL, Chu C, Carter NP, Latif F, Maher ER. Characterization of a 3;6 translocation associated with renal cell carcinoma. Genes Chromosomes Cancer. 2007;46(4):311–7.
6. Komai Y, Fujiwara M, Fujii Y, Mukai H, Yonese J, Kawakami S, Yamamoto S, Migita T, Ishikawa Y, Kurata M, Nakamura T, Fukui I. Adult Xp11 translocation renal cell carcinoma diagnosed by cytogenetics and immunohistochemistry. Clin Cancer Res. 2009;15(4):1170–6.
7. Zhong M, De Angelo P, Osborne L, Paniz-Mondolfi AE, Geller M, Yang Y, Linehan WM, Merino MJ, Cordon-Cardo C, Cai D. Translocation renal cell carcinomas in adults: a single-institution experience. Am J Surg Pathol. 2012;36(5):654–62.
8. Hora M, Urge T, Travnicek I, Ferda J, Chudacek Z, Vanecek T, Michal M, Petersson F, Kuroda N, Hes O. MiT translocation renal cell carcinomas: two subgroups of tumors with translocations involving 6p21 [t(6;11)] and Xp11.2 [t(X;1 or X or 17)]. SpringerPlus. 2014;3:245.
9. de Jong B, Molenaar IM, Leeuw JA, Idenberg VJ, Oosterhuis JW. Cytogenetics of a renal adenocarcinoma in a 2-year-old child. Cancer Genet Cytogenet. 1986;21(2):165–9.
10. Tomlinson GE, Nisen PD, Timmons CF, Schneider NR. Cytogenetics of a renal cell carcinoma in a 17-month-old child: evidence for Xp11.2 as a recurring breakpoint. Cancer Genet Cytogenet. 1991;57(1):11–7.
11. Ramphal R, Pappo A, Zielenska M, Grant R, Ngan BY. Pediatric renal cell carcinoma: clinical, pathologic, and molecular abnormalities associated with the members of the mit transcription factor family. Am J Clin Pathol. 2006;126(3):349–64.
12. Altinok G, Kattar MM, Mohamed A, Poulik J, Grignon D, Rabah R. Pediatric renal carcinoma associated with Xp11.2 translocations/TFE3 gene fusions and clinicopathologic associations. Pediatr Dev Pathol. 2005;8(2):168–80.
13. Wu A, Kunju LP, Cheng L, Shah RB. Renal cell carcinoma in children and young adults: analysis of clinicopathological, immunohistochemical and molecular characteristics with an emphasis on the spectrum of Xp11.2 translocation-associated and unusual clear cell subtypes. Histopathology. 2008;53(5):533–44.
14. Pflueger D, Sboner A, Storz M, Roth J, Comperat E, Bruder E, Rubin MA, Schraml P, Moch H. Identification of molecular tumor markers in renal cell carcinomas with TFE3 protein expression by RNA sequencing. Neoplasia. 2013;15(11):1231–40.
15. Argani P, Laé M, Ballard ET, Amin M, Manivel C, Hutchinson B, Reuter VE, Ladanyi M. Translocation carcinomas of the kidney after chemotherapy in childhood. J Clin Oncol. 2006;24(10):1529–34.
16. Argani P, Olgac S, Tickoo SK, Goldfischer M, Moch H, Chan DY, Eble JN, Bonsib SM, Jimeno M, Lloreta J, Billis A, Hicks J, De Marzo AM, Reuter VE, Ladanyi M. Xp11 translocation renal cell carcinoma in adults: expanded clinical, pathologic, and genetic spectrum. Am J Surg Pathol. 2007;31(8):1149–60.
17. Argani P, Antonescu CR, Illei PB, Lui MY, Timmons CF, Newbury R, Reuter VE, Garvin AJ, Perez-Atayde AR, Fletcher JA, Beckwith JB, Bridge JA, Ladany M. Primary renal neoplasms with the ASPL-TFE3 gene fusion of alveolar soft part sarcoma: a distinctive tumor entity previously included among renal cell carcinomas of children and adolescents. Am J Pathol. 2001;159(1):179–92.
18. Meyer PN, Clark JI, Flanigan RC, Picken MM. Xp11.2 translocation renal cell carcinoma with very aggressive course in five adults. Am J Clin Pathol. 2007;128(1):70–9.
19. Inamura K, Fujiwara M, Togashi Y, Nomura K, Mukai H, Fujii Y, Yamamoto S, Yonese J, Fukui I, Ishikawa Y. Diverse fusion patterns and heterogeneous pathologic features of renal cell carcinoma with t(6;11) translocation. Am J Surg Pathol. 2012;36(1):35–42.
20. Petersson F, Vanecek T, Michael M, Martignoni G, Brunelli M, Halbhuber Z, Spagnolo D, Kuroda N, Yang X, Cabrero IA, Hora M, Branzovsky J, Trivunic S, Kacerovska D, Steiner P, Hes O. A distinctive

translocation carcinoma of the kidney; "rosette forming", t(6;11), HMB45-positive renal tumor: a histomorphologic, immunohistochemical, ultrastructural, and molecular genetic study of 4 cases. Hum Pathol. 2012;43(5):726–36.

21. Blute ML, Itano NB, Cheville JC, Weaver AL, Lohse CM, Zincke H. The effect of bilaterality, pathological features and surgical outcome in nonhereditary renal cell carcinoma. J Urol. 2003;169(4): 1276–81.

22. Cohen AJ, Li FP, Berg S, Marchetto DJ, Tsai S, Jacobs SC, Brown RS. Hereditary renal-cell carcinoma associated with a chromosomal translocation. N Engl J Med. 1979;301(11):592–5.

23. Linehan WM. Genetic basis of kidney cancer: role of genomics for the development of disease-based therapeutics. Genome Res. 2012;22(11):2089–100.

24. Sidhar SK, Clark J, Gill S, Hamoudi R, Crew AJ, Gwilliam R, Ross M, Linehan WM, Birdsall S, Shipley J, Cooper CS. The t(X;1)(p11.2;q21.2) translocation in papillary renal cell carcinoma fuses a novel gene PRCC to the TFE3 transcription factor gene. Hum Mol Genet. 1996;5(9):1333–8.

25. Ross H, Argani P. Xp11 translocation renal cell carcinoma. Pathology. 2010;42(4):369–73.

26. Tsuda M, Davis IJ, Argani P, Shukla N, McGill GG, Nagai M, Salto T, Lae M, Fisher DE, Ladanyi M. TFE3 fusions activate MET signaling by transcriptional up-regulation, defining another class of tumors as candidates for therapeutic MET inhibition. Cancer Res. 2007;67(3):919–29.

27. Parikh J, Coleman T, Messias N, Brown J. Temsirolimus in the treatment of renal cell carcinoma associated with Xp11.2 translocation/TFE gene fusion proteins: a case report and review of literature. Rare Tumors. 2009;1(2):164–6.

28. Argani P, Lal P, Hutchinson B, Reuter VE, Ladanyi M. Aberrant nuclear immunoreactivity for TFE3 in neoplasms with TFE3 gene fusions: a sensitive and specific immunohistochemical assay. Am J Surg Pathol. 2003;27(6):750–61.

29. Kim SH, Choi Y, Jeong HY, Lee K, Chae JY, Moon KC. Usefulness of a break-apart FISH assay in the diagnosis of Xp11.2 translocation renal cell carcinoma. Virchows Arch. 2011;459(3):299–306.

30. Boldog FL, Gemmill RM, Wilke CM, Glover TW, Nilsson AS, Chandrasekharappa SC, Brown RS, Li FP, Drabkin HA. Positional cloning of the hereditary renal carcinoma 3;8 chromosome translocation breakpoint. Proc Natl Acad Sci U S A. 1993;90(18): 8509–13.

31. Kuroda N, Mikami S, Pan CC, Cohen RJ, Hes O, Michal M, Nagashima Y, Tanaka Y, Inoue K, Shuin T, Lee GH. Review of renal carcinoma associated with Xp11.2 translocations/TFE3 gene fusions with focus on pathobiological aspect. Histol Histopathol. 2012;27(2):133–40.

32. Koo HJ, Choi HJ, Kim MH, Cho KS. Radiologic-pathologic correlation of renal cell carcinoma associated with Xp11.2 translocation. Acta Radiol. 2013; 54(7):827–34.

33. Liu K, Xie P, Peng W, Zhou Z. Renal carcinomas associated with Xp11.2 translocations/TFE3 gene fusions: findings on MRI and computed tomography imaging. J Magn Reson Imaging. 2014;40:440–7.

34. Prasad SR, Humphrey PA, Catena JR, Narra VR, Srigley JR, Cortez AD, Dalrymple NC, Chintapalli KN. Common and uncommon histologic subtypes of renal cell carcinoma: imaging spectrum with pathologic correlation. RadioGraphics. 2006;6(26):1795–806.

35. Klatte T, Streubel B, Wrba F, Remzi M, Krammer B, de Martino M, Waldert M, Marberger M, Susani M, Haitel A. Renal cell carcinoma associated with transcription factor E3 expression and Xp11.2 translocation. Am J Clin Pathol. 2012;137(5):761–8.

36. Jonasch E, Matin SF, Pagliaro LC, Wood CG, Tannir NM. Renal cell carcinoma. In: Kantarjian HM, Wolff RA, Koller CA, editors. The MD Anderson manual of medical oncology. 2nd ed. New York: McGraw-Hill; 2011.

37. Zhan HQ, Wang CF, Zhu XZ, Xu XL. Renal cell carcinoma with t(6;11) translocation: a patient case with a novel alpha-TFEB fusion point. J Clin Oncol. 2010;28(34):e709–13.

38. Rao Q, Liu B, Cheng L, Zhu Y, Shi QL, Wu B, Jiang SJ, Wang Y, Wang X, Yu B, Zhang RS, Ma HH, Lu ZF, Tu P, Wang JD, Zhou XJ. Renal cell carcinomas with t(6;11)(p21;q12): a clinicopathologic study emphasizing unusual morphology, novel alpha-TFEB gene fusion point, immunobiomarkers, and ultrastructural features, as well as detection of the gene fusion by fluorescence in sit hybridization. Am J Surg Pathol. 2012;36(9):1327–38.

39. Stolle C, Glenn G, Zbar B, Humphrey JS, Choyke P, Walther M, Pack S, Hurley K, Andrey C, Klausner R, Linehan WM. Improved detection of germline mutations in the von Hippel-Lindau disease tumor suppressor gene. Hum Mutat. 1998;12(6):417–23.

40. Kim WY, Kaelin WG. Role of VHL gene mutation in human cancer. J Clin Oncol. 2004;22(24):4991–5004.

41. Maher ER. Von Hippel-Lindau disease. Curr Mol Med. 2004;4(8):833–42.

42. Ritchey ML, Shamberger RC. Pediatric urologic oncology. In: Wein AJ, Kavoussi LR, Novick AC, Partin AW, Peters CA, editors. Campbell-Walsh urology. 10th ed. Philadelphia: Elsevier Saunders; 2012.

43. Laguna MP, Kümmerlin I, Rioja J, de la Rosette JJ. Biopsy of a renal mass: where are we now? Curr Opin Urol. 2009;19(5):447–53.

44. Aoyagi T, Shinohara N, Kubota-Chikai K, Kuroda N, Nonomura K. Long-term survival in a patient with node-positive adult-onset Xp11.2 translocation renal cell carcinoma. Urol Int. 2011;86(4):487–90.

45. Hung CC, Pan CC, Lin CC, Lin AT, Chen KK, Chang YH. Xp11.2 translocation renal cell carcinoma: clinical experience of Taipei Veterans General Hospital. J Chin Med Assoc. 2011;74(11):500–4.

46. Numakura K, Tsuchiya N, Yuasa T, Saito M, Obara T, Tsuruta H, Narita S, Horikawa Y, Satoh S, Habuchi T. A case study of metastatic Xp11.2 translocation renal cell carcinoma effectively treated with sunitinib. Int J Clin Oncol. 2011;16(5):577–80.

47. Malouf GG, Camparo P, Oudard S, Schleiermacher G, Theodore C, Rustine A, Dutcher J, Billemont B, Rixe O, Bompas E, Guillot A, Boccon-Gibod L, Couturier J, Molinie V, Escudler B. Targeted agents in metastatic Xp11 translocation/TFE3 gene fusion renal cell carcinoma (RCC): a report from the juvenile RCC network. Ann Oncol. 2010;21(9):1834–8.
48. Choueiri TK, Lim ZD, Hirsch MS, Tamboli P, Jonasch E, McDermott DF, Dal Cin P, Corn P, Vaishampayan U, Heng DY, Tannir NM. Vascular endothelial growth factor-targeted therapy for the treatment of adult metastatic Xp11.2 translocation renal cell carcinoma. Cancer. 2010;116(22):5219–25.
49. Dutcher AP. Recent developments in the treatment of renal cell carcinoma. Ther Adv Urol. 2013;5(6): 338–53.
50. Wagner AJ, Goldberg JM, Dubois SG, Choy E, Rosen L, Pappo A, Geller J, Judson I, Hogg D, Senzer N, Davis IJ, Chai F, Waghorne C, Schwartz B, Demetri GD. Tivantinib (ARQ 197), a selective inhibitor of MET, in patients with microphthalmia transcription factor-associated tumors: results of a multicenter phase 2 trial. Cancer. 2012;118(23):5894–902.
51. Kuiper RP, Schepens M, Thijssen J, van Asseldonk M, van den Berg E, Bridge J, Schuuring E, Schoenmakers EF, van Kessel AG. Upregulation of the transcription factor (TFEB) in t(6;11)(p21;q13)-positive renal carcinomas due to promoter substitutions. Hum Mol Genet. 2003;12(14):1661–9.
52. Argani P, Hawkins A, Griffin CA, Goldstein JD, Haas M, Beckwith JB, Mankinen CB, Perlman EJ. A distinctive pediatric renal neoplasm characterized by epithelioid morphology, basement membrane production, focal HMB45 immunoreactivity, and t(6;11) (p21.1;q12) chromosome translocation. Am J Pathol. 2001;158(6):2089–95.
53. Argani P, Lae M, Hutchinson B, Reuter VE, Collins MH, Perentesis J, Tomaszewski JE, Brooks JS, Acs JA, Vargas SO, Davis IJ, Fisher DE, Ladanyi M. Renal carcinomas with the t(6;11)(p21;q12): clinicopathologic features demonstration of the specific alpha-TEFB fusion gene by immunohistochemistry, RT-PCR, and DNA PCR. Am J Surg Pathol. 2005;29(2):230–40.
54. Pecciarini L, Cangi MG, Lo Cunsolo C, Macri E, Dal Cin E, Martignoni G, Doglioni C. Characterization of t(6;11)(p21;q12) in a renal-cell carcinoma of an adult patient. Genes Chromosomes Cancer. 2007;46(5): 419–26.
55. Camparo P, Vasiliu V, Molinie V, Couturier J, Dykema KJ, Petillo D, Furge KA, Comperat EM, Lae M, Bouvier R, Boccon-Gibod L, Denoux Y, Ferlicot S, Forest E, Fromont G, Hintzy MC, Laghouati M, Sibony M, Tucker ML, Weber N, Teh BT, Vieillefond A. Renal translocation carcinomas: clinicopathologic, immunohistochemical and gene expression profiling analysis of 31 cases with a review of the literature. Am J Surg Pathol. 2008;32(5):656–70.
56. Hora M, Hes O, Urge T, Eret V, Klecka J, Michal M. A distinctive translocation carcinoma of the kidney ["rosette-like forming", t(6;11), HMB45-positive renal tumor]. Int Urol Nephrol. 2009;41(3):553–7.
57. Suarez-Vilela D, Izquierdo-Garcia F, Mendez-Alvarez JR, Miguelez-Garcia E, Dominguez-Iglesias F. Renal translocation carcinoma expression of TFEB: presentation of a case with distinctive histological and immunohistochemical features. Int J Surg Pathol. 2009;19(4):506–9.
58. Srinivasan R, Linehan WM. Treatment of advanced renal cell carcinoma. In: Wein AJ, Kavoussi LR, Novick AC, Partin AW, Peters CA, editors. Campbell-Walsh urology. 10th ed. Philadelphia: Elsevier Saunders; 2012.
59. Kavolius JP, Mastorakos DP, Pavlovich C, Russo P, Burt ME, Brady MS. Resection of metastatic renal cell carcinoma. J Clin Oncol. 1998;16(6):2261–6.
60. Murthy SC, Kim K, Rice TW, Rajeswaran J, Bukowski R, DeCamp MM, Blackstone EH. Can we predict long-term survival after pulmonary metastasectomy for renal cell carcinoma? Ann Thorac Surg. 2005;79(3):996–1003.
61. Chin AI, Lam JS, Figlin RA, Belldegrun AS. Surveillance strategies for renal cell carcinoma patients following nephrectomy. Rev Urol. 2006;8(1):1–7.
62. Klaassen Z, Tatem A, Burnette JO, Donohoe JM, Terris MK. Adult Xp11 translocation associated renal cell carcinoma: time to recognize. Urology. 2012;80(5):965–8.
63. Motzer RJ, Jonasch E, Agarwal N, Beard C, Bhayani S, Bolger GB, Chang SS, Choueiri TK, Derweesh IH, Gupta S, Hancock SL, Kim JJ, Kuzel TM, Lam ET, Lau C, Levine EG, Lin DW, Margolin KA, Michaelson MD, Olencki T, Pili R, Plimack ER, Rampersaud EN, Redman BG, Ryan CJ, Sheinfeld J, Sircar K, Somer B, Wang J, Wilder RB, Dwyer MA, Kumar R. Kidney cancer, version 2.2014. J Natl Compr Canc Netw. 2014;12(2):175–82.

# Collecting Duct Carcinoma and Renal Medullary Carcinoma

Jamie Koo, Christopher P. Filson, Jiaoti Huang, and Allan J. Pantuck

## Introduction

Collecting duct carcinoma (CDC), also called "carcinoma of collecting ducts of Bellini," is a rare renal epithelial malignancy first described in 1949 and later recognized as a distinct subtype of renal cell carcinoma (RCC) in 1986. Renal medullary carcinoma (RMC) was initially described in 1995 as a rare and unique renal malignancy occurring in a distinct population of patients, specifically in young African American patients with sickle cell hemoglobinopathy, thus prompting the authors to call it the "seventh sickle cell nephropathy" [1]. These two tumors are similar in that both are rare and aggressive neoplasms that are thought to arise from the distal segment of the collecting ducts in the renal medullary pyramids, yet some distinct clinical and pathologic features can aid in distinguishing these two entities.

## Epidemiology, Clinical Features, and Radiographic Features of Collecting Duct and Renal Medullary Carcinoma

### Epidemiology and Clinical Features

CDC accounts for <1 % of renal malignancies [2] and occurs in patients with a median age of 63 years (range 53–72.5), with a male predominance of about 2:1, and more frequently in Caucasians (71 %) than in African Americans (23 %) based on recent analysis of the Surveillance, Epidemiology, and End Results (SEER) database [3]. Over 50 % of patients are symptomatic at presentation with gross hematuria, abdominal/back pain, or general malaise [4, 5]. Patients with CDC generally present at higher stage than patients with clear cell RCC, as evidenced by a higher rate of locally advanced (T3–T4) disease (33 % vs. 18 %, respectively), nodal involvement (15 % vs. 2 %, respectively), and distant metastasis (28 % vs. 17 %, respectively) [6]. One and 3-year disease-specific survival rates for CDC are 70 % and 58 %, respectively, which is significantly worse when compared to patients with clear cell RCC [6].

J. Koo, M.D. • J. Huang, M.D., Ph.D.
Department of Pathology and Laboratory Medicine, David Geffen School of Medicine at UCLA, 10833 Le Conte Ave, 13-229 CHS, Los Angeles, CA 90095, USA
e-mail: jakoo@mednet.ucla.edu; jiaotihuang@mednet.ucla.edu

C.P. Filson, M.D., M.S.
A.J. Pantuck, M.D., M.S. (✉)
Department of Urology, Institute of Urologic Oncology, David Geffen School of Medicine at UCLA, 924 Westwood Blvd., Suite 1050, Los Angeles, CA 90024, USA
e-mail: cfilson@mednet.ucla.edu; apantuck@mednet.ucla.edu

© Springer Science+Business Media New York 2016
D.E. Hansel et al. (eds.), *The Kidney*, DOI 10.1007/978-1-4939-3286-3_8

RMC is a rare tumor with less than 200 cases reported in the literature since its original description in 1995 by Davis [1]. The mean age at diagnosis is 19 years (range 5–69) with a male predominance of about 2:1. The overwhelming majority of patients are African American, with few cases occurring in Caucasian, Hispanic, and Asian Indian patients [5, 7]. Almost all patients have a sickle cell hemoglobinopathy, most commonly sickle cell trait and less commonly SC disease or sickle cell disease (SS disease), with only very rare cases reported in Caucasian patients without hemoglobinopathy [5, 8]. Most patients present with symptoms such as hematuria, flank pain, and weight loss and have evidence of metastatic disease at presentation, which can involve lymph nodes, lungs, liver, bones, or adrenal glands [5, 9]. Median cancer-specific survival for RMC is reported to be about 5 months (Fig. 8.1) [3, 5].

When patient and tumor characteristics between CDC and RMC are compared, RMC patients are significantly younger, more often African American, and more likely to have lymph node involvement and distant metastatic disease at presentation, and median cancer-specific survival is significantly shorter [3]. Distinguishing clinical features in CDC and RMC are summarized in Table 8.1.

## Radiographic Features

The usual CT findings of CDC are of a solid renal mass located in the medulla with involvement of the renal sinus, infiltrative growth, preserved renal contour, and a cystic component [10]. Weak and heterogeneous enhancement due to areas of necrosis, hemorrhage, and calcification can be seen [11]. RMC is also characterized by an infiltrative, medullary-based solid renal mass with heterogeneity due to areas of hemorrhage and necrosis, and caliectasis is often present [11, 12]. Regional lymphadenopathy and metastasis are frequently seen in both CDC and RMC at initial diagnosis. These findings are nonspecific and do not allow for differentiation from more common types of RCC by imaging.

## Pathologic Characteristics of Collecting Duct and Renal Medullary Carcinoma

## Collecting Duct Carcinoma

### Gross Pathology

On gross examination, CDCs are white to grey, firm, multinodular tumors with infiltrative borders and focal areas of tumor necrosis (Fig. 8.2), but without significant areas of hemorrhage, making them grossly distinct from the more usual types of RCCs. When small, the tumors appear centered in the renal medulla; however, this may be difficult to appreciate in larger tumors, which can extend into the renal cortex, renal pelvis, perinephric fat, or renal hilum [7, 13]. Tumors average about 6 cm in diameter and can range from 1 to 15 cm [4].

### Microscopic Pathology

Histologically, CDC is essentially a high-grade poorly differentiated adenocarcinoma and most commonly shows tubules or tubulopapillary structures with irregular, angulated glands infiltrating the renal parenchyma (Fig. 8.3). However, other architectural patterns may be admixed in varying proportions, including solid cords, sheets, papillary formations with fibrovascular cores, a "hobnail" pattern, cystically dilated spaces, and cribriform histology [13]. At higher power, tumor cells have moderate to abundant eosinophilic cytoplasm with large hyperchromatic, pleomorphic nuclei and prominent nucleoli (Fig. 8.4) [2, 13]. As in other types of RCC, sarcomatoid differentiation and rhabdoid change can be seen (Fig. 8.5). Mitotic figures are frequently present. Both intraluminal and intracytoplasmic mucin may be seen, which can be highlighted with mucicarmine or Alcian blue stains. An additional characteristic feature of CDC is the presence of a pronounced desmoplastic stromal reaction, which can range in appearance from loose, myxoid, and collagenous to dense, eosinophilic, and fibrosclerotic. Associated inflammatory infiltrates, which are predominantly lymphocytic but occasionally mixed, are seen within the areas of desmoplasia (Fig. 8.6)

**Fig. 8.1** Cancer-specific survival among patients diagnosed with CDC or RMC as reported by Abern et al. The *x*-axis represents the proportion of patients surviving and the *y*-axis represents time in months. Patients with RMC had nearly three times the hazard of dying compared to CDC patients [3]. *CSS* cancer-specific survival (permission granted by Elsevier. Abern et al. [3])

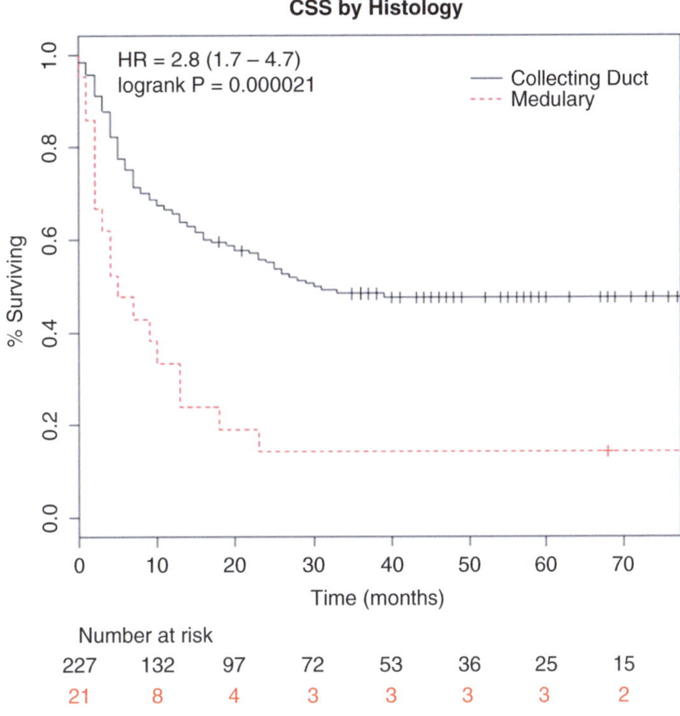


**Table 8.1** Distinguishing clinical features in collecting duct carcinoma versus renal medullary carcinoma

| Feature | Collecting duct carcinoma | Renal medullary carcinoma |
|---|---|---|
| Average age | 63 years | 19 years |
| Race | | |
|   Caucasian | 71 % | 5 % |
|   African American | 23 % | 90 % |
| Association with sickle cell hemoglobinopathy | No | Yes |
| Metastatic at presentation | 28 % | 71 % |
| Median survival | 30 months | 5 months |

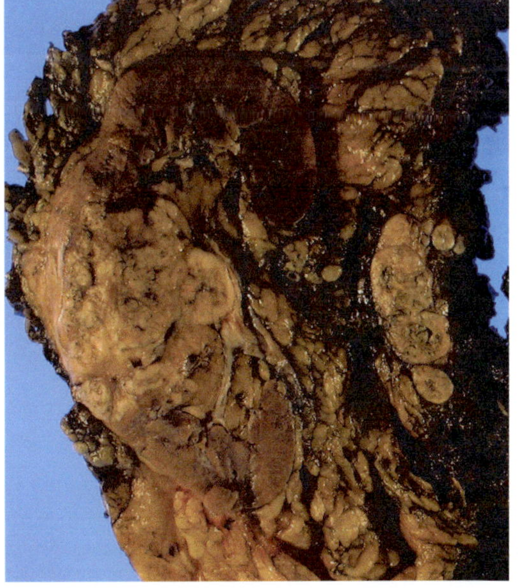

**Fig. 8.2** Grossly, collecting duct carcinomas are firm, white-grey tumors with ill-defined, infiltrative borders, often with multinodularity. Note the separate tumor nodules in the hilar fat

[13]. Areas of geographic tumor necrosis and microscopic angiolymphatic invasion are also frequently present.

Dysplasia of the adjacent renal tubular epithelium is another feature of CDC that can be helpful in making the diagnosis (Fig. 8.7), but can also occasionally be seen in urothelial carcinomas of the renal pelvis and in renal tubules adja-

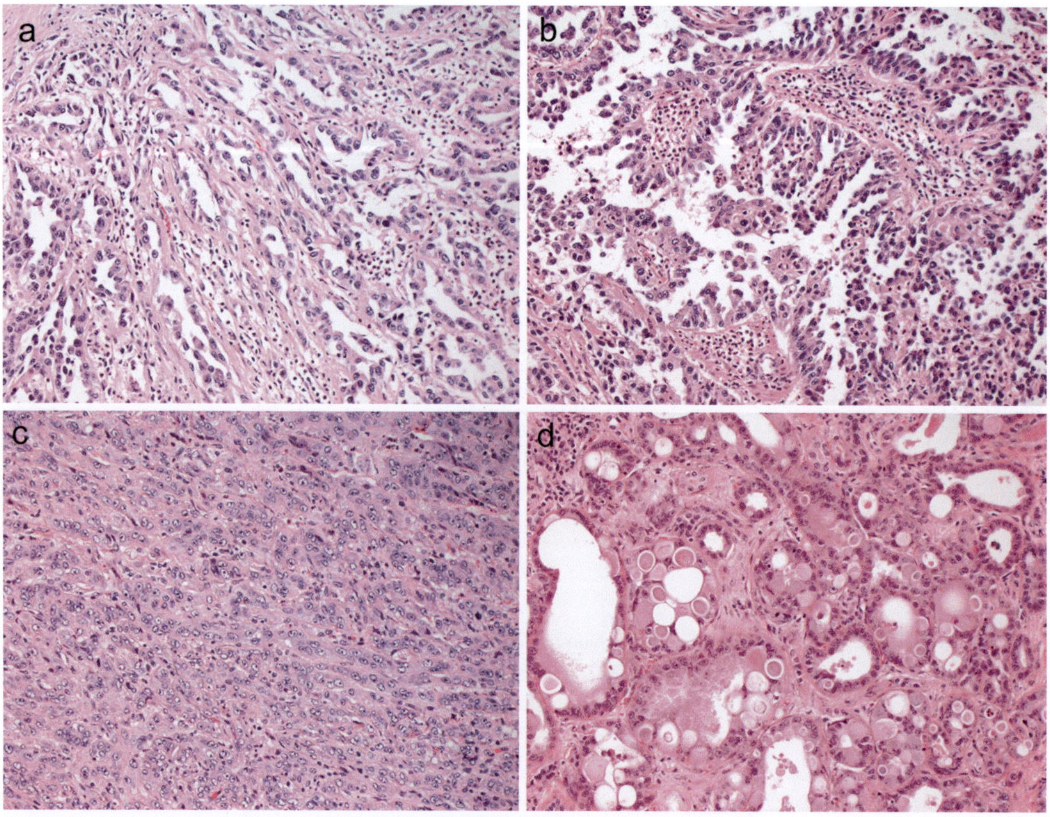

**Fig. 8.3** Histologically, collecting duct carcinomas commonly show tubular (**a**) or tubulopapillary architecture with other admixed patterns, including papillary with true fibrovascular cores (**b**), solid cords and sheets (**c**), and cribriform (**d**)

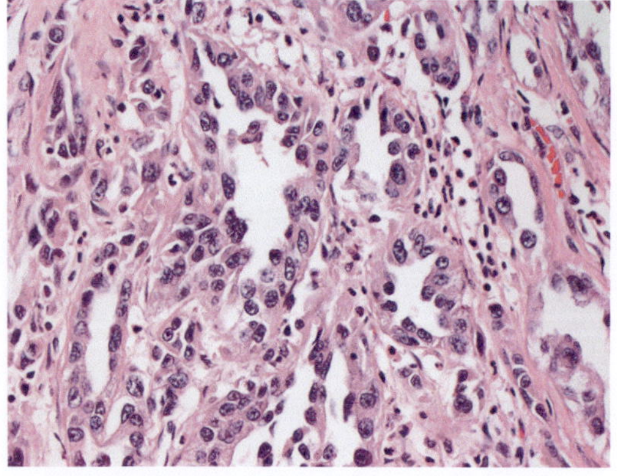

**Fig. 8.4** High-grade cytologic features in collecting duct carcinoma, including high nuclear to cytoplasmic ratio, nuclear enlargement and irregularity, pleomorphism, and prominent nucleoli

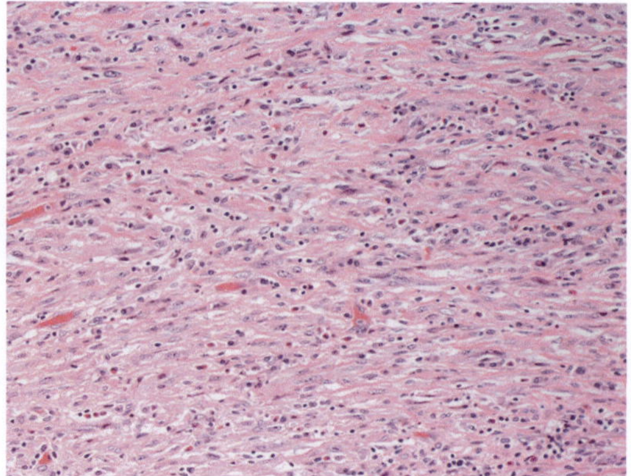

**Fig. 8.5** Sarcomatoid differentiation as evidenced by high-grade, malignant spindle cells can also be seen in collecting duct carcinoma

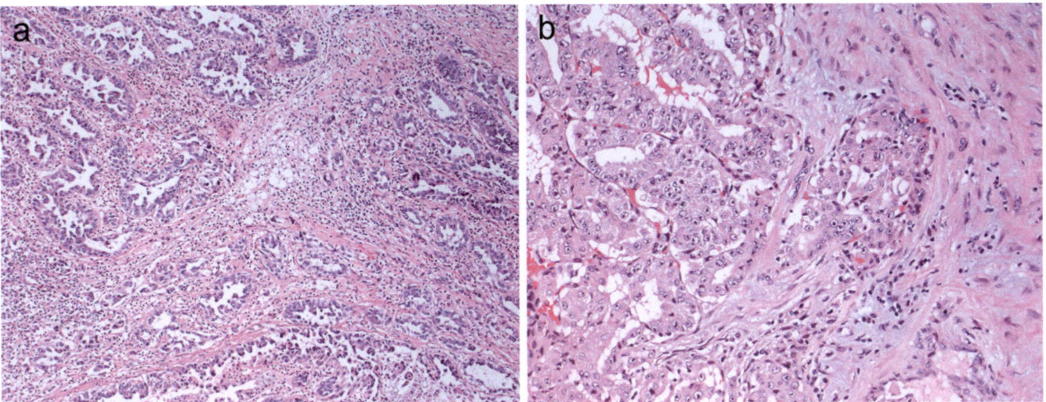

**Fig. 8.6** Pronounced desmoplastic stromal response in collecting duct carcinoma, which can be dense and fibrosclerotic (**a**) to myxoid (**b**). Associated lymphocytic inflammatory infiltrates are also present

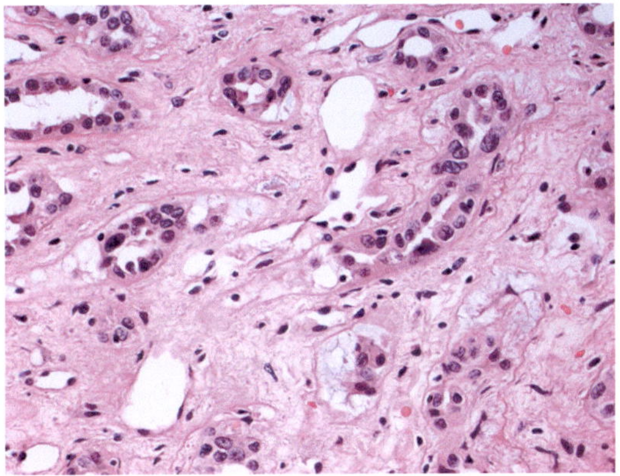

**Fig. 8.7** Dysplastic tubules in areas adjacent to a collecting duct carcinoma can be a helpful diagnostic feature

cent to other types of RCC [7, 14]. Other more typical RCC patterns, urothelial carcinoma, or urothelial carcinoma in situ of the renal pelvis should not be present and would exclude the diagnosis of CDC [7].

Recently, the International Society of Urological Pathology (ISUP) has recommended the following histologic criteria for the diagnosis of CDC: (1) at least some of the lesion involves the medullary region; (2) there is a predominant formation of tubules; (3) a desmoplastic stromal reaction should be present; (4) cytologic features are high grade; (5) growth pattern is infiltrative; and (6) there is an absence of other typical RCC subtypes or urothelial carcinoma [15]. Because CDCs are by definition high-grade tumors, it has also been recommended that CDCs should not be assigned a grade (i.e., Fuhrman grade).

## Immunohistochemistry

The immunohistochemical profile of CDC is reflective of the tumor's origin from the cells of the collecting ducts in the renal medulla. Tumors are usually positive with lectins such as *Ulex europaeus* agglutinin-1 (UEA1) and peanut lectin. CDCs are also generally positive for low molecular weight cytokeratin (LMWCK), epithelial membrane antigen (EMA), PAX8, c-KIT/CD117, and vimentin, and a smaller number are positive for high molecular weight cytokeratin (HMWCK), CK7, CK20, and PAX2 [13, 16, 17]. In contrast, markers typically positive in proximal renal tubules such as CD10, alpha-methylacyl-CoA racemase (AMACR), and RCC antigen are negative [18], as is p63, a commonly used marker of urothelial differentiation [17].

In contrast to RMCs, which show complete loss of staining for INI1 by immunohistochemistry (discussed below), only 15 % (3 of 20 cases) of CDC showed complete loss of INI1 staining in one study, and only 5 % (1 of 22 cases) in another study [19, 20]. Loss of INI1 staining in CDC does not portend a worse clinical outcome [19].

## Cytogenetic and Molecular Findings

There are only limited data on the cytogenetic abnormalities seen in CDC, with no consistent genetic abnormality being identified to date. By conventional cytogenetics, CDCs show complex karyotypes with numerical and structural abnormalities involving multiple chromosomes [21–24]. More common abnormalities include loss of chromosomes 1, 13, 14, and 22. Loss of heterozygosity of 1q, 6p, 8p, 13q, and 21q by microsatellite analysis has also been reported in CDC [25, 26], while the characteristic loss of chromosome 3p commonly seen in clear cell RCC is not seen in CDC. Her2neu amplification was seen in about 50 % of CDC in a small series of cases [27].

## Differential Diagnosis

The histologic differential diagnosis of CDC includes invasive urothelial carcinoma, papillary RCC, metastatic adenocarcinoma, unclassified RCC, and renal medullary carcinoma (summarized in Tables 8.2 and 8.3).

Urothelial carcinoma involving the renal pelvis can be challenging to differentiate from CDC, especially if glandular differentiation and invasion of the renal parenchyma with desmoplasia are present. Identification of an associated urothelial papillary surface component, urothelial carcinoma in situ (CIS), squamous differentiation, or a predominance of other more typical patterns of urothelial carcinoma such as nested growth would essentially exclude the diagnosis of CDC [13, 18]. Immunohistochemistry can be helpful in this distinction, with PAX8 positivity seen in virtually all CDCs and only in 9 % of upper tract urothelial carcinomas [17]. Additionally, p63 positivity is seen in almost all upper tract urothelial carcinomas and in 14 % of CDCs. Further, when these two markers are interpreted together, the PAX8+/p63− profile gives a 100 % positive predictive value for CDC, and the PAX8−/p63+ profile gives a 100 % positive predictive value for urothelial carcinoma [17]. It should be noted that CK20 can be positive in a small number of CDC [13] and UEA1 is positive in both CDC and urothelial carcinoma [16]. Distinguishing between these two tumors has significant clinical implications, since CDC generally has an unfavorable prognosis, and patients with urothelial carcinoma generally require further evaluation of their urinary tract for additional urothelial lesions.

Papillary RCC may mimic CDC because of its predominant papillary or tubulopapillary architecture, especially if it is of high grade (papillary RCC, type 2). However, papillary RCCs are usually well circumscribed and encapsulated, in contrast to CDCs, which are grossly and histologically infiltrative. Papillary RCC also does not exhibit the desmoplastic stroma and angulated tubules of CDC. Immunohistochemistry can also distinguish between these two entities, as papillary RCC is usually positive for CD10, RCC antigen, and AMACR, while CDC is usually negative for these markers.

Metastatic adenocarcinoma, most commonly of colorectal or lung origin, is an important consideration in the differential diagnosis of CDC, as it also displays a marked desmoplastic stromal reaction. Generally, metastatic lesions tend to be multifocal, small, and relatively circumscribed. A previous history of malignancy would obviously be helpful in this distinction and could guide the selection of lineage-specific immunohistochemical markers such as TTF-1 and CDX2 to prove the metastatic nature of these lesions.

If a tumor of renal origin with infiltrative growth and desmoplasia is proven not to be urothelial or metastatic carcinoma and shows an absence of angulated glands with high-grade nuclear cytologic features, the diagnosis of unclassified RCC should be made [13]. Generally, these high-grade unclassified carcinomas are predominated by sheetlike, nested, and solid patterns. However, if there is any component of the tumor that meets the ISUP criteria for CDC (see above), it is recommended that the diagnosis should be "poorly differentiated CDC" and not "unclassified RCC" [15].

Renal medullary carcinoma shows overlapping histologic features with CDC and is considered by some to represent an especially aggressive variant of CDC [7]. However, there are subtle features that can help differentiate between the two (summarized in Table 8.3; also see below for detailed description of RMC). First, CDC typically shows angulated tubules, glands, and tubulopapillary structures, while RMC commonly demonstrates a reticular pattern composed of anastomosing tubules and cords with irregular microcystic spaces. Both

**Table 8.2** Features helpful in distinguishing collecting duct carcinoma from other entities in the differential diagnosis

| Feature | Collecting duct carcinoma | Urothelial carcinoma | Papillary renal cell carcinoma | Metastatic carcinoma |
|---|---|---|---|---|
| Circumscription/encapsulation | No | No | Often both | Often circumscribed |
| Focality | Unifocal | Unifocal | Unifocal | Multifocal |
| Multinodularity | Often | Sometimes | No | No |
| Desmoplastic stroma | Yes, prominent | Yes | No | Yes |
| Other | Associated lymphocytic inflammation | Associated papillary lesion, urothelial CIS | Sometimes foam cells in papillary cores | Clinical history of other malignancies |
| Immunohistochemistry | | | | |
| Positive | PAX8, UEA1 | p63, UEA1, CK20 | PAX8, CD10, RCC, AMACR | Possibly other lineage markers (e.g., TTF1, CDX2) |
| Negative | p63, CK20 (rare +), CD10, RCC, AMACR | PAX8 | UEA1 | PAX8, RCC |

**Table 8.3** Distinguishing histologic features in collecting duct carcinoma versus renal medullary carcinoma

| Feature | Collecting duct carcinoma | Renal medullary carcinoma |
|---|---|---|
| Dominant histologic pattern | Tubular, tubulopapillary architecture with angulated glands | Reticular composed of tubules, cords, and microcysts; irregular cribriform structures |
| Inflammatory infiltrate | Predominantly lymphocytic to mixed | Predominantly neutrophilic to mixed |
| Necrosis | Coagulative, geographic | Microabscess-like foci |
| Sickled red blood cells in tissue | No | Yes |

tumors show desmoplastic stroma with associated inflammatory infiltrates, but the inflammatory infiltrates in CDC are predominantly lymphocytic, in contrast to the neutrophilic to polymorphous infiltrates seen in RMC [13]. Additionally, CDC often shows areas of coagulative necrosis, while RMC will occasionally show distinctive microabscess-like areas of suppurative necrosis. Importantly, RMC clinically affects younger patients with sickle cell hemoglobinopathy who are commonly African American. Immunohistochemistry appears to have a limited role in distinguishing these two tumors since both are consistently positive for vimentin and UEA1 and variably positive for HMWCK, CK7, and PAX2 [13]. RMC consistently shows complete loss of immunohistochemical staining with INI1, but since a minority of CDC also shows this pattern of staining, it appears that INI1 immunohistochemistry cannot reliably distinguish these two tumors [15].

## Renal Medullary Carcinoma

### Gross Pathology

RMC shows a similar gross appearance to CDC, as these tumors are also white-grey to tan, firm to rubbery, poorly circumscribed with infiltrative borders, and centered in the renal medulla with variable hemorrhage and necrosis. There are often satellite nodules in the adjacent renal parenchyma corresponding to areas of lymphovascular invasion in large caliber vessels, as well as diffuse infiltration into the renal parenchyma, perinephric fat, or renal hilum [1, 7]. Tumors average 7 cm in diameter and can range from 4 to 18 cm [1, 28, 29]. Interestingly, RMC occurs more commonly in the right kidney (>75 %), but the reason for this is unclear [1, 18].

### Microscopic Pathology

The most distinct and consistent histologic growth pattern seen in RMC is a reticular pattern formed by anastomosing tubules and cords with irregular microcytic spaces, imparting a resemblance to testicular yolk sac tumor (Fig. 8.8) [1, 13]. Often there is an admixture of architectural growth patterns including infiltrating cords, solid sheets, trabeculae, cribriform structures, and papillary with true fibrovascular cores [13]. Compact cribriform structures with rigid round spaces simulating adenoid cystic carcinoma can also be present. Tumor cells have moderate to abundant eosinophilic cytoplasm and high-grade nuclear features with prominent nucleoli. Areas demonstrating rhabdoid and sarcomatoid features may be present focally. Intracytoplasmic or intraluminal mucin is seen in a majority of cases.

A prominent desmoplastic stromal reaction is also a characteristic and tends to have a myxoid, edematous, hypocellular, loose, basophilic appearance. Focal areas with dense, eosinophilic, collagenous desmoplastic stroma are usually also appreciated. The associated inflammatory infiltrate can be quite striking and ranges from predominantly neutrophilic to polymorphous, including a mixture of neutrophils, lymphocytes, and eosinophils [7, 13]. Geographic and microabscess-like areas of necrosis can be seen.

As RMC almost invariably occurs in patients with sickle cell hemoglobinopathy, most commonly sickle cell trait, sickled red blood cells are frequently seen, both in the main tumor and within capillaries in the adjacent renal parenchyma (Fig. 8.9). In addition, the red blood cells may appear clustered or agglutinated within capillaries [14].

## Immunohistochemistry

By immunohistochemistry, RMC is consistently positive for cytokeratin AE1/AE3, LMWCK, EMA, vimentin, cytokeratin 7, CEA, and PAX8 [9, 13, 28–31]. Tumors also show variable positivity with HMWCK, cytokeratin 20, UEA-1, OCT3/4, and PAX2.

Complete loss of INI1/SMARCB1 expression in RMC by immunohistochemistry was first reported in 5 cases by Cheng et al. and has now been confirmed in 13 additional cases of RMC [20, 30] (details and significance discussed below). In RMC, INI1 is completely negative in tumor cells, while moderate to strong staining is present in inflammatory, stromal, and adjacent nonneoplastic collecting duct epithelial cells. Although this pattern of INI1 staining is not necessarily associated with rhabdoid cytologic features in RMC, most urothelial carcinomas and RCC are positive for immunohistochemical expression for INI1 even when rhabdoid features are present [31]. As mentioned above, a minority of CDC cases also show complete loss of INI1 expression. Thus, INI1 immunohistochemistry can be useful in distinguishing RMC from urothelial carcinomas and other RCCs, but is of more limited value in distinguishing RMC from CDC [15].

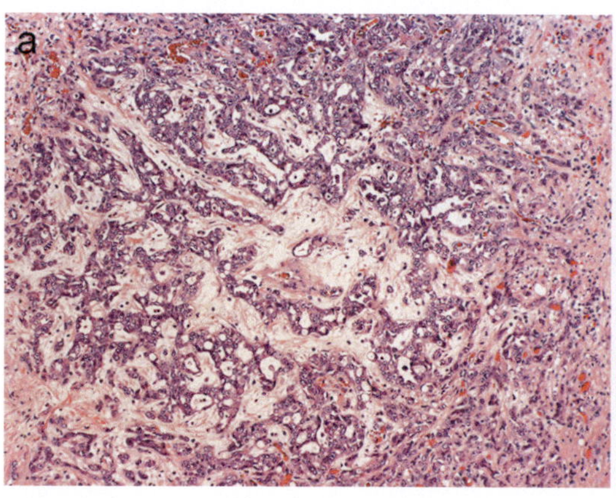
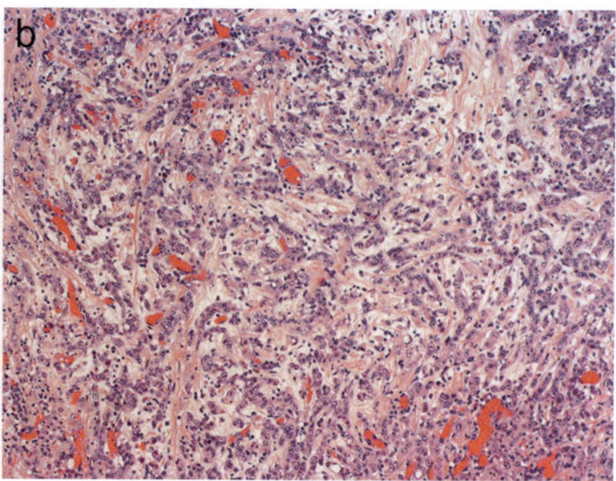
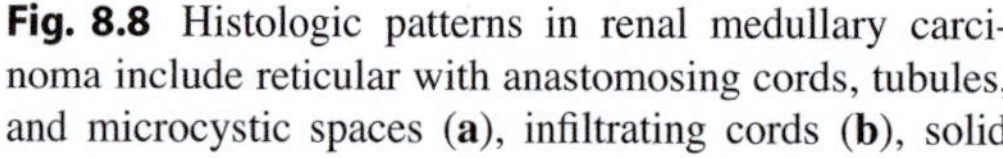

**Fig. 8.8** Histologic patterns in renal medullary carcinoma include reticular with anastomosing cords, tubules, and microcystic spaces (**a**), infiltrating cords (**b**), solid nests, and cribriform. Note associated hypocellular, hyalinized desmoplastic stroma (photos provided by Dr. Liang Cheng, Indiana University)

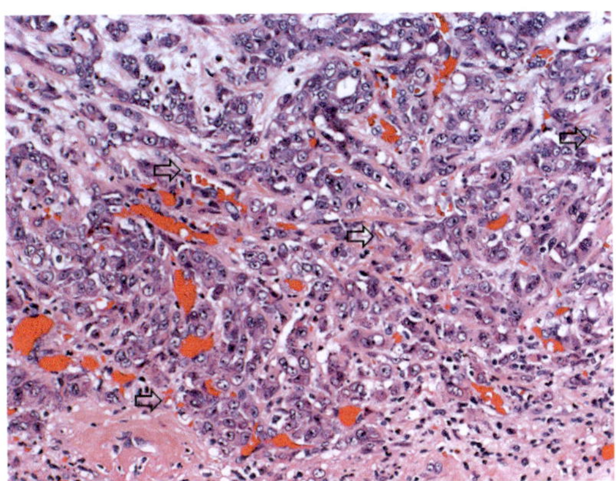

**Fig. 8.9** Sickled red blood cells (*arrows*) are seen in capillaries of renal medullary carcinoma, as well as clusters of agglutinated red blood cells (photo provided by Dr. Liang Cheng, Indiana University)

## Cytogenetic and Molecular Findings

A small number of RMCs have been studied by conventional cytogenetics, which have generally shown complex karyotypes with a variety of insertions, deletions, and/or balanced translocations, but no recurrent genetic abnormalities have been identified [8]. Of note, one case showed the presence of a t(9;22) bcr-abl translocation, which was confirmed by fluorescence in situ hybridization (FISH) [32], and a subsequent study demonstrated *ABL* amplification in three tumors by FISH, but no bcr-abl translocation [5]. Comparative genomic hybridization analysis has shown an overall lack of genetic gains and losses in RMC, with only one case demonstrating loss of chromosome 22 [29].

Based on the results of immunohistochemistry studies, it has been suggested that TP53, hypoxia inducible factor (HIF), and vascular endothelial growth factor (VEGF) may play a role in the pathogenesis of RMC [29]. Molecular analysis of two RMC cases occurring in Caucasian patients without hemoglobinopathy has shown mutations in *fumarate hydratase* and *von Hippel-Lindau* (*VHL*) genes [8]. These findings suggest that a common underlying hypoxic cellular environment, either due to sickle cell trait/disease or mutations affecting hypoxia-sensing pathways, may subsequently lead to activation of HIF pathways and contribute to the development of RMC.

Two small studies have demonstrated that topoisomerase II alpha (TopoII), a nuclear enzyme involved in cell cycle progression and DNA repair, is overexpressed in RMC based on immunohistochemistry and whole-genome microarray analysis [33, 34]. However, there was no evidence of TopoII gene amplification by FISH, suggesting that some other mechanisms such as transcriptional or posttranslational modification are responsible for this overexpression [34].

Most recently, absence of INI1 (known also as SMARCB1) expression has been reported in all tested cases of RMC. *INI1* is a tumor suppressor gene located on 22q11.23 that encodes a component of the SWI/SNF complex, which regulates transcription of target genes in an ATP-dependent manner. Loss of INI1 expression is seen in tumors with rhabdoid histology, such as pediatric renal and extrarenal malignant rhabdoid tumors and atypical teratoid/rhabdoid tumors of the central nervous system, and is now also reported in RMC. In addition to complete absence of INI1 expression by immunohistochemistry (described above), hemizygous *INI1* gene deletions detected by comparative genomic hybridization [20] and loss of heterozygosity of INI1 with polymerase chain reaction-based microsatellite analysis [30] have been documented in RMC, suggesting that inactivation of the *INI1* gene may have an important role in RMC pathogenesis. Interestingly, the presence or absence of rhabdoid histology in RMC does not appear to influence the pattern of INI1 staining, as both areas with rhabdoid and non-rhabdoid histology are negative for INI1 [31].

## Differential Diagnosis

The histologic differential diagnosis for RMC includes invasive urothelial carcinoma and CDC. Since RMC is known to occur in a specific patient population (young African American patients with sickle cell trait), clinical information such as age, race, and hemoglobinopathy status are invaluable; sickle cell trait is not known to be associated with either urothelial carcinoma or CDC. In the absence of relevant clinical information, identification of some histologic features may distinguish RMC from other entities. As discussed previously, findings that would support the diagnosis of urothelial carcinoma include identification of a papillary urothelial lesion involving the renal pelvis, urothelial CIS, or other more conventional growth patterns of urothelial carcinoma. The differential between RMC and CDC is discussed above and summarized in Table 8.3.

# Clinical Management of Patients with Collecting Duct and Renal Medullary Carcinoma

Due the relative rarity of CDC and RMC, most of the data related to treatment are limited to small case series and case reports. Furthermore, most series are retrospective in nature, and strong conclusions related to survival associated with various treatments are limited by selection bias. In the next section, we will review the treatment options for patients with tumors having these two histology types.

## Collecting Duct Carcinoma

### Surgical Management

As described above, CDC typically presents in an advanced stage, with nodal involvement and metastatic spread present at the time of diagnosis. Nevertheless, most patients with CDC undergo surgical excision of the primary tumor (either by radical or partial nephrectomy) [3, 6, 35, 36]. In rare cases when a CDC is localized to the kidney, radical nephrectomy alone may result in cure [37]. Also, individual case reports indicate that CDC patients with localized T1 tumors can be treated with partial nephrectomy and have a prolonged cancer-specific and overall survival [38–40]. However, compared to clear cell RCC, patients with more advanced, locoregional CDC (i.e., T3a or better) treated with surgery still have over twice the risk of cancer-specific mortality [3].

There is also a paucity of data regarding performance of lymphadenectomy at the time of nephrectomy for patients with CDC. For patients with clear cell RCC, a randomized trial did not show a survival benefit associated with performance of extended lymphadenectomy [41]. Although a recent study using SEER registry data suggested a survival benefit associated with more extensive lymphadenectomy for node-positive kidney cancer patients [42], others have raised concerns that these results suffer from biases related to imputation of missing data [43]. In general, excision of enlarged lymph nodes (on radiographic imaging) would be recommended, with the decision to perform a more extended dissection left to the discretion of the surgeon.

As many patients with collecting duct carcinoma present with metastatic disease, it would be helpful to know whether cytoreductive nephrectomy (i.e., radical nephrectomy in the setting of metastases) would be beneficial for patients with CDC. Unfortunately, the data remain mixed and limited to small case series. One large retrospective series found the patients with metastatic CDC had longer cancer-specific survival when treated with cytoreductive radical nephrectomy, compared to those patients not undergoing radical nephrectomy (with or without retroperitoneal lymphadenectomy) [3]. This series suffers from possible surgical selection bias. In general, among patients with metastatic RCC and tumors amenable to nephron sparing surgery, SEER registry data suggests a survival advantage associated with treatment with partial nephrectomy [44]. However, again as with any retrospective study, these results are subject to selection bias and only included 19 patients with CDC [44]. On the other hand, at a population level, surgical removal of the primary tumor had no effect on survival among patients with metastatic CDC [6]. In addition, another series demonstrated extremely poor prognosis among five patients with metastatic CDC treated with radical nephrectomy, with 60 % of the patients experiencing death in the immediate postoperative period [45].

## Systemic Therapy
### Cytotoxic Chemotherapy

Metastatic CDC is typically resistant to systemic cytotoxic chemotherapy. The largest series of Japanese CDC patients showed that among 17 patients who received chemotherapy, only one patient showed a partial response to gemcitabine and carboplatin [4]. Motzer et al. reported one partial response to gemcitabine and cisplatin among 30 patients receiving systemic chemotherapy or novel agents on a clinical trial [35]. In 2007, results from a phase II trial assessing use of gemcitabine plus a platinum-based agent (carboplatin or cisplatin) were published; they reported a 26 % response rate with a median progression-free survival of 7.1 months [46]. A number of case reports exist that describe responses to other cytotoxic agents, including salvage paclitaxel [47] or combination of paclitaxel and carboplatin [48].

## Immunotherapy

Based on evidence from clinical trials, interleukin-2 (IL-2) [49] and interferon-alpha (IFN-α) [50] can have a role in metastatic clear cell RCC. However, the activity of these agents in treating metastatic CDC has not been studied extensively. In the series reported by Motzer et al., none of the 15 patients with CDC who were treated with cytokine therapy had a clinical response [35]. Furthermore, none of the 34 CDC patients in the large Japanese series had a clinical response to either IFN-α or IL-2 treatments [4]. Evidence of clinical efficacy of cytokine therapy for this disease is limited to a solitary case report of a CDC patient responding to IL-2 therapy [51].

## Targeted Therapy

After phase III trials confirmed their efficacy in improving progression-free survival, a number of "targeted therapies" have been approved for the treatment of metastatic clear cell RCC, including sunitinib [52], sorafenib [53], temsirolimus [54], everolimus [55], and pazopanib [56]. However, the use of these therapies has been limited to subgroups in phase II trials or individual case reports. Within a phase II trial looking at the efficacy of sunitinib among advanced non-clear cell RCC patients, there were six patients with CDC. None of these patients had an objective response to sunitinib therapy and the median progression-free survival was just over 3 months [57]. A case series of two CDC patients who had progression after surgery and gemcitabine/cisplatin chemotherapy reported no objective response to additional sunitinib therapy [58]. However, there is one case report describing a partial response to sunitinib therapy in a CDC patient with lung and skeletal metastases [59]. Ansari et al. reported a single case of a partial response to sorafenib therapy for a patient with metastatic CDC with a durable 13-month progression-free survival [60]. Among metastatic RCC patients treated with everolimus, two patients with CDC did not exhibit a response with treatment [61]. Another case series of seven patients with metastatic CDC showed that two patients were able to have stable disease with either sequential sorafenib followed by sunitinib (for 49 months) or temsirolimus followed by sunitinib (for 19 months) [62]. Another case series did not observe any radiographic treatment response among four CDC patients treated with mTOR inhibitors [63]. Overall the quantity and quality of data limit any overall conclusion in regard to the effectiveness of any systemic therapy for this subtype.

## Renal MedullaryCarcinoma

As with CDC, patients with RMC harbor an abysmal prognosis in general. Furthermore, the rarity of the disease makes it difficult to assess optimal treatment for patients with this malignancy. The two largest case series include nine patients treated in the United States, reported by Hakimi et al. [64], and seven patients treated in Brazil, described by Watanabe et al. [9]. Seven and four patients in each series underwent radical nephrectomy. Another multicenter series reported outcomes from six patients in the United States; five of six patients were treated with radical nephrectomy and overall survival ranged from 1 to 7 months [65].

A number of chemotherapy regimens have been reported in the literature, with typically poor responses. The longest reported survival after diagnosis was 24 months; this was seen in an 11-year-old who had a complete response with carboplatin, gemcitabine, and paclitaxel [66]. Another series described the use of high-dose-intensity methotrexate-vinblastine-doxorubicin-cisplatin (MVAC) in three patients, where all three patients had partial responses and overall survival ranged from 3.5 to 16 months [67]. Outcomes from selected case reports and series are summarized in Table 8.4.

**Table 8.4** Select case reports and series of patients with medullary renal carcinoma

| Patient | Treatment received | Chemotherapy regimen | Objective response | Survival (months) | Reference |
|---|---|---|---|---|---|
| 13 y/o F | Chemotherapy | 5-FU | No | 1 | [68] |
| 23 y/o M | Radical nephrectomy, radiation, chemotherapy | Vincristine + actinomycin-D; salvage doxorubicin | No | 17 | [69] |
| 26 y/o F | Radical nephrectomy | None | N/A | 1.7 | [69] |
| 35 y/o M | Radical nephrectomy, chemotherapy, IFN-a and IL-2 | 5-FU | No | 4 | [69] |
| 12 y/o M | Radical nephrectomy, chemotherapy | MVAC; salvage ifosfamide, etoposide, carboplatin, topotecan | No | 15 | [70] |
| 18 y/o F | Chemotherapy | MVAC | Partial | 1 | [71] |
| 14 y/o M | Radical nephrectomy, chemotherapy | MVAC; salvage etoposide, carboplatin | Complete | 11.5 | [32] |
| 28 y/o M | Radical nephrectomy | None | N/A | 2 | [72] |
| 31 y/o F | Radical nephrectomy, chemotherapy | MVAC | No | 3 | [72] |
| 21 y/o F | Radical nephrectomy, chemotherapy, bortezomib | Gemcitabine, cisplatin | Partial | 6 | [73] |
| 20 y/o M | Radical nephrectomy, chemotherapy | NR | No | 10 | [73] |
| 15 y/o F | Chemotherapy | Etoposide; cisplatin, gemcitabine, paclitaxel; salvage MVAC | Partial | 10 | [74] |
| 17 y/o M | Radical nephrectomy, chemotherapy, radiation | Carboplatin, gemcitabine, paclitaxel | Complete | 12 | [74] |
| 25 y/o M | Radical nephrectomy, chemotherapy | MVAC | NR | 4 | [9] |
| 11 y/o M | Radical nephrectomy, chemotherapy | Etoposide, doxorubicin, cyclophosphamide, vincristine | NR | 9 | [9] |
| 19 y/o M | Chemotherapy | Gemcitabine, cisplatin, radiation | NR | 6 | [9] |
| 8 y/o M | Radical nephrectomy | None | N/A | 72 | [9] |
| 17 y/o M | Radical nephrectomy, chemotherapy | High-dose-intensity MVAC | Partial | 12 | [67] |
| 30 y/o M | Chemotherapy | High-dose-intensity MVAC | Partial | 3.5 | [67] |
| 48 y/o F | Radical nephrectomy, chemotherapy, sunitinib | High-dose-intensity MVAC | Partial | At least 16 | [67] |
| 11 y/o M | Radical nephrectomy, chemotherapy | Carboplatin, paclitaxel, gemcitabine | Complete | 24 | [66] |

*MVAC* methotrexate-vinblastine-doxorubicin-cisplatin, *N/A* not applicable, *NR* no response

Overall, it is clear that a diagnosis of either CDC or RMC imparts a poor prognosis. Although individual case reports demonstrate occasional success stories with multimodality treatment, it is clear that improvements in survival for these patient populations will require continued translational research and enrollment in clinical trials.

## References


1. Davis CJ, Mostofi FK, Sesterhenn IA. Renal medullary carcinoma. The seventh sickle cell nephropathy. Am J Surg Pathol. 1995;19(1):1–11.
2. Srigley JR, Moch H. Carcinoma of the collecting ducts of Bellini. In: Eble JN, Sauter G, Epstein JI, Sesterhenn IA, editors. World Health Organization classification of tumors pathology and genetics: tumors of the urinary system and male genital organs. Lyon: IARC; 2004. p. 33–4.
3. Abern MR, Tsivian M, Polascik TJ, Coogan CL. Characteristics and outcomes of tumors arising from the distal nephron. Urology. 2012;80(1):140–6.
4. Tokuda N, Naito S, Matsuzaki O, Nagashima Y. Collecting duct (Bellini duct) renal cell carcinoma: a nationwide survey in Japan. J Urol. 2006;176(1):40–3.
5. Simpson L, He X, Pins M, Huang X, Campbell S, Yang X, et al. Renal medullary carcinoma and abl gene amplification. J Urol. 2005;173(6):1883–8.
6. Wright JL, Risk MC, Hotaling J, Lin DW. Effect of collecting duct histology on renal cell cancer outcome. J Urol. 2009;182(6):2595–600.
7. Srigley JR, Eble JN. Collecting duct carcinoma of kidney. Semin Diagn Pathol. 1998;15(1):54–67.
8. Gatalica Z, Lilleberg SL, Monzon FA, Koul MS, Bridge JA, Knezetic J, et al. Renal medullary carcinomas: histopathologic phenotype associated with diverse genotypes. Hum Pathol. 2011;42(12):1979–88.
9. Watanabe IC, Billis A, Guimarães MS, Alvarenga M, de Matos AC, Cardinalli IA, et al. Renal medullary carcinoma: report of seven cases from Brazil. Mod Pathol. 2007;20(9):914–20.
10. Yoon SK, Nam KJ, Rha S-H, Kim JK, Cho K-S, Kim B, et al. Collecting duct carcinoma of the kidney: CT and pathologic correlation. Eur J Radiol. 2006;57(3):453–60.
11. Prasad SR, Humphrey PA, Catena JR, Narra VR, Srigley JR, Cortez AD, et al. Common and uncommon histologic subtypes of renal cell carcinoma: imaging spectrum with pathologic correlation. Radiographics. 2006;26(6):1795–806.
12. Blitman NM, Berkenblit RG, Rozenblit AM, Levin TL. Renal medullary carcinoma: CT and MRI features. Am J Roentgenol. 2005;185(1):268–72.
13. Gupta R, Billis A, Shah RB, Moch H, Osunkoya AO, Jochum W, et al. Carcinoma of the collecting ducts of Bellini and renal medullary carcinoma. Am J Surg Pathol. 2012;36(9):1265–78.
14. Tickoo AK, Reuter VE. Collecting duct carcinoma and renal medullary carcinoma. In: Amin MB, McKenney JK, Tickoo SK, editors. Diagnostic pathology: genitourinary. Manitoba: Amirsys; 2010. p. 64–75.
15. Srigley JR, Delahunt B, Eble JN, Egevad L, Epstein JI, Grignon D, et al. The International Society of Urological Pathology (ISUP) Vancouver classification of renal neoplasia. Am J Surg Pathol. 2013;37(10):1469–89.
16. Kobayashi N, Matsuzaki O, Shirai S, Aoki I, Yao M, Nagashima Y. Collecting duct carcinoma of the kidney: an immunohistochemical evaluation of the use of antibodies for differential diagnosis. Hum Pathol. 2008;39(9):1350–9.
17. Albadine R, Schultz L, Illei P, Ertoy D, Hicks J, Sharma R, et al. PAX8 (+)/p63 (−) Immunostaining pattern in renal collecting duct carcinoma (CDC). Am J Surg Pathol. 2010;34(7):965–9.
18. Srigley JR, Delahunt B. Uncommon and recently described renal carcinomas. Mod Pathol. 2009;22:S2–23.
19. Elwood H, Chaux A, Schultz L, Illei PB, Baydar DE, Billis A, et al. Immunohistochemical analysis of SMARCB1/INI-1 expression in collecting duct carcinoma. Urology. 2011;78(2):474.e1–e5.
20. Calderaro J, Moroch J, Pierron G, Pedeutour F, Grison C, Maillé P, et al. SMARCB1/INI1 inactivation in renal medullary carcinoma. Histopathology. 2012;61(3):428–35.
21. Fuzesi L, Cober M, Mittermayer CH. Collecting duct carcinoma: cytogenetic characterization. Histopathology. 1992;21(2):155–60.
22. Cavazzana AO, Prayer-Galetti T, Tirabosco R, Macciomei MC, Stella M, Lania L, et al. Bellini duct carcinoma. A clinical and in vitro study. Eur Urol. 1996;30(3):340–4.
23. Antonelli A, Portesi E, Cozzoli A, Zanotelli T, Tardanico R, Balzarini P, et al. The collecting duct carcinoma of the kidney: a cytogenetical study. Eur Urol. 2003;43(6):680–5.
24. Gregori-Romero MA, Morell-Quadreny L, Llombart-Bosch A. Cytogenetic analysis of three primary Bellini duct carcinomas. Genes Chromosomes Cancer. 1996;15(3):170–2.
25. Schoenberg M, Cairns P, Brooks JD, Marshall FF, Epstein JI, Isaacs WB, et al. Frequent loss of chromosome arms 8p and 13q in collecting duct carcinoma (CDC) of the kidney. Genes Chromosomes Cancer. 1995;12(1):76–80.
26. Polascik TJ, Cairns P, Epstein JI, Fuzesi L, Ro JY, Marshall FF, et al. Distal nephron renal tumors: microsatellite allelotype. Cancer Res. 1996;56(8):1892–5.
27. Selli C, Amorosi A, Vona G, Sestini R, Travaglini F, Bartoletti R, et al. Retrospective evaluation of c-erbB-2 oncogene amplification using competitive PCR in collecting duct carcinoma of the kidney. J Urol. 1997;158(1):245–7.
28. Rao P, Tannir NM, Tamboli P. Expression of OCT3/4 in renal medullary carcinoma represents a potential diagnostic pitfall. Am J Surg Pathol. 2012;36(4):583–8.
29. Swartz MA, Karth J, Schneider DT, Rodriguez R, Beckwith JB, Perlman EJ. Renal medullary carcinoma: clinical, pathologic, immunohistochemical, and genetic analysis with pathogenetic implications. Urology. 2002;60(6):1083–9.

30. Liu Q, Galli S, Srinivasan R, Linehan WM, Tsokos M, Merino MJ. Renal medullary carcinoma: molecular, immunohistochemistry, and morphologic correlation. Am J Surg Pathol. 2013;37(3):368–74.

31. Cheng JX, Tretiakova M, Gong C, Mandal S, Krausz T, Taxy JB. Renal medullary carcinoma: rhabdoid features and the absence of INI1 expression as markers of aggressive behavior. Mod Pathol. 2008;21(6):647–52.

32. Stahlschmidt J, Cullinane C, Roberts P, Picton SV. Renal medullary carcinoma: prolonged remission with chemotherapy, immunohistochemical characterisation and evidence of bcr/abl rearrangement. Med Pediatr Oncol. 1999;33(6):551–7.

33. Schaeffer EM, Guzzo TJ, Furge KA, Netto G, Westphal M, Dykema K, et al. Renal medullary carcinoma: molecular, pathological and clinical evidence for treatment with topoisomerase-inhibiting therapy. BJU Int. 2009;106(1):62–5.

34. Albadine R, Wang W, Brownlee NA, Toubaji A, Billis A, Argani P, et al. Topoisomerase II α status in renal medullary carcinoma: immuno-expression and gene copy alterations of a potential target of therapy. J Urol. 2009;182(2):735–40.

35. Motzer RJ, Bacik J, Mariani T, Russo P, Mazumadar M, Reuter V. Treatment outcome and survival associated with metastatic renal cell carcinoma of non-clear-cell histology. J Clin Oncol. 2002;20(9):2376–81.

36. Karakiewicz PI, Trinh Q-D, Rioux-Leclercq N, La Taille DA, Novara G, Tostain J, et al. Collecting duct renal cell carcinoma: a matched analysis of 41 cases. Eur Urol. 2007;52(4):1140–6.

37. Chao D, Zisman A, Pantuck AJ, Gitlitz BJ, Freedland SJ, Said JW, et al. Collecting duct renal cell carcinoma: clinical study of a rare tumor. J Urol. 2002;167(1):71–4.

38. Matsumoto H, Wada T, Aoki A, Hoshii Y, Takahashi M, Aizawa S, et al. Collecting duct carcinoma with long survival treated by partial nephrectomy. Int J Urol. 2001;8(7):401–3.

39. Yoshida K, Kinoshita H, Taniguti H, Chizaki R, Nishida T, Hiura Y, et al. Bellini duct carcinoma of the kidney: a case report. Hinyokika Kiyo. 2007;53(2):121–4.

40. Vazquez-Lavista LG, Uribe-Uribe N, Gabilondo-Navarro F. Collecting duct renal cell carcinoma: two different clinical stages, two different clinical outcomes. Urol Int. 2008;81(1):116–8.

41. Blom JHM, van Poppel H, Maréchal JM, Jacqmin D, Schröder FH, de Prijck L, et al. Radical nephrectomy with and without lymph-node dissection: final results of European Organization for Research and Treatment of Cancer (EORTC) randomized phase 3 trial 30881. Eur Urol. 2009;55(1):28–34.

42. Whitson JM, Harris CR, Reese AC, Meng MV. Lymphadenectomy improves survival of patients with renal cell carcinoma and nodal metastases. J Urol. 2011;185(5):1615–20.

43. Sun M, Trinh Q-D, Bianchi M, Hansen J, Abdollah F, Tian Z, et al. Extent of lymphadenectomy does not improve the survival of patients with renal cell carcinoma and nodal metastases: biases associated with the handling of missing data. BJU Int. 2013;113(1):36–42.

44. Hellenthal NJ, Mansour AM, Hayn MH, Schwaab T. Is there a role for partial nephrectomy in patients with metastatic renal cell carcinoma? Urol Oncol. 2013;31(1):36–41.

45. Mejean A, Roupret M, Larousserie F, Hopirtean V, Thiounn N, Dufour B. Is there a place for radical nephrectomy in the presence of metastatic collecting duct (Bellini) carcinoma? J Urol. 2003;169(4):1287–90.

46. Oudard S, Banu E, Vieillefond A, Fournier L, Priou F, Medioni J, et al. Prospective multicenter phase II study of gemcitabine plus platinum salt for metastatic collecting duct carcinoma: results of a GETUG (Groupe d'Etudes des Tumeurs Uro-Génitales) study. J Urol. 2007;177(5):1698–702.

47. Bagrodia A, Gold R, Handorf C, Liman A, Derweesh IH. Salvage paclitaxel chemotherapy for metastatic collecting duct carcinoma of the kidney. Can J Urol. 2008;15(6):4425–7.

48. Gollob JA, Upton MP, DeWolf WC, Atkins MB. Long-term remission in a patient with metastatic collecting duct carcinoma treated with taxol/carboplatin and surgery. Urology. 2001;58(6):1058.

49. Fyfe G, Fisher RI, Rosenberg SA, Sznol M, Parkinson DR, Louie AC. Results of treatment of 255 patients with metastatic renal cell carcinoma who received high-dose recombinant interleukin-2 therapy. J Clin Oncol. 1995;13(3):688–96.

50. Pyrhönen S, Salminen E, Ruutu M, Lehtonen T, Nurmi M, Tammela T, et al. Prospective randomized trial of interferon alfa-2a plus vinblastine versus vinblastine alone in patients with advanced renal cell cancer. J Clin Oncol. 1999;17(9):2859–67.

51. Upton MP, Parker RA, Youmans A, McDermott DF, Atkins MB. Histologic predictors of renal cell carcinoma response to interleukin-2-based therapy. J Immunother. 2005;28(5):488–95.

52. Motzer RJ, Rini BI, Bukowski RM, Curti BD, George DJ, Hudes GR, et al. Sunitinib in patients with metastatic renal cell carcinoma. JAMA. 2006;295(21):2516–24.

53. Escudier B, Eisen T, Stadler WM, Szczylik C, Oudard S, Siebels M, et al. Sorafenib in advanced clear-cell renal cell carcinoma. N Engl J Med. 2007;356(2):125–34.

54. Hudes G, Carducci M, Tomczak P, Dutcher J, Figlin R, Kapoor A, et al. Temsirolimus, interferon alfa, or both for advanced renal cell carcinoma. N Engl J Med. 2007;356(22):2271–81.

55. Motzer RJ, Escudier B, Oudard S, Hutson TE, Porta C, Bracarda S, et al. Efficacy of everolimus in advanced renal cell carcinoma: a double-blind, randomised, placebo-controlled phase III trial. Lancet. 2008;372(9637):449–56.

56. Sternberg CN, Davis ID, Mardiak J, Szczylik C, Lee E, Wagstaff J, et al. Pazopanib in locally advanced or metastatic renal cell carcinoma: results of a randomized phase III trial. J Clin Oncol. 2010;28(6):1061–8.

57. Tannir NM, Plimack E, Ng C, Tamboli P, Bekele NB, Xiao L, et al. A phase 2 trial of sunitinib in patients with advanced non–clear cell renal cell carcinoma. Eur Urol. 2012;62(6):1013–9.

58. Staehler M, Schöppler G, Haseke N, Stadler T, Karl A, Siebels M, et al. Carcinoma of the collecting ducts of Bellini of the kidney: adjuvant chemotherapy followed by multikinase inhibition with sunitinib. Clin Genitourin Cancer. 2009;7(1):58–61.

59. Miyake H, Haraguchi T, Takenaka A, Fujisawa M. Metastatic collecting duct carcinoma of the kidney responded to sunitinib. Int J Clin Oncol. 2010;16(2):153–5.

60. Ansari J, Fatima A, Chaudhri S, Bhatt RI, Wallace M, James ND. Sorafenib induces therapeutic response in a patient with metastatic collecting duct carcinoma of kidney. Onkologie. 2009;32(1–2):44–6.

61. Koh Y, Lim HY, Ahn JH, Lee JL, Rha SY, Kim YJ, et al. Phase II trial of everolimus for the treatment of nonclear-cell renal cell carcinoma. Ann Oncol. 2013;24(4):1026–31.

62. Procopio G, Verzoni E, Iacovelli R, Colecchia M, Torelli T, Mariani L. Is there a role for targeted therapies in the collecting ducts of Bellini carcinoma? Efficacy data from a retrospective analysis of 7 cases. Clin Exp Nephrol. 2012;16(3):464–7.

63. Voss MH, Bastos DA, Karlo CA, Ajeti A, Hakimi AA, Feldman DR, et al. Treatment outcome with mTOR inhibitors for metastatic renal cell carcinoma with nonclear and sarcomatoid histologies. Ann Oncol. 2014;25(3):663–8.

64. Hakimi AA, Koi PT, Milhoua PM, Blitman NM, Li M, Hugec V, et al. Renal medullary carcinoma: the Bronx experience. Urology. 2007;70(5):878–82.

65. Avery RA, Harris JE, Davis CJ, Borgaonkar DS. Renal medullary carcinoma: clinical and therapeutic aspects of a newly described tumor. Cancer. 1996;78(1):128–32.

66. Walsh A, Kelly DR, Vaid YN, Hilliard LM, Friedman GK. Complete response to carboplatin, gemcitabine, and paclitaxel in a patient with advanced metastatic renal medullary carcinoma. Pediatr Blood Cancer. 2010;55(6):1217–20.

67. Rathmell WK, Monk JP. High-dose-intensity MVAC for advanced renal medullary carcinoma: report of three cases and literature review. Urology. 2008;72(3):659–63.

68. Kalyanpur A, Schwartz DS, Fields JM. Renal medulla carcinoma in a white adolescent. AJR Am J Roentgenol. 1997;169(4):1037–8.

69. Coogan CL, McKiel Jr CF, Flanagan MJ, Bormes TP, Matkov TG. Renal medullary carcinoma in patients with sickle cell trait. Urology. 1998;51(6):1049–50.

70. Pirich LM, Chou P, Walterhouse DO. Prolonged survival of a patient with sickle cell trait and metastatic renal medullary carcinoma. J Pediatr Hematol Oncol. 1999;21(1):67.

71. Warren KE, Gidvani-Diaz V, Duval-Arnould B. Renal medullary carcinoma in an adolescent with sickle cell trait. Pediatrics. 1999;103(2), e22.

72. Figenshau RS, Basler JW, RItter JH, Siegel CL, Simon JA, Dierks SM. Renal medullary carcinoma. J Urol. 1998;159(3):711–3.

73. Yang XJ, Sugimura J, Tretiakova MS, Furge K, Zagaja G, Sokoloff M, et al. Gene expression profiling of renal medullary carcinoma. Cancer. 2004;100(5):976–85.

74. Strouse JJ, Spevak M, Mack AK, Arceci RJ, Small D, Loeb DM. Significant responses to platinum-based chemotherapy in renal medullary carcinoma. Pediatr Blood Cancer. 2005;44(4):407–11.

Leili Mirsadraei, Michelle S. Hirsch,
Christopher J. Kane, and Donna E. Hansel


## Mucinous Tubular and Spindle Cell Carcinoma (MTSCC)

### Introduction

Mucinous tubular and spindle cell carcinoma (MTSCC) is an uncommon, low-grade renal epithelial tumor [5, 6]. It was initially believed to derive from the collecting duct and was originally considered the well-differentiated variant of collecting duct carcinoma [6, 7]. This neoplasm has been previously reported under different names: renal cell carcinoma originating from the distal loop of Henle, renal cell carcinoma of distal nephron origin, loopoma, and low-grade collecting duct


L. Mirsadraei, M.D. • D.E. Hansel, M.D., Ph.D. (✉)
Department of Pathology, University of California at San Diego, San Diego, CA, USA
e-mail: lmirsadraei@ucsd.edu; dhansel@ucsd.edu

M.S. Hirsch, M.D., Ph.D.
Department of Pathology, Brigham and Women's Hospital, Harvard Medical School, Boston, MA 02115, USA
e-mail: mhirsch1@partners.org

C.J. Kane, M.D., F.A.C.S.
Department of Urology, University of California San Diego, San Diego, CA 92093, USA
e-mail: ckane@ucsd.edu


(Bellini) carcinoma [8]. MTSCC occurs more commonly in females (female-to-male ratio of 2:1 to 3:1) and encompasses a broad age range (17–82 years) [7–9].

### Clinical Presentation

Most patients with MTSCC are asymptomatic, although some may experience flank pain and hematuria [5]. A subset of patients may present with renal stones [10]. A common clinical finding is the presence of and associated staghorn renal calculus in approximately 50 % of the cases [5]. MSTCC is often found incidentally when imaging for other indications; however, imaging modalities cannot definitively distinguish MTSCC from other RCC subtes [11, 12]. Reported cases have been found in the subcapsular, corticomedullary, and medullary areas of the kidney, with the majority presenting as clinical stage pT1 [6, 9].

### Pathology

On gross evaluation, MTSCC is typically small but can vary in size, is often localized to the cortex or corticomedullary junction, and appears well defined with a tan-white homogenous cut surface [13]. Occasionally, mucin-containing areas may appear gelatinous in nature [5].


© Springer Science+Business Media New York 2016
D.E. Hansel et al. (eds.), *The Kidney*, DOI 10.1007/978-1-4939-3286-3_9

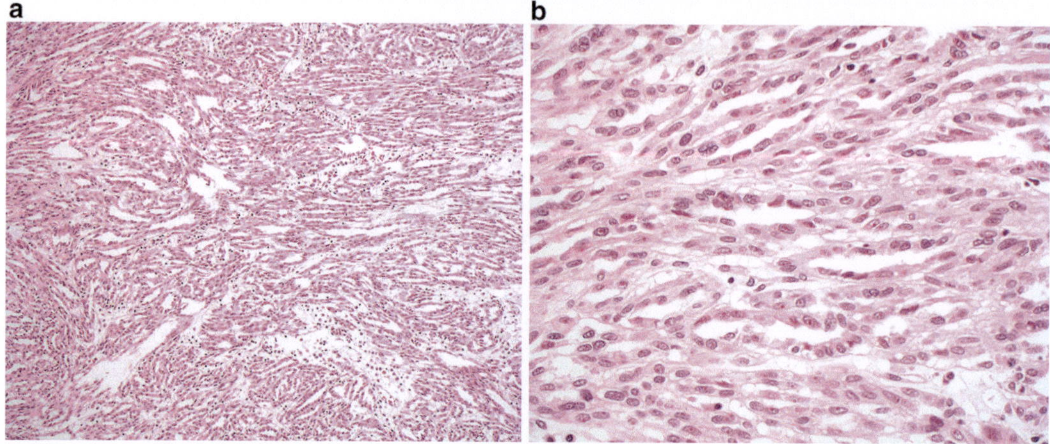

**Fig. 9.1** Mucinous and tubular spindle cell carcinoma. (**a**) Inter-anastomosing cords of cells in a mucinous background are seen at low magnification. (**b**) Tumor cells show relatively uniform nuclei with minimal atypia

At low magnification, three distinct components are generally identifiable: a mucinous background, monomorphic spindle cells present in sheets, and cystic, elongated, and compressed tubules lined by a single layer of cuboidal cells (Fig. 9.1a). At higher magnification, the tumor cells are well differentiated and show low-grade morphology and minimal variation in cytologic appearance (Fig. 9.1b). Nuclei are commonly low grade in appearance with a round to oval shape, smooth chromatin, and occasional small nucleoli. The cytoplasm may be eosinophilic, and an admixture of inflammatory cells might be seen [5, 11]. Less common features include papillary architecture, oncocytic change, presence of clear cells, and calcifications (psammoma bodies). Rarely, sarcomatoid change has been described in association with MTSCC [14, 15]. If papillary structures are seen, the main differential diagnosis includes conventional papillary RCC; however, the presence of a mucinous background and the absence of characteristic chromosomal alterations associated with papillary RCC support the diagnosis of MTSCC.

MTSCC has been shown to harbor multiple chromosomal alterations, including 1, 4, 8, 9, 13, 14, 15, and 22 [16]. The genetic changes characteristic of papillary RCC, namely, trisomy 7 and 17 and loss of the Y chromosome, are not identified in MTSCC [17].

Most MTSCC lesions express markers that are reminiscent of distal nephron differentiation, including EMA, AE1/3, CK7, E-cadherin, and α-methylacyl CoA racemase. RCC antigen is positive in the majority of cases. The proximal tubular marker CD10 is positive in only 10–15 % of MTSCC cases [18, 19]. The immunohistochemical profile of MTSCC is nonspecific and partially overlaps with papillary RCC with the absence of CD10 being the most supportive immunohistochemical biomarker for the former [6].

## Prognosis and Clinical Management

MTSCC is often indolent and surgery is curative in most cases [20–22]. A small subset of cases may recur or be associated with regional lymph node metastases [13, 16, 22, 23]. Sarcomatoid transformation is associated with an increased likelihood of distant metastases and risk of death from disease [14, 24, 25].

## Clear Cell Papillary RCC

### Introduction

Clear cell papillary RCC (also referred to by some as "clear cell tubulopapillary RCC") is reported to account for less than 5 % of renal epithelial neoplasms; however, this incidence is likely an underestimation due to the misclassification of this tumor as a clear cell or less frequently a papillary, RCC. Clear cell papillary RCC affects men and women equally, and the age distribution ranges from 18 to 88 years [26–28]. Clear cell papillary RCC may occur sporadically or may be associated with end-stage renal disease [29–33].

## Clinical Presentation

The majority of clear cell papillary RCC cases are discovered incidentally, although a subset of patients may present with hematuria or flank pain [27].

## Pathology

Clear cell papillary RCC is primarily a cortical lesion. On gross evaluation, these tumors are well circumscribed, encapsulated, and relatively small in size (0.6–5.5 cm) [28, 31]. Cystic change may be present. The cut surface ranges from yellow to tan to brown in appearance. These tumors are commonly unifocal, although bilateral and multifocal tumors have been described.

Microscopically, several architectural patterns may be present and include cystic and solid structures as well as branching glands [27, 31, 34]. A defining characteristic of these tumors is the presence of tubular and papillary structures lined by clear cells (Fig. 9.2a). Occasional eosinophilic luminal secretions may be seen. Tumor cells show clear cytoplasm, and the nuclei are uniform and small and lack nucleoli (Fig. 9.2b). Prominent nuclear polarization toward the luminal surface is striking in these cases [27, 31, 35]. The intervening stroma is often fibrous or hyalinized but may contain smooth muscle.

Genetic analysis shows these tumors to be distinct from clear cell RCC and papillary RCC. Specifically, clear cell papillary RCC lacks chromosome 3p deletions or *VHL* gene alteration characteristic of clear cell RCC, as well as extra copies of chromosomes 7 and 17 as is seen in papillary RCC [30, 31, 36–39]. Some molecular differences have been reported between clear cell papillary RCC that occurs in the sporadic and the ESRD settings [31, 40, 41].

Immunohistochemistry is helpful in the diagnosis of this entity by distinguishing it from both clear cell RCC and papillary RCC. Clear cell papillary RCC shows positive immunoreactivity for CK7; carbonic anhydrase IX (CAIX), PAX2, and PAX8; and high-molecular-weight cytokeratin (34βE12) [26, 29, 42]. Immunostains for AMACR (racemase) and RCC antigen are negative, and CD10 is negative or only focally positive. In contrast, clear cell RCC is typically negative for CK7 and positive for CD10, RCC antigen, and CAIX and may show variable AMACR staining. Papillary RCC is typically positive for CK7, AMACR, and CD10; RCC antigen may be variable and CAIX should be negative.

## Prognosis and Clinical Management

All cases reported to date in the literature have shown indolent behavior, without recurrence or metastatic spread [1, 32, 33, 42].

## Tubulocystic Carcinoma

### Introduction

Tubulocystic carcinoma is an uncommon form of RCC described in numerous case reports and small case series [6, 43–46]. Tubulocystic carcinoma was initially described by Amin et al. [43] in 2009; however, earlier descriptions of similar tumors date back to1956, when it was included with Bellini (collecting duct) carcinomas, and later described as the low-grade collecting duct carcinoma [47, 48]. However, more recent studies have demonstrated that tubulocystic carcinomas are more likely related to papillary RCC instead of collecting duct carcinoma [43, 44]. Tubulocystic carcinoma affects adults over a broad age range of 29–94 years of age [49, 50]. There is a strong male predominance (male-to-female ratio of 7:1) [47, 51]. Based on

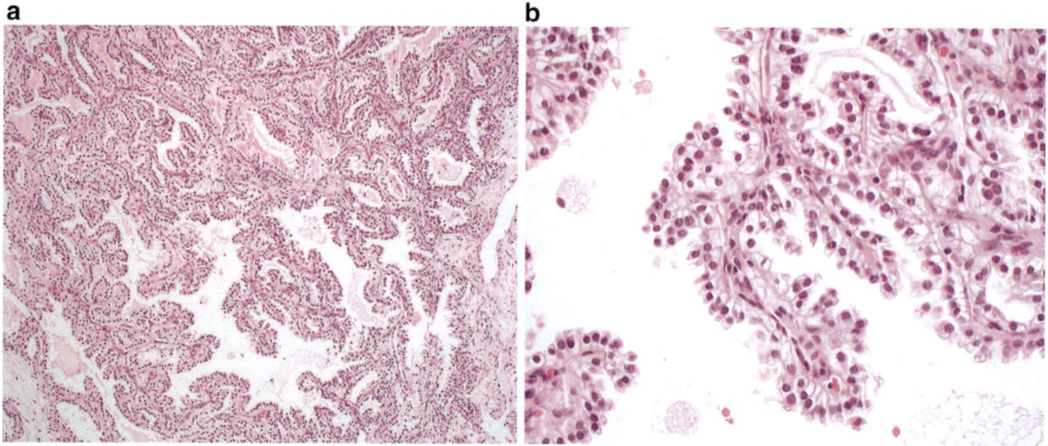

**Fig. 9.2** Clear cell papillary renal cell carcinoma. (**a**) A combination of papillary and nested patterns is identifiable in this example. Uniform alignment of the nuclei to the luminal surface is evident even at low magnification. (**b**) Papillary fronds lined by clear cells are a characteristic feature of this lesion

immunohistochemical staining pattern, ultrastructural features, and gene expression profiling, tubulocystic carcinoma is favored to originate from either the proximal convoluted tubule or intercalated tubule [6, 43, 51].

## Clinical Presentation

Patients are often asymptomatic, although some may present with abdominal pain, distension, and hematuria. Tubulocystic carcinoma is usually solitary and often involves the left kidney [51]; however, multifocal tumors have been described in approximately 23 % of patients [44, 47]. Tubulocystic carcinoma should be considered in the differential diagnosis of a renal lesion with a cystic component on radiological examination.

## Pathology

On gross examination, tubulocystic carcinoma is usually solitary and well circumscribed and has a tan-gray, spongy appearance; the latter is due to numerous cysts/microcysts [47]. Tubulocystic carcinoma varies in size from 0.2 to 17 cm [48, 51]. Multifocal tumors may be present, which can include multiple distinct tubulocystic carcinomas or tubulocystic carcinoma associated with a concurrent second renal neoplasm, most frequently a papillary RCC [47, 48]. Tumors are most commonly located in the cortex, although up to a third can be present at the corticomedullary junction [6].

Microscopically, tubulocystic carcinoma is composed of many cystic structures that are small to medium in size, which are separated by thin fibrous septa (Fig. 9.3a). Solid growth is not seen. The cells lining the cysts are cuboidal, columnar, or hobnail in appearance with abundant eosinophilic or amphophilic cytoplasm which characteristically contain large nuclei with prominent red nucleoli (Fig. 9.3b) [47]. Rarely, sarcomatoid features may be seen in association with this tumor but only in the presence of solid growth (i.e., an associated component of high-grade papillary RCC) [1, 52]. On ultrastructural examination, the tumors show abundant microvilli with brush border organization suggestive of proximal convoluted tubules, with some features resembling intercalated cells of the collecting ducts [51].

Genetic analysis of these tumors report a similar profile to papillary RCC, which include gains of chromosome 7 and 17 and loss of the Y chromosome. However, classic features associated with "low-grade" papillary RCC are typically not

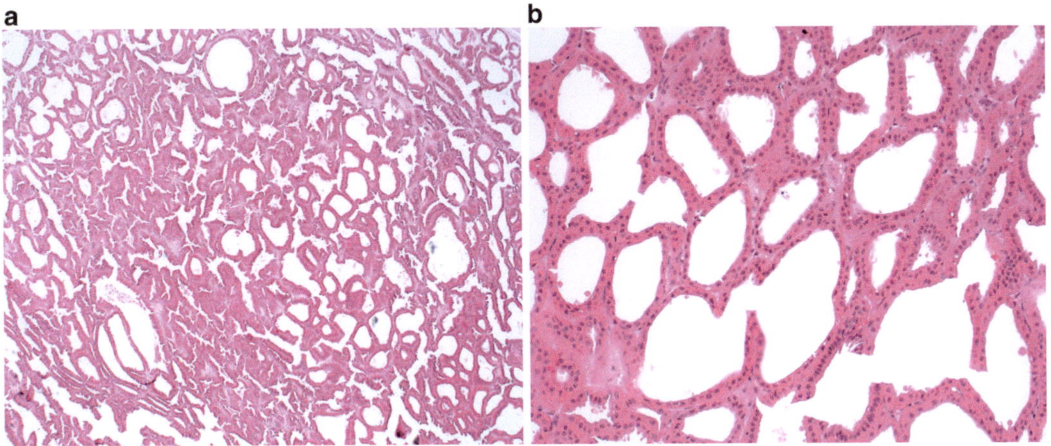

**Fig. 9.3** Tubulocystic renal cell carcinoma. (**a**) Multiple cystic structures of variable size are present at low magnification. (**b**) Cysts are lined by a single layer of cells with eosinophilic cytoplasm, large nuclei, and prominent nucleoli

seen in this entity; in contrast, high-grade tumors with solid and papillary growth patterns and similar nuclear and immunophenotypic features can be seen [44, 45, 53]

Immunohistochemical studies demonstrate immunoreactivity for cytokeratins 8, 18, and 19 [6, 44]. CD10 and P504S (racemase) are positive in greater than 90 % of cases. Diffuse and strong AMACR positivity, positive to variable CK7 expression, and staining for kidney-specific cadherin and PAX2 have been reported [44, 47]. Tubulocystic carcinoma is negative for high-molecular-weight cytokeratin (34BE12) [47, 48].

The main differential diagnoses include other tumors with a multiloculated gross appearance, including multiloculated clear cell RCC, cystic clear cell tubulopapillary RCC, cystic nephroma, mixed epithelial and stromal tumor, and cystic oncocytoma [47, 51, 54, 55]. Distinction between these entities is primarily based on light microscopic evaluation, rather than use of ancillary studies.

## Prognosis and Clinical Management

Whereas the majority of reported cases of tubulocystic carcinoma demonstrate indolent behavior, recurrence and metastases to regional and distant sites such as the bone and liver have been reported

in rare cases; the latter is associated with tumors that demonstrate solid and papillary growth patterns [44, 45, 47, 51, 56].

# Acquired Cystic Disease-Associated RCC

## Introduction

Cystic change occurs in the majority of patients with end-stage renal disease (ESRD) who undergo dialysis and is termed "acquired renal cystic disease" (ARCD) [5, 6]. Patients with ARCD have increased risk of developing RCC comparing to normal population [6, 57, 58], with an RCC incidence rate of 10 % in ARCD patients [5, 6, 37, 59]. A direct correlation between the duration of dialysis and RCC development in ESRD patients has been suggested in some studies [5, 6, 29, 60]. Multiple types of renal neoplasms may arise in the background of ESRD, including clear cell RCC, papillary RCC, clear cell papillary RCC, and chromophobe RCC [5, 61–63], although acquired cystic disease-associated RCC represents up to 36 % of all renal neoplasms in this setting [29]. Similar to non-ESRD RCC, acquired cystic disease-associated RCC occurs most commonly in men between the ages of 55 and 65 years [5, 30, 40, 61].

## Clinical Presentation

Most cases are found as an incidental finding on nephrectomy specimens removed for ESRD [5]. However, a subset of patients undergoing dialysis may have pain or demonstrate hematuria. In addition, imaging may identify an incidental lesion in the background of cystic renal parenchyma [6, 62].

## Pathology

On gross examination, acquired cystic disease-associated RCC is well circumscribed and tan/yellow in appearance and may show focal hemorrhage or necrosis [5, 6]. The background renal parenchyma shows multiple variably sized cysts, with the neoplasm appearing to arise in association with a cyst wall or from one of the connecting trabecular areas. Multifocal tumors occur approximately 50 % of cases, and bilateral tumors are found in up to 20 % of patients [1, 29].

At low magnification, acquired cystic disease-associated RCC shows a distinct "sieve-like" appearance (Fig. 9.4a). At higher magnification, multiple growth patterns that include acinar, alveolar, solid, cystic, and papillary regions may be identified. The tumor cells show granular, eosinophilic cytoplasm and contain large nuclei with prominent nucleoli [6]. Intratumoral calcium

oxalate crystal is a relatively specific feature in this entity, although may be lacking a minority of cases (Fig. 9.4b) [6, 29, 59]. Rhabdoid and sarcomatoid features have been reported in a small number of cases [29, 61, 64].

Fluorescence in situ hybridization (FISH) and comparative genomic hybridization performed on nine cases showed variable combined gains of chromosomes 3, 7, 16, 17, and Y [6, 60].

Acquired cystic disease-associated RCC shows immunoreactivity for a-methylacyl-coenzyme A racemase (AMACR), CD10, RCC antigen, and glutathione S-transferase A [6, 60]. CK7 is often negative but can show focal immunoreactivity [6].

The main differential diagnosis includes papillary renal cell carcinoma. Immunostains for CK7 and chromosomal analysis can be used to distinguish these two entities in most cases, if required.

## Prognosis and Clinical Management

Most cases of acquired cystic renal disease-associated RCC typically show indolent behavior, which may reflect early detection in patients with ESRD [6, 62]. As anticipated, the minority of tumors that show rhabdoid or sarcomatoid features may behave more aggressively and be associated with metastatic spread [1, 29, 64, 65].

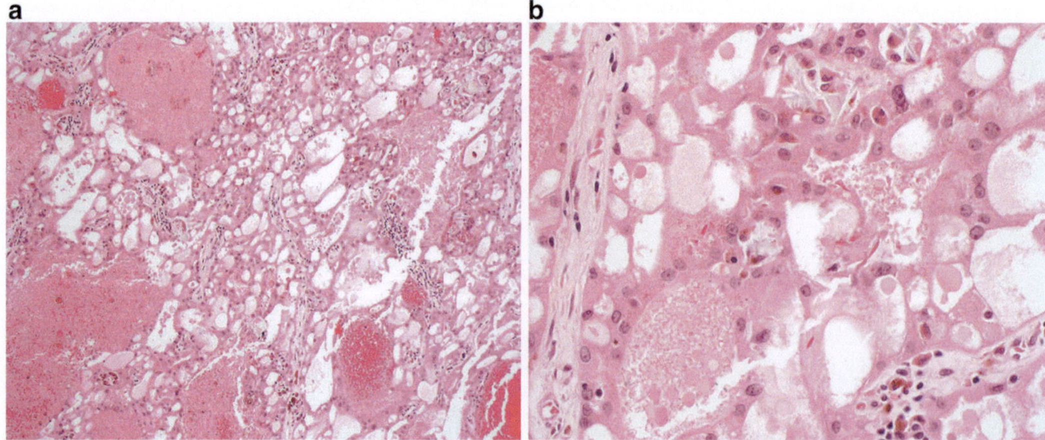

**Fig. 9.4** Acquired cystic disease-associated renal cell carcinoma. (**a**) A sieve-like pattern is evident at low magnification. (**b**) Crystals may be seen in a subset of cases

## Neuroblastoma-Associated RCC

### Introduction

Neuroblastoma-associated RCC is a unique entity that occurs 3–35 years after diagnosis and treatment of childhood or adult neuroblastoma [5, 6, 66, 67]. It is a rare tumor, accounting for less than 1 % of all cases of RCC and approximately 2.5 % of the cases of RCC in children [5, 11]. Males and females have an equal risk of involvement [63]. Some reports suggest a relationship between the treatment for neuroblastoma and development of neuroblastoma-associated RCC [11]. However, a small number of patients develop RCC in the absence of radiation or chemotherapy, suggesting a possible underlying germ line susceptibility for these lesions [67].

### Clinical Presentation

Neuroblastoma-associated RCC can be unilateral or bilateral [11]. Rare cases showing multifocal tumors have also been reported. No specific radiologic findings have been associated with this entity. The diagnosis may be suggested based on a history of treatment for neuroblastoma [11].

### Pathology

On gross evaluation, tumors range in size from 1 to 8 cm [5, 63]. Neuroblastoma-associated RCC is histologically heterogeneous [11]. The most common appearance is that of an oncocytic tumor that shows solid and papillary architecture and occasional vacuolization of the cytoplasm [5, 53, 63, 68]. Variable nuclear size and medium-sized nucleoli are present, and mitotic figures may be identified. One should note that other forms of RCC, including Xp11.2 translocation-associated carcinoma and classic clear cell RCC, can also occur in a subset of patients following neuroblastoma [5, 63, 69].

Due to the small number of cases described to date, the genetic profile of this tumor has not been well defined, although chromosomal altera-tions affecting 14q31 and 20q13 have been reported [5, 70].

Immunohistochemistry shows neuroblastoma-associated RCC to be frequently positive for EMA, vimentin, and cytokeratins 8, 18, and 20 and negative for cytokeratins 7, 14, 19, 20, S100, and HMB45 [5, 63]. The main differential diagnosis includes oncocytoma and chromophobe RCC in the oncocytic subtype of neuroblastoma-associated RCC. Clinical history is critical in this differential diagnosis.

### Prognosis and Clinical Management

The oncocytic subtype of neuroblastoma-associated RCC behaves in an indolent manner. Outcomes associated with clear cell RCC and Xp11-associated RCC are likely similar to their de novo counterparts. Awareness of this entity is important to ensure close follow-up and frequent assessment of survivors of neuroblastoma in order to detect RCC early in the course of disease.

## Thyroid-Like Follicular Carcinoma of the Kidney (TLFCK)

### Introduction

Thyroid-like follicular carcinoma of the kidney (TLFCK) is a rare renal neoplasm. To date, only a limited number of TLFCK cases have been reported in the literature [1, 6, 71–75]. This tumor occurs over a broad range of 29–83 years, with an equal gender distribution [1, 6, 73, 75]. This entity has not yet been classified as a distinct renal neoplasm by the World Health Organization.

### Clinical Presentation

Most of these carcinomas are identified as an incidental finding on radiologic imaging, although a subset of patients present with abdominal pain, flank pain, hematuria, and relapsing urinary infection [6, 71, 75].

## Pathology

On gross examination, these tumors are well defined and encapsulated, with a solid or cystic and yellow-tan cut surface [71, 75]. Focal areas of hemorrhage or necrosis may be seen. Microscopically, TLFCK shows variably sized follicular structures containing both microfollicular and macrofollicular patterns (Fig. 9.5a). The follicles contain pink colloid-like material and are lined by a single layer of cuboidal to columnar cells with moderate amphophilic to eosinophilic cytoplasm (Fig. 9.5b) [71, 73]. Nuclei are typically round to oval and may demonstrate nuclear grooves, similar to that seen in thyroid neoplasms. Lymphocytic infiltrates with or without reactive germinal centers can be present [71].

Given the low incidence, the genetic profile of TLFCK has not been well defined.

The immunohistochemical profile of TLFCK shows positive immunoreactivity for PAX8, EMA, CK7, and vimentin, with a subset of cases reported to express CD10 and PAX2 [71, 76]. The colloid-like material in TLFCK is composed of Tamm-Horsfall glycoprotein, the most abundant protein in normal urine [71, 77]. The main differential diagnosis is metastatic follicular carcinoma of the thyroid; however, TLFCK is negative for thyroid markers TTF-1 and thyroglobulin [6, 71]. The diagnosis of TLFCK is strengthened by the absence of lesions in the thyroid or other locations by imaging [6, 73]. TLFCK should also be distinguished from thyroidization of the kidney, which is characterized by atrophic distal tubules or collecting ducts, with colloid-like hyaline casts that mimic normal thyroid parenchyma. Thyroidization is a benign, widespread, and usually bilateral process that occurs in patients with a history of chronic pyelonephritis, obstructive uropathy, or end-stage renal disease. In contrast, TLFCK presents as a well-circumscribed tumor in a background of unremarkable kidney and is often in patients with no history of renal disease [71].

## Prognosis and Clinical Management

Although most cases of TLFCK remain localized, one case of TLFCK metastasized to the renal hilar lymph nodes and a second showed widespread metastases to the lungs and retroperitoneal lymph nodes [71, 73].

## Succinate Dehydrogenase-Deficient RCC

### Introduction

Succinate dehydrogenase (SDH)-deficient renal cell carcinoma is a recently described entity that is not yet widely recognized due to its morphologic

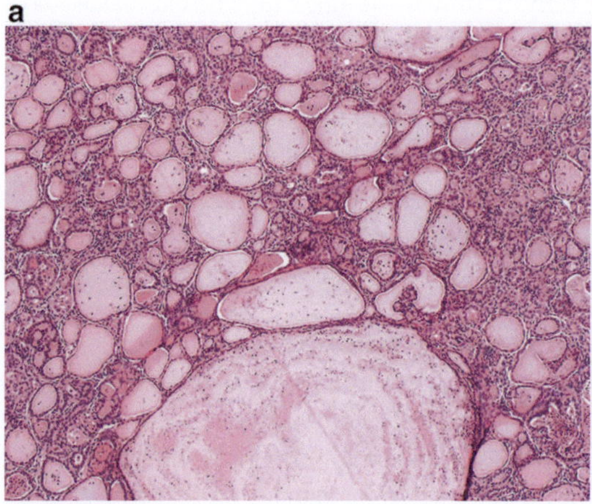

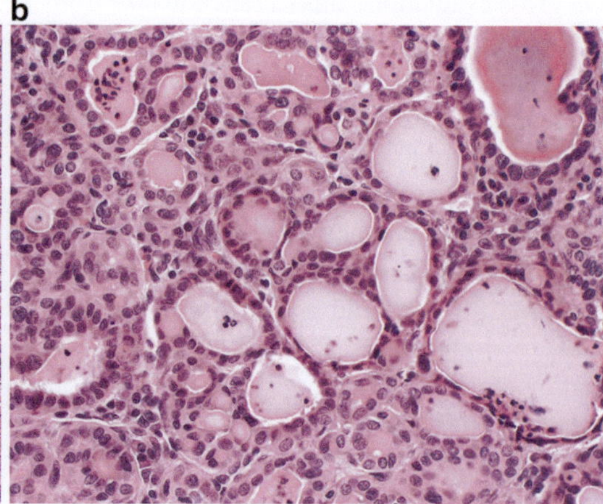

**Fig. 9.5** Thyroid-like follicular carcinoma of the kidney. (**a**) A combination of variably sized follicular structures filled with colloid-like material and small nests may be seen in this entity. (**b**) The follicular structures are lined by a single layer of cuboidal to columnar cells with eosinophilic cytoplasm and minimal nuclear atypia

overlap with other oncocytic renal neoplasms. Nevertheless, SDH-deficient RCC has been accepted as a provisional entity in the 2013 International Society of Urological Pathology Vancouver Classification of renal tumors, as it represents a distinct renal neoplasm, defined by loss of IHC staining for the B subunit of the SDH mitochondrial complex (the entire complex consists of four subunits: A, B, C, and D) [1, 78, 79]. The tumor is rare, estimated as less than 1 % of all renal epithelial tumors [79], and it occurs in individuals with germ line mutations of the genes that encode the SDH complex [1, 78]. SDH-deficient RCC has been reported more commonly in men, with the mean age of 40 years [78, 79]. Patients with germ line mutation in a SDH subunit gene are also prone to develop paraganglioma/pheochromocytoma, gastrointestinal stromal tumor (GIST), and pituitary adenoma [1, 78–80].

## Clinical Presentation

Due to the low incidence of this renal cancer, clinical presentation has yet not been described in detail. Some patients have reported episodic headache and palpitation associated with paraganglioma-related hypertension, with an incidental renal mass discovered on imaging during work-up [81]. Bilateral tumors have been reported [79].

## Pathology

On gross examination, this tumor is well circumscribed with a tan to red cut surface [78, 79]. Hemorrhage and microcystic change may be present [78, 79]. Tumor diameter ranges from 2.0 to 20 cm [78]. Both unifocal, multifocal, and bilateral tumors have been described [78, 79].

Microscopically, cells are arranged in solid or nested patterns that contain uniform neoplastic cells with eosinophilic, variably granular cytoplasm [1, 78, 79, 81]. The most distinctive histological feature is the presence of perinuclear cytoplasmic vacuoles and inclusion-like spaces, some of which contain pink flocculent-like material (Fig. 9.6) [78, 79, 81]. Nuclei are typically

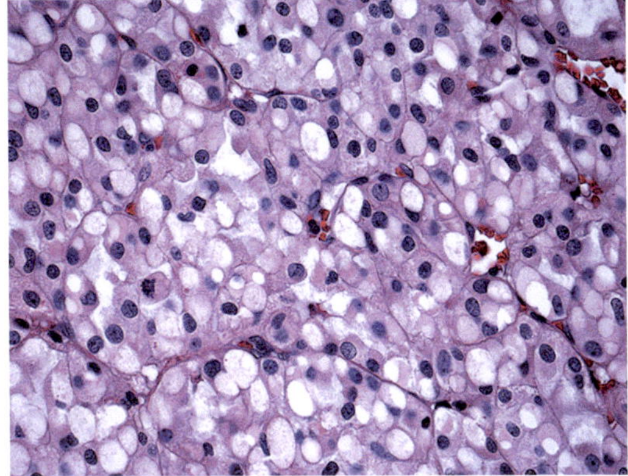

**Fig. 9.6** SDHB-associated renal cell carcinoma. Distinctive features include perinuclear cytoplasmic vacuoles and inclusion-like spaces filled with *pink secretions*

round with smooth boarders, finely clumped chromatin, and small or inconspicuous nucleoli [78]. Benign tubules or glomeruli are often entrapped at the edges of the tumors [81]. Stromal hemorrhage, fibrosis, and hyalinization are commonly seen [78]. Intratumoral mast cells and aggregates of lymphocytes, as well as necrosis, may be present [78]. Sarcomatoid change has been described [79].

By immunohistochemistry, the characteristic and pathognomonic finding is loss of SDHB; however, this can occur when any of the four SDH complex components (A, B, C, or D) are mutated. In SDHB-mutated RCC, the SDHA antibody will highlight the perinuclear cytoplasmic inclusions which contain the mutated mitochondria [78, 79]. Immunohistochemistry beyond loss of expression with SDH antibodies is nonspecific: neoplastic cells are positive for PAX8 (confirming renal origin), EMA, and S100 and negative for RCC; labeling for CAM5.2, AE1/AE3, cytokeratin 7, CD10, and AMCR is variable, and C-KIT highlights intratumoral mast cells but is negative in the tumor cells [78, 79].

The differential diagnosis of SDH-deficient RCC includes oncocytoma, chromophobe RCC, and the "granular variant" of clear cell RCC. Loss of staining for SDHB is a definitive confirmation of the diagnosis. Also, SDH-deficient RCC commonly shows negative or focal cytokeratin reactivity [79].

## Prognosis and Clinical Management

Metastatic disease to the liver, lung, ribs, vertebrae, adrenal gland, and lymph nodes has been reported. Concurrent paragangliomas may also be observed [78, 79, 81]. Tumor progression and death from disease have been reported [78, 79, 81].

## TCEB1-Mutated (Monosomy-8) Renal Cell Carcinoma

Renal cell tumor with TCEB1 mutations and loss of heterozygosity of chromosome 8 are a recently described renal tumor variant that has morphologic overlap with clear cell RCC and clear cell papillary RCC [82, 83]. This emerging renal neoplasm was identified through common mutations in the TCEB1 gene (which encodes elongin, a member of the VHL complex) and by loss of chromosome 8 with conventional G-band karyotyping and fluorescence in situ hybridization. To date, only 17 tumors have been reported [82–84]. Alterations of TCEB1 impact VHL-pathway signaling, a commonly altered pathway in clear cell renal cell carcinoma, but in a mechanism that is independent of direct VHL mutation [82, 84].

## Clinical Presentation

All but one reported TCEB1-mutated RCCs reported to date have been small (stage pT1) and therefore likely to present incidentally, although nonspecific symptoms typically associated with other renal masses (pain and hematuria) may be present.

## Pathology

Grossly, tumors are typically small, tan/yellow, and well circumscribed. A prominent thick fibrous capsule is almost invariably present. Microscopically, TCEB1-mutated tumors show nests and tubule of clear cells with occasional focal papillary structures. Cells contain abundant clear cytoplasm and pink amorphous material within tubule lumens [82, 83] (Fig. 9.7a). Nuclei are low grade but typically larger than is seen in clear cell tubulopapillary RCC; nucleoli are absent (i.e., size suggestive of Fuhrman nuclear grades 2–3, but absence of nucleoli is more in keeping with Fuhrman nuclear grade 2). There is a hint of nuclear polarization but not to the extent seen in clear cell papillary RCC. A relatively distinct and reproducible feature is the presence of thick fibromuscular bands that dissect through the mass (Fig. 9.7b).

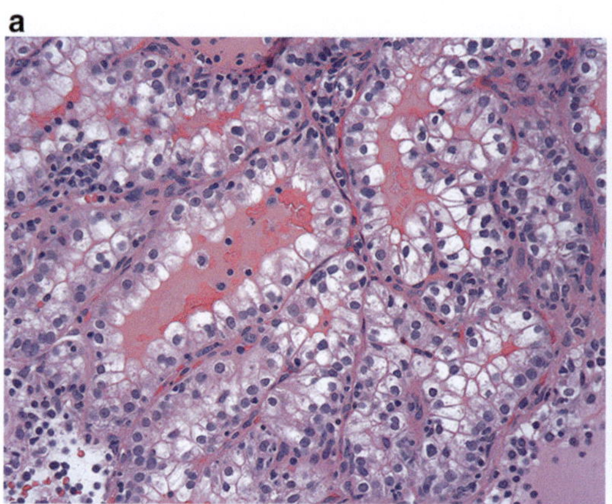
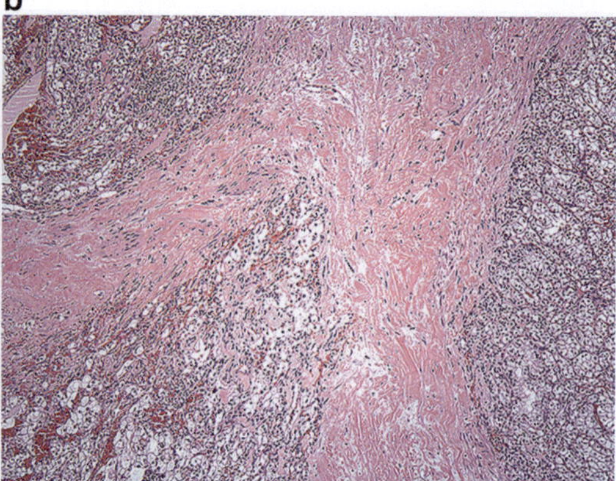

**Fig. 9.7** TCEB1-mutated renal cell carcinoma. (**a**) Tubular structures lined by clear cells with abundant clear cytoplasm. *Pink amorphous material* is present in the tubule lumen. (**b**) A unique feature is the presence of thick fibromuscular bands within the lesion

Immunohistochemistry shows immunoreactivity for CAIX and HIF-1-alpha, as well as CK-7; the latter distinguishes it from most clear cell RCCs. Tumor cells are negative for high-molecular-weight cytokeratin (34BE12) [82], and unlike clear cell tubulopapillary RCC, TCEB1-mutated tumors show variable staining for AMACR, CD-10, and RCC antigen [83]. Of note, the cuplike staining pattern described for CAIX in clear cell papillary RCC is not present in TCEB1-mutated RCC; instead a membranous pattern, similar to clear cell RCC, is observed.

The differential diagnosis includes both clear cell renal cell carcinoma and clear cell papillary renal cell carcinoma. Although morphological features can be very suggestive and immunohistochemistry can be supportive, definitive diagnosis requires molecular analysis to show mutations in the TCEB1 gene and/or loss of heterozygosity at the chromosomal region that contains TCEB1 (8q21.11). Clinically, the use of G-band karyotyping (fresh tissue required) or FISH analysis (possible with formalin-fixed tissue) can be used to demonstrate a loss of chromosome 8. The short arms of chromosome 3 should be intact to make a diagnosis of a TCEB1-mutated RCC.

## Prognosis and Clinical Management

All cases reported thus far have been low stage (pT1), except one pT3a case. During a median 48-month follow-up period, no patient was reported to develop metastatic disease. However, further evaluation on a larger number of tumors with extended follow-up is needed to determine outcomes relative to conventional clear cell RCC.

## Renal Carcinoid Tumor

## Introduction

Less than 1 % of carcinoid tumors arise in the genitourinary system, with the testes and ovaries being the most common locations, followed by the kidneys [85]. Primary renal carcinoid tumor of the kidney is very rare, and less than 100 cases are reported in the literature [5, 86]. Age of diagnosis is broad, ranging from 13 to 79 years [86, 87]. There is an equal male-to-female distribution [5]. Intrinsic neuroendocrine cells in normal kidneys have not been reported previously; however, the pathogenesis of renal carcinoid tumors is controversial [86]. Carcinoid tumors in the kidney have been suggested to occur in patients with underlying renal congenital or acquired anomalies such as horseshoe kidney and mature teratoma [86, 88, 89]. These tumors demonstrate distinct morphological features from small cell carcinoma, which have also been reported to occur in pure form in the renal cortex [90, 91] or associated with invasive urothelial carcinoma of the renal pelvis [92].

## Clinical Presentation

Patients may present with abdominal pain or fullness, gross hematuria, and evidence of carcinoid syndrome, including serotonin-related flushing, edema, and less frequently diarrhea [5, 86, 93]. The diagnosis of primary renal carcinoid tumor is incidental in 25–30 % of cases [86, 94]. Imaging studies show a heterogeneous tumor, with solid and cystic components. Calcification has been reported in ~1/4 of cases [86, 95]. The tumors show minimal enhancement by CT imaging [86, 96].

## Pathology

On gross evaluation, renal carcinoid tumor is well circumscribed and soft and shows a homogenous white-yellow cut surface. Calcifications, hemorrhage, and cystic change may be present [5, 86]. On microscopic review, tumor cells can show ribbonlike, trabecular, rosette-like, and rarely nested patterns (Fig. 9.8a) [5, 86]. Tumor cells have a monotonous appearance. Nuclei are relatively uniform and round and contain finely

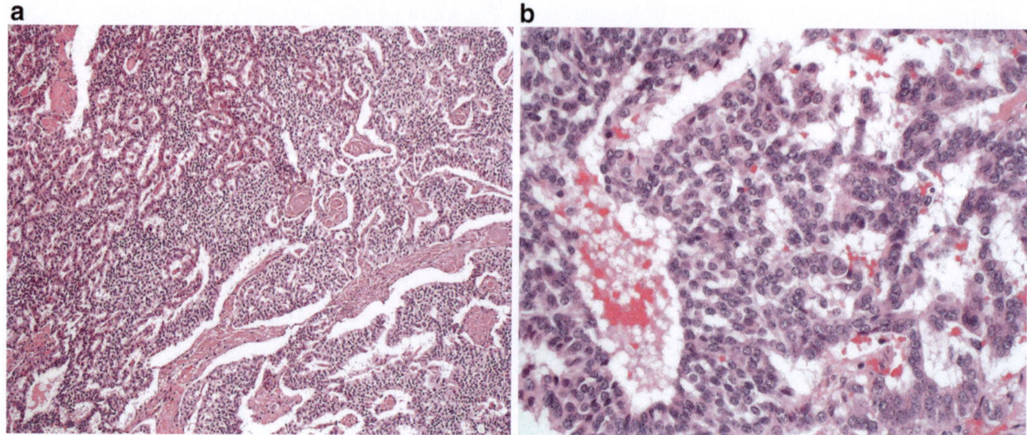

**Fig. 9.8** Renal carcinoid tumor. (**a**) This example shows both trabecular and nested growth patterns. (**b**) Nuclei show the characteristic granular chromatin pattern associated with carcinoid lesions

granular chromatin (Fig. 9.8b) [5, 86, 89]. Rarely, moderate nuclear atypia or mitotic figures can be identified.

The genetic profile of renal carcinoid tumor has not been defined due to a small number of cases studied. One study has reported heterozygosity of 3p21 [5, 97].

The immunohistochemical profile of renal carcinoid is similar to neuroendocrine tumors in other locations. Synaptophysin and chromogranin are positive in the majority of tumors [5, 89, 98]. In addition, tumor cells can show dot-like immunoreactivity for CAM5.2 and may be positive for vimentin and cytokeratin 7 [89]. Renal carcinoid tumor is negative for TTF-1, WT-1, PAX2, and PAX8 [5, 89, 98].

Renal carcinoid tumor should be differentiated from other lesions that demonstrate neuroendocrine features, including small cell carcinoma, primitive neuroectodermal tumor (PNET), pheochromocytoma, and neuroblastoma. Small cell carcinoma is distinguished by the presence of classic features that include frequent mitotic features, apoptotic debris, necrosis, and nuclear molding. Morphology and clinical information is most helpful, as CD99, and typical neuroendocrine markers will not distinguish these entities [89, 98]. S100 immunostain may be helpful when neuroblastoma

and pheochromocytoma (sustentacular cells) are in the differential diagnosis. Metastases from other primary sites (such as the gastrointestinal tract) should be clinically excluded. Of note, PAX8 expression supports the diagnosis of a metastatic carcinoid as primary renal carcinoids have been shown to be negative for PAX8, whereas a subset of GI primary carcinoid tumors are positive for polyclonal PAX8 [98–100].

## Prognosis and Clinical Management

Distant metastases to the liver, bone, and orbit have been reported [82, 85, 86, 89].

## References


1. Srigley JR, Delahunt B, Eble JN, Egevad L, Epstein JI, Grignon D, et al. The International Society of Urological Pathology (ISUP) Vancouver classification of renal neoplasia. Am J Surg Pathol. 2013;37(10):1469–89.
2. Eble J, Sauter G, Epstein J, et al. Pathology and genetics of tumours of the urinary system and male genital organs. Lyon: IARC; 2004.
3. Motzer RJ, Jonasch E, Agarwal N, Beard C, Bhayani S, Bolger GB, et al. Kidney cancer, version 3.2015. J Natl Compr Canc Netw. 2015;13(2):151–9.

4. Motzer RJ, Hutson TE, Tomczak P, Michaelson MD, Bukowski RM, Rixe O, et al. Sunitinib versus interferon alfa in metastatic renal-cell carcinoma. N Engl J Med. 2007;356(2):115–24.

5. Hansel DE, Zhou M. Practical renal pathology, a diagnostic approach. 1st ed. Philadelphia: Elsevier Saunders; 2013. p. 1–22.

6. Crumley SM, Divatia M, Truong L, Shen S, Ayala AG, Ro JY. Renal cell carcinoma: evolving and emerging subtypes. World J Clin Cases. 2013;1(9):262–75.

7. MacLennan GT, Bostwick DG. Tubulocystic carcinoma, mucinous tubular and spindle cell carcinoma, and other recently described rare renal tumors. Clin Lab Med. 2005;25(2):393–416.

8. MacLennan GT, Farrow GM, Bostwick DG. Low-grade collecting duct carcinoma of the kidney: report of 13 cases of low-grade mucinous tubulocystic renal carcinoma of possible collecting duct origin. Urology. 1997;50(5):679–84.

9. Eble JN. Mucinous tubular and spindle cell carcinoma and post-neuroblastoma carcinoma: newly recognised entities in the renal cell carcinoma family. Pathology. 2003;35(6):499–504.

10. Hes O, Hora M, Perez-Montiel DM, Suster S, Curík R, Sokol L, et al. Spindle and cuboidal renal cell carcinoma, a tumor having frequent association with nephrolithiasis: report of 11 cases including a case with hybrid conventional renal cell carcinoma/ spindle and cuboidal renal cell carcinoma components. Histopathology. 2002;41(6):549–55.

11. Prasad SR, Humphrey PA, Catena JR, Narra VR, Srigley JR, Cortez AD, et al. Common and uncommon histologic subtypes of renal cell carcinoma: imaging spectrum with pathologic correlation. Radiographics. 2006;26(6):1795–806.

12. Sahni VA, Hirsch MS, Sadow CA, Silverman SG. Mucinous tubular and spindle cell carcinoma of the kidney: imaging features. Cancer Imaging. 2012;12:66–71.

13. Ursani NA, Robertson AR, Schieman SM, Bainbridge T, Srigley JR. Mucinous tubular and spindle cell carcinoma of kidney without sarcomatoid change showing metastases to liver and retroperitoneal lymph node. Hum Pathol. 2011;42(3):444–8.

14. Bulimbasic S, Ljubanovic D, Sima R, Michal M, Hes O, Kuroda N, et al. Aggressive high-grade mucinous tubular and spindle cell carcinoma. Hum Pathol. 2009;40(6):906–7.

15. Pillay N, Ramdial PK, Cooper K, Batuule D. Mucinous tubular and spindle cell carcinoma with aggressive histomorphology – a sarcomatoid variant. Hum Pathol. 2008;39(6):966–9.

16. Rakozy C, Schmahl GE, Bogner S, Störkel S. Low-grade tubular-mucinous renal neoplasms: morphologic, immunohistochemical, and genetic features. Mod Pathol. 2002;15(11):1162–71.

17. Cossu-Rocca P, Eble JN, Delahunt B, Zhang S, Martignoni G, Brunelli M, et al. Renal mucinous tubular and spindle carcinoma lacks the gains of chromosomes 7 and 17 and losses of chromosome Y that are prevalent in papillary renal cell carcinoma. Mod Pathol. 2006;19(4):488–93.

18. Ferlicot S, Allory Y, Comperat E, Mege-Lechevalier F, Dimet S, Sibony M, et al. Mucinous tubular and spindle cell carcinoma: a report of 15 cases and a review of the literature. Virchows Arch. 2005;447(6):978–83.

19. Paner GP, Srigley JR, Radhakrishnan A, Cohen C, Skinnider BF, Tickoo SK, et al. Immunohistochemical analysis of mucinous tubular and spindle cell carcinoma and papillary renal cell carcinoma of the kidney: significant immunophenotypic overlap warrants diagnostic caution. Am J Surg Pathol. 2006;30(1):13–9.

20. Kuroda N, Toi M, Hiroi M, Shuin T, Enzan H. Review of mucinous tubular and spindle-cell carcinoma of the kidney with a focus on clinical and pathobiological aspects. Histol Histopathol. 2005;20(1):221–4.

21. Parwani AV, Husain AN, Epstein JI, Beckwith JB, Argani P. Low-grade myxoid renal epithelial neoplasms with distal nephron differentiation. Hum Pathol. 2001;32(5):506–12.

22. Shen SS, Ro JY, Tamboli P, Truong LD, Zhai Q, Jung SJ, et al. Mucinous tubular and spindle cell carcinoma of kidney is probably a variant of papillary renal cell carcinoma with spindle cell features. Ann Diagn Pathol. 2007;11(1):13–21.

23. Thway K, du Parcq J, Larkin JM, Fisher C, Livni N. Metastatic renal mucinous tubular and spindle cell carcinoma. Atypical behavior of a rare, morphologically bland tumor. Ann Diagn Pathol. 2012;16(5):407–10.

24. Kuroda N, Hes O, Michal M, Nemcova J, Gal V, Yamaguchi T, et al. Mucinous tubular and spindle cell carcinoma with Fuhrman nuclear grade 3: a histological, immunohistochemical, ultrastructural and FISH study. Histol Histopathol. 2008;23(12):1517–23.

25. Simon RA, di Sant'agnese PA, Palapattu GS, Singer EA, Candelario GD, Huang J, et al. Mucinous tubular and spindle cell carcinoma of the kidney with sarcomatoid differentiation. Int J Clin Exp Pathol. 2008;1(2):180–4.

26. Williamson SR, Eble JN, Cheng L, Grignon DJ. Clear cell papillary renal cell carcinoma: differential diagnosis and extended immunohistochemical profile. Mod Pathol. 2013;26(5):697–708.

27. Zhou H, Zheng S, Truong LD, Ro JY, Ayala AG, Shen SS. Clear cell papillary renal cell carcinoma is the fourth most common histologic type of renal cell carcinoma in 290 consecutive nephrectomies for renal cell carcinoma. Hum Pathol. 2014;45(1):59–64.

28. Alexiev BA, Drachenberg CB. Clear cell papillary renal cell carcinoma: incidence, morphological features, immunohistochemical profile, and biologic behavior—a single institution study. Pathol Res Pract. 2014;210(4):234–41.

29. Tickoo SK, de Peralta-Venturina MN, Harik LR, Worcester HD, Salama ME, Young AN, et al.

Spectrum of epithelial neoplasms in end-stage renal disease: an experience from 66 tumor-bearing kidneys with emphasis on histologic patterns distinct from those in sporadic adult renal neoplasia. Am J Surg Pathol. 2006;30:141–53.

30. Gobbo S, Eble JN, Grignon DJ, Martignoni G, MacLennan GT, Shah RB, et al. Clear cell papillary renal cell carcinoma: a distinct histopathologic and molecular genetic entity. Am J Surg Pathol. 2008;32:1239–45.

31. Aydin H, Chen L, Cheng L, Vaziri S, He H, Ganapathi R, et al. Clear cell tubulopapillary renal cell carcinoma: a study of 36 distinctive low-grade epithelial tumors of the kidney. Am J Surg Pathol. 2010;34(11):1608–21.

32. Aron M, Chang E, Herrera L, Hes O, Hirsch MS, Comperat E, et al. Clear cell-papillary renal cell carcinoma of the kidney not associated with end-stage renal disease: clinicopathologic correlation with expanded immunophenotypic and molecular characterization of a large cohort with emphasis on relationship with renal angiomyoadenomatous tumor. Am J Surg Pathol. 2015;39(7):873–88.

33. Deml KF, Schildhaus HU, Compérat E, von Teichman A, Storz M, Schraml P, et al. Clear cell papillary renal cell carcinoma and renal angiomyoadenomatous tumor: two variants of a morphologic, immunohistochemical, and genetic distinct entity of renal cell carcinoma. Am J Surg Pathol. 2015;39(7):889–901.

34. Park JH, Lee C, Suh JH, Moon KC. Clear cell papillary renal cell carcinoma: a report of 15 cases including three cases of concurrent other-type renal cell carcinomas. Korean J Pathol. 2012;46(6):541–7.

35. Michal M, Hes O, Nemcova J, Sima R, Kuroda N, Bulimbasic S, et al. Renal angiomyoadenomatous tumor: morphologic, immunohistochemical, and molecular genetic study of a distinct entity. Virchows Arch. 2009;454(1):89–99.

36. Fisher KE, Yin-Goen Q, Alexis D, Sirintrapun JS, Harrison W, Benjamin Isett R, et al. Gene expression profiling of clear cell papillary renal cell carcinoma: comparison with clear cell renal cell carcinoma and papillary renal cell carcinoma. Mod Pathol. 2014;27(2):222–30.

37. Rohan SM, Xiao Y, Liang Y, Dudas ME, Al-Ahmadie HA, Fine SW, et al. Clear-cell papillary renal cell carcinoma: molecular and immunohistochemical analysis with emphasis on the von Hippel-Lindau gene and hypoxia-inducible factor pathway-related proteins. Mod Pathol. 2011;24:1207–20.

38. Munari E, Marchionni L, Chitre A, Hayashi M, Martignoni G, Brunelli M, et al. Clear cell papillary renal cell carcinoma: micro-RNA expression profiling and comparison with clear cell renal cell carcinoma and papillary renal cell carcinoma. Hum Pathol. 2014;45(6):1130–8.

39. Lawrie CH, Larrea E, Larrinaga G, Goicoechea I, Arestin M, Fernandez-Mercado M, et al. Targeted next-generation sequencing and non-coding RNA expression analysis of clear cell papillary renal cell carcinoma suggests distinct pathological mechanisms from other renal tumour subtypes. J Pathol. 2014;232(1):32–42.

40. Adam J, Couturier J, Molinié V, Vieillefond A, Sibony M. Clear-cell papillary renal cell carcinoma: 24 cases of a distinct low-grade renal tumour and a comparative genomic hybridization array study of seven cases. Histopathology. 2011;58:1064–71.

41. Inoue T, Matsuura K, Yoshimoto T, Nguyen LT, Tsukamoto Y, Nakada C, et al. Genomic profiling of renal cell carcinoma in patients with end-stage renal disease. Cancer Sci. 2012;103(3):569–76.

42. Kuroda N, Ohe C, Kawakami F, Mikami S, Furuya M, Matsuura K, et al. Clear cell papillary renal cell carcinoma: a review. Int J Clin Exp Pathol. 2014;7(11):7312–8.

43. Osunkoya AO, Young AN, Wang W, Netto GJ, Epstein JI. Comparison of gene expression profiles in tubulocystic carcinoma and collecting duct carcinoma of the kidney. Am J Surg Pathol. 2009;33:1103–6.

44. Yang XJ, Zhou M, Hes O, Shen S, Li R, Lopez J, et al. Tubulocystic carcinoma of the kidney: clinicopathologic and molecular characterization. Am J Surg Pathol. 2008;32:177–87.

45. Zhou M, Yang XJ, Lopez JI, Shah RB, Hes O, Shen SS, et al. Renal tubulocystic carcinoma is closely related to papillary renal cell carcinoma: implications for pathologic classification. Am J Surg Pathol. 2009;33:1840–9.

46. Quiroga-Garza G, Piña-Oviedo S, Cuevas-Ocampo K, Goldfarb R, Schwartz MR, Ayala AG, et al. Synchronous clear cell renal cell carcinoma and tubulocystic carcinoma: genetic evidence of independent ontogenesis and implications of chromosomal imbalances in tumor progression. Diagn Pathol. 2012;7:21.

47. Bhullar JS, Varshney N, Bhullar AK, Mittal VK. A new type of renal cancer-tubulocystic carcinoma of the kidney: a review of the literature. Int J Surg Pathol. 2013;22(4):297–302.

48. Hora M, Michal M, Hes O. Cystic nephroma and mixed epithelial and stromal tumour of the kidney: opposite ends of the spectrum of the same entity? Eur Urol. 2008;54:1237–46.

49. Kryvenko ON, Jorda M, Argani P, Epstein JI. Diagnostic approach to eosinophilic renal neoplasms. Arch Pathol Lab Med. 2014; 138(11):1531–41.

50. Alexiev BA, Drachenberg CB. Tubulocystic carcinoma of the kidney: a histologic, immunohistochemical, and ultrastructural study. Virchows Arch. 2013;462(5):575–81.

51. Amin MB, MacLennan GT, Gupta R, Grignon D, Paraf F, Vieillefond A, et al. Tubulocystic carcinoma of the kidney: clinicopathologic analysis of 31 cases of a distinctive rare subtypeof renal cell carcinoma. Am J Surg Pathol. 2009;33:384–92.

52. Bhullar JS, Thamboo T, Esuvaranathan K. Unique case of tubulocystic carcinoma of the kidney with sarcomatoid features: a new entity. Urology. 2011;78(5):1071–2.

53. Chen N, Nie L, Gong J, Chen X, Xu M, Chen M, et al. Gains of chromosomes 7 and 17 in tubulocystic carcinoma of kidney: two cases with fluorescence in situ hybridisation analysis. J Clin Pathol. 2014;67(11):1006–9.

54. Azoulay S, Vieillefond A, Paraf F, et al. Tubulocystic carcinoma of the kidney: a new entity among renal tumors. Virchows Arch. 2007;451:905–9.

55. Eble JN, Bonsib SM. Extensively cystic renal neoplasms: cystic nephroma, cystic partially differential nephroblastoma, multi-locular cyst renal cell carcinoma, and cystic hamartoma of renal pelvis. Semin Diagn Pathol. 1998;15:2–20.

56. Al-Hussain TO, Cheng L, Zhang S, Epstein JI. Tubulocystic carcinoma of the kidney with poorly differentiated foci: a series of 3 cases with fluorescence in situ hybridization analysis. Hum Pathol. 2013;44(7):1406–11.

57. Denton MD, Magee CC, Ovuworie C, Mauiyyedi S, Pascual M, Colvin RB, et al. Prevalence of renal cell carcinoma in patients with ESRD pre-transplantation: a pathologic analysis. Kidney Int. 2002;61:2201–9.

58. Hughson MD, Buchwald D, Fox M. Renal neoplasia and acquired cystic kidney disease in patients receiving longterm dialysis. Arch Pathol Lab Med. 1986;110:592–601.

59. Sule N, Yakupoglu U, Shen SS, Krishnan B, Yang G, Lerner S, et al. Calcium oxalate deposition in renal cell carcinoma associated with acquired cystic kidney disease: a comprehensive study. Am J Surg Pathol. 2005;29:443–51.

60. Pan CC, Chen YJ, Chang LC, Chang YH, Ho DM. Immunohistochemical and molecular genetic profiling of acquire cystic disease-associated renal cell carcinoma. Histopathology. 2009;55:145–53.

61. Kuroda N, Tamura M, Taguchi T, Tominaga A, Hes O, Michal M, et al. Sarcomatoid acquired cystic disease-associated renal cell carcinoma. Histol Histopathol. 2008;23:1327–31.

62. Ishikawa I, Saito Y, Asaka M, Tomosugi N, Yuri T, Watanabe M, et al. Twenty-year follow-up of acquired renal cystic disease. Clin Nephrol. 2003;59:153–9.

63. Medeiros LJ, Palmedo G, Krigman HR, et al. Oncocytoid renal cell carcinoma after neuroblastoma: a report of four cases of a distinct clinicopathologic entity. Am J Surg Pathol. 1999;23(7):772–80.

64. Kuroda N, Tamura M, Hamaguchi N, Mikami S, Pan CC, Brunelli M, et al. Acquired cystic disease-associated renal cell carcinoma with sarcomatoid change and rhabdoid features. Ann Diagn Pathol. 2011;15(6):462–6.

65. Bhatnagar R, Alexiev BA. Renal-cell carcinomas in end-stage kidneys: a clinicopathological study with emphasis on clear-cell papillary renal-cell carcinoma and acquired cystic kidney disease-associated carcinoma. Int J Surg Pathol. 2012;20(1):19–28.

66. Fleitz JM, Wootton-Gorges SL, Wyatt-Ashmead J, McGavran L, Koyle M, West DC, et al. Renal cell carcinoma in long-term survivors of advanced stage neuroblastoma in early childhood. Pediatr Radiol. 2003;33(8):540–5.

67. Altinok G, Kattar MM, Mohamed A, Poulik J, Grignon D, Rabah R. Pediatric renal carcinoma associated with Xp11.2 translocations/TFE3 gene fusions and clinicopathologic associations. Pediatr Dev Pathol. 2005;8(2):168–80.

68. Koyle MA, Hatch DA, Furness PD, et al. Long-term urological complications in survivors younger than 15 months of advanced stage abdominal neuroblastoma. J Urol. 2001;166(4):1455–8.

69. Hedgepeth RC, Zhou M, Ross J. Rapid development of metastatic Xp11 translocation renal cell carcinoma in a girl treated for neuroblastoma. J Pediatr Hematol Oncol. 2009;31(8):602–4.

70. Vogelzang NJ, Yang X, Goldman S, et al. Radiation induced renal cell cancer: a report of 4 cases and review of the literature. J Urol. 1998;160(6 Pt 1):1987–90.

71. Ghaouti M, Roquet L, Baron M, Pfister C, Sabourin JC. Thyroid-like follicular carcinoma of the kidney: a case report and review of the literature. Diagn Pathol. 2014;9:186.

72. Jung SJ, Chung JI, Park SH, Ayala AG, Ro JY. Thyroid follicular carcinoma-like tumor of kidney: a case report with morphologic, immunohistochemical, and genetic analysis. Am J Surg Pathol. 2006;30:411–5.

73. Amin MB, Gupta R, Ondrej H, McKenney JK, Michal M, Young AN, et al. Primary thyroidlike follicular carcinoma of the kidney: report of 6 cases of a histologically distinctive adult epithelial neoplasm. Am J Surg Pathol. 2009;33:393–400.

74. Khoja HA, Almutawa A, Binmahfooz A, Aslam M, Ghazi AA, Almaiman S. Papillary thyroid carcinoma-like tumor of the kidney: a case report. Int J Surg Pathol. 2012;20:411–5.

75. Malde S, Sheikh I, Woodman I, Fish D, Bilagi P, Sheriff MK. Primary thyroid-like follicular renal cell carcinoma: an emerging entity. Case Rep Pathol. 2013;2013:687427.

76. Argani P, Olgac S, Tickoo SK, Goldfischer M, Moch H, Chan DY, et al. Xp11 translocation renal cell carcinoma in adults: expanded clinical, pathologic, and genetic spectrum. Am J Surg Pathol. 2007;31:1149–60.

77. Srigley J. Mucinous tubular and spindle cell carcinoma. In: Eble J, Sauter G, Epstein J, Sesterhenn I, editors. Pathology and genetics of tumours of the urinary system and male genital organs. Lyon: IARC; 2004. p. 40.

78. Williamson SR, Eble JN, Amin MB, Gupta NS, Smith SC, Sholl LM, et al. Succinate dehydrogenase-deficient renal cell carcinoma: detailed characterization

of 11 tumors defining a unique subtype of renal cell carcinoma. Mod Pathol. 2015;28(1):80–94.

79. Gill AJ et al. Succinate dehydrogenase (SDH)-deficient renal carcinoma: a morphologically distinct entity: a clinicopathologic series of 36 tumors from 27 patients. Am J Surg Pathol. 2014;38(12):1588–602.

80. Henderson A, Douglas F, Perros P, et al. SDHB-associated renal oncocytoma suggests a broadening of the renal phenotype in hereditary paragangliomatosis. Fam Cancer. 2009;8:257–60.

81. Gill AJ, Pachter NS, Chou A, et al. Renal tumors associated with germline SDHB mutation show distinctive morphology. Am J Surg Pathol. 2011;35:1578–85.

82. Hakimi AA, Tickoo SK, Jacobsen A, Sarungbam J, Sfakianos JP, Sato Y, et al. TCEB1-mutated renal cell carcinoma: a distinct genomic and morphological subtype. Mod Pathol. 2015;28(6):845–53.

83. Hirsch MS, Barletta J, Gorman M, Dal Cin P. Renal cell carcinoma with monosomy 8 and CAIX expression: a distinct entity or another member or the clear cell tubulopapillary RCC/RAT family. Mod Pathol. 2015;28(S2):229A.

84. Sato Y, Yoshizato T, Shiraishi Y, Maekawa S, Okuno Y, Kamura T, et al. Integrated molecular analysis of clear-cell renal cell carcinoma. Nat Genet. 2013;45(8):860–7.

85. Parikh D, Shinder R. Primary renal carcinoid metastatic to the orbit. Ophthal Plast Reconstr Surg. 2015;31(2):e37–8.

86. Tanaka T, Yamamoto H, Imai A, Shingo H, Yoneyama T, Koie T, et al. A case of primary renal carcinoid tumor. Case Rep Urol. 2015;2015:736213.

87. Krishnan B, Truong LD, Saleh G, Sirbasku DM, Slawin KM. Horseshoe kidney is associated with an increased relative risk of primary renal carcinoid tumor. J Urol. 1997;157(6):2059–66.

88. McCaffrey JA, Reuter V, Herr HW, Macapinlac HA, Russo P, Motzer RJ. Carcinoid tumor of the kidney: the use of somatostatin receptor scintigraphy in diagnosis and management. Urol Oncol. 2000;5(3):108–11.

89. Hansel DE, Epstein JI, Berbescu E, Fine SW, Young RH, Cheville JC. Renal carcinoid tumor: a clinicopathologic study of 21 cases. Am J Surg Pathol. 2007;31(10):1539–44.

90. Si Q, Dancer J, Stanton ML, Tamboli P, Ro JY, Czerniak BA, et al. Small cell carcinoma of the kidney: a clinicopathologic study of 14 cases. Hum Pathol. 2011;42(11):1792–8.

91. Kuroda N, Imamura Y, Hamashima T, Ohe C, Mikami S, Nagashima Y, et al. Review of small cell carcinoma of the kidney with focus on clinical and pathobiological aspects. Pol J Pathol. 2014;65(1):15–9.

92. Miller RJ, Holmäng S, Johansson SL, Lele SM. Small cell carcinoma of the renal pelvis and ureter: clinicopathologic and immunohistochemical features. Arch Pathol Lab Med. 2011;135(12):1565–9.

93. Raslan WF, Ro JY, Ordonez NG, et al. Primary carcinoid of the kidney. Immunohistochemical and ultrastructural studies of five patients. Cancer. 1993;72(9):2660–6.

94. Murali R, Kneale K, Lalak N, Delprado W. Carcinoid tumors of the urinary tract and prostate. Arch Pathol Lab Med. 2006;130(11):1693–706.

95. Romero FR, Rais-Bahrami S, Permpongkosol S, Fine SW, Kohanim S, Jarrett TW. Primary carcinoid tumors of the kidney. J Urol. 2006;176(6):2359–66.

96. Kurl S, RytkÅNonen H, Farin P, Ala-Opas M, Soimakallio S. A primary carcinoid tumor of the kidney: a case report and review of the literature. Abdom Imaging. 1996;21(5):464–7.

97. El-Naggar AK, Troncoso P, Ordonez NG. Primary renal carcinoid tumor with molecular abnormality characteristic of conventional renal cell neoplasms. Diagn Mol Pathol. 1995;4(1):48–53.

98. Jeung JA, Cao D, Selli BW, Clapp WL, Oliai BR, Parwani AV, et al. Primary renal carcinoid tumors: clinicopathologic features of 9 cases with emphasis on novel immunohistochemical findings. Hum Pathol. 2011;42(10):1554–61.

99. Long KB, Srivastava A, Hirsch MS, Hornick JL. PAX8 expression in well-differentiated pancreatic endocrine tumors: correlation with clinicopathologic features and comparison with gastrointestinal and pulmonary carcinoid tumors. Am J Surg Pathol. 2010;34(5):723–9.

100. Sangoi AR, Ohgami RS, Pai RK, Beck AH, McKenney JK, Pai RK. PAX8 expression reliably distinguishes pancreatic well-differentiated neuroendocrine tumors from ileal and pulmonary well-differentiated neuroendocrine tumors and pancreatic acinar cell carcinoma. Mod Pathol. 2011;24(3):412–24.

Chad R. Ritch, Giovanna A. Giannico,
Lan L. Gellert, Peter E. Clark, and Omar Hameed


## Introduction

The International Society of Urological Pathology (ISUP)/Vancouver classification of renal neoplasms lists over 50 histologic types of non-epithelial neoplasms. [1] These primarily include mesenchymal, hematopoietic, and neuro-endocrine neoplasms, as well as a few others of different origin/histogenesis. In this chapter, we present a subset of the more common of these lesions, with emphasis on differential treatment when relevant.


C.R. Ritch, M.D., M.B.A.
Department of Urology, University of Miami, Miami, FL 33129, USA
e-mail: critch@miami.edu

G.A. Giannico, M.D. • L.L. Gellert, M.D., Ph.D.
Department of Pathology, Microbiology and Immunology, Vanderbilt University Medical Center, Nashville, TN 37232, USA
e-mail: giovanna.giannico@vanderbilt.edu;
Lan.Gellert@vanderbilt.edu

P.E. Clark, M.D.
Department of Urologic Surgery, Vanderbilt University Medical Center, Nashville, TN 37232, USA
e-mail: peter.clark@vanderbilt.edu

O. Hameed, M.D. (✉)
Department of Pathology, Microbiology and Immunology, Vanderbilt University Medical Center, Nashville, TN 37232, USA

Department of Urologic Surgery, Vanderbilt University Medical Center, Nashville, TN 37232, USA
e-mail: omar.hameed@vanderbilt.edu


## Mesenchymal Neoplasms

Mesenchymal tumors in the kidney, similar to other parts of the body, cover a wide spectrum with characteristic morphogenesis, histological findings, and variable behaviors [2]. These have been classified into those predominantly occurring in children (see Chap. 11) and those predominantly in adults [1]. The latter include mostly benign neoplasms such as angiomyolipoma, leiomyoma, hemangioma, lymphangioma, juxtaglomerular cell tumor, renomedullary interstitial cell tumor, schwannoma and solitary fibrous tumor, as well as malignant neoplasms that include leiomyosarcoma, angiosarcoma, rhabdomyosarcoma, malignant fibrous histiocytoma, osteosarcoma, and synovial sarcoma [1, 3]. The clinical presentation of non-epithelial neoplasms is related to both the histological type and size, although the majority of these neoplasms are regardless detected incidentally by imaging, usually with computed tomography (CT) scan imaging as the diagnostic modality of choice.


© Springer Science+Business Media New York 2016
D.E. Hansel et al. (eds.), *The Kidney*, DOI 10.1007/978-1-4939-3286-3_10

## Benign Mesenchymal Tumors

### Angiomyolipoma (AML)

Sporadic renal angiomyolipoma (AML) is usually solitary and has been described in 0.3–2.1 % of kidneys in autopsy studies [4], whereas they tend to be multiple and develop in approximately 55–75 % of patients with tuberous sclerosis complex (TSC) [5]. TSC is an autosomal dominant multiorgan genetic disease caused by mutations in either the *TSC1* (chromosome 9q) or *TSC2* (chromosome 16p) tumor suppressor genes and associated loss of their respective gene products, hamartin and tuberin, which through the mTOR pathway result in growth/progression of TSC lesions. AML is more common in females, occurring at approximately 50 years of age and about two decades earlier in patients with TSC. Angiomyolipomas are often asymptomatic, although larger angiomyolipomas can be associated with bleeding that results in anemia and, in severe acute cases, hemodynamic instability.

On imaging, the classic appearance is that of a solid enhancing lesion with contrast injection; however, this is not always the case. Unless liposarcoma is in the differential diagnosis (often suggested by the presence of a large, rapidly growing mass), the latter finding is considered pathognomonic for AML. However, roughly 4 % may not have macroscopic fat and may be indistinguishable from renal cell carcinoma (RCC) [6]. Pixel mapping is a technique which may be applied on CT to distinguish minimal fat containing AML from RCC [7]. The general principle involves outlining the region of interest on CT to analyze the attenuation levels of each pixel in that region, and if the range of pixel attenuation falls within −30 to −120HU, the diagnosis of AML might be suspected. While there is no standard on the number of pixels to make the diagnosis, Simpfendorfer et al. demonstrated that 20 or more pixels with less than −20HU and 5 pixels with less than −30HU have a positive predictive value of 100 % [7]. However, others have found that pixel mapping may not be reliable in distinguishing AML from RCC [8]. On sonography, AML appears as a uniformly hyperechoic lesion without a hypoechoic rim and may have increased vascularity [6]. Loss of signal intensity on magnetic resonance imaging during the fat sequence may help demonstrate the presence of macroscopic fat and support the diagnosis of AML [6].

On gross examination, AML is usually well circumscribed but not encapsulated and varies in size from 0.5 to 25 cm. Microscopically, AML is a triphasic neoplasm containing varying amounts of adipose tissue, smooth muscle, and abnormally structured blood vessels. Vessels typically show smooth muscle hypertrophy and eccentric lumina and lack a well-developed internal elastic lamina (Fig. 10.1). Monomorphic (spindle cell/fat-poor) (Fig. 10.2) or predominantly lipomatous (Fig. 10.3) forms may occur. Lymphatic, vascular, and lymph node involvement can be present and has not been shown to be of prognostic significance [9, 10]. Other morphologic variants of AML include oncocytoma-like angiomyolipoma [11], angiomyolipoma with epithelial cysts [12], microscopic angiomyolipoma, and so-called intraglomerular microlesions [13]. The few reported examples of such variants have been associated with benign outcomes.

Immunohistochemically, AMLs express melanocytic markers (HMB-45, Melan-A/MART-1, microphthalmia transcription factor, and tyrosinase), smooth muscle markers (smooth muscle actin, h-caldesmon), and cathepsin K and are typically negative for keratins or other epithelial markers and PAX8. This immunoprofile is very useful in the distinction of AML from other differential diagnostic considerations.

Classic AML is associated with a benign outcome. Treatment consists primarily of surgical resection, although percutaneous renal biopsy can be used to establish a diagnosis and potentially obviate the need for surgery.

### Epithelioid Angiomyolipoma

Epithelioid angiomyolipoma is identified on histological review and is characterized by the presence of plump epithelioid stromal cells. Two major morphologic patterns, which may occur pure or in combination, have been described: (a) carcinoma-like

**Fig. 10.1** Classic angiomyolipoma with various amounts of adipose tissue, smooth muscle, and thickened vessels (Hematoxylin eosin, 20×)

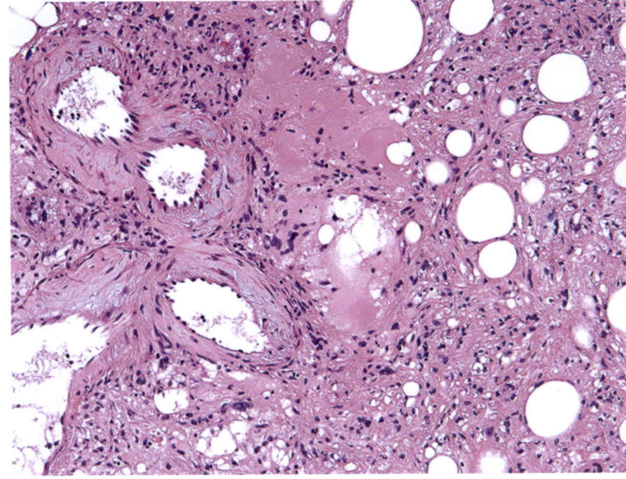

**Fig. 10.2** Spindle cell variant of angiomyolipoma with a predominant smooth muscle component without significant fat (Hematoxylin eosin, 20×)

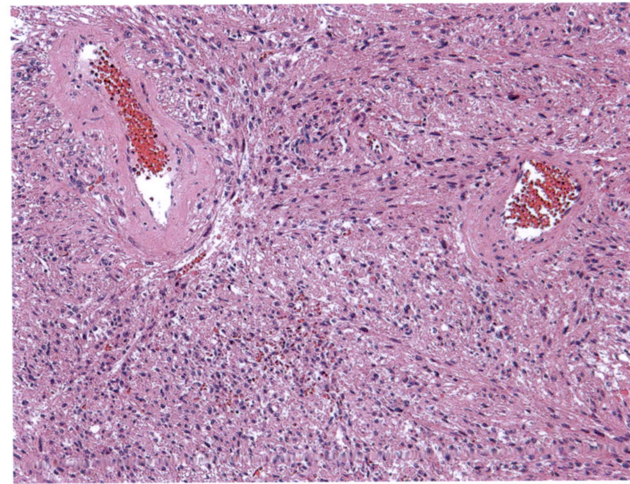

**Fig. 10.3** Predominantly lipomatous angiomyolipoma (Hematoxylin eosin, 10×)

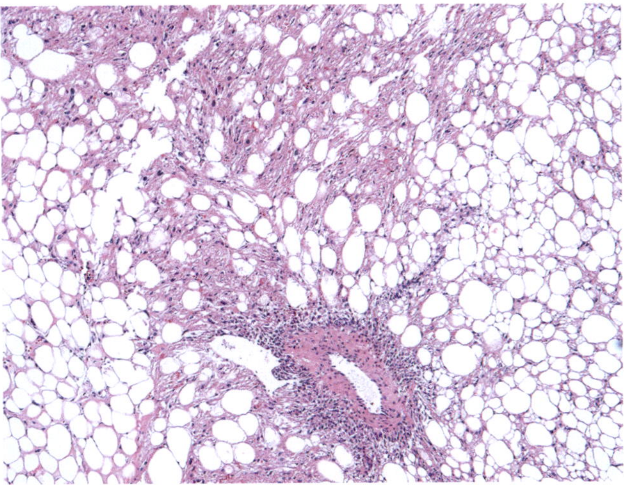

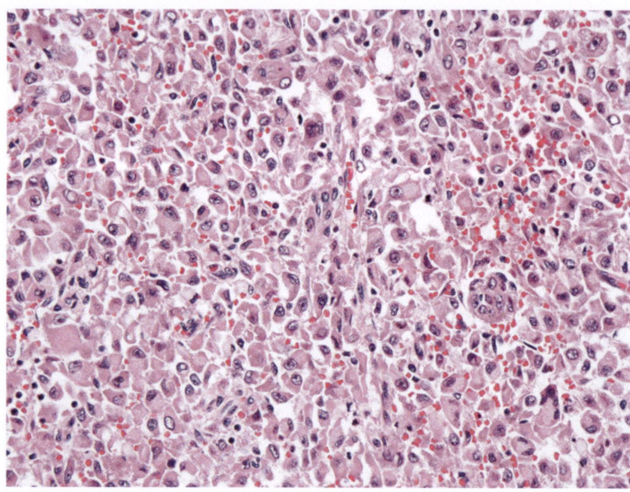

**Fig. 10.4** Epithelioid angiomyolipoma with diffuse sheets of discohesive, plump, epithelioid cells (Hematoxylin eosin, 20×)

growth, characterized by large cells arranged in cohesive nests, alveoli, and sheets with intervening thin fibrovascular septa, and (b) epithelioid and plump spindle cells in diffuse growth [14] (Fig. 10.4). Compared to tumors with predominant spindle histology, epithelioid AML tends to show less smooth muscle marker expression with more widespread melanocytic marker expression as well as estrogen receptor expression [15].

In contrast to classic AML, a series of 34 cases of epithelioid AML with available follow-up showed malignant behavior in 26 % of cases [16]. Another study of 31 cases showed recurrence or metastasis in 17 and 49 % of patients, respectively [14]. Larger tumor size, invasion outside the kidney, a carcinoma-like growth pattern, significant/diffuse nuclear atypia, and necrosis were among the factors associated with disease progression [14, 16].

## Leiomyoma

Leiomyomas may arise from the renal capsule (most common), from muscularis of the renal pelvis, or from cortical vascular smooth muscle [17–19]. Most patients are adults and can present with pain or an abdominal/flank mass. Tumor size is variable, with one series reporting an average of 12 cm [18], while the morphology is quite bland with sparse mitotic activity. Calcification and cystic change have been described, but necrosis should not be present. As expected, leiomyomas express smooth muscle markers, but not melanocytic markers. The latter is of value in the distinction from the more common lipid-poor AMLs.

## Hemangioma

Hemangiomas occasionally arise in the kidney and appear as capillary [20, 21] or cavernous blood-filled vascular spaces lined by a single layer of endothelial cells. Although certain hemangiomas can exhibit an infiltrative growth pattern, they lack the mitosis and nuclear pleomorphism seen in angiosarcoma.

## Solitary Fibrous Tumor

Frequently arising in extrathoracic sites, this tumor can occasionally arise in the kidney. It characteristically exhibits fibroblastic differentiation with a prominent staghorn-like branching vascular pattern and areas of collagen deposition. In contrast to solitary fibrous tumors elsewhere that can be malignant, almost all of those arising in the kidney have reportedly behaved in a benign fashion [22, 23].

## Juxtaglomerular Cell Tumor (JG Tumor)

This is a benign neoplasm that often affects adolescents and young adults. JG tumors secrete renin, and as such this entity may be suspected in patients with severe poorly controlled hypertension and marked hypokalemia. Headaches and polyuria have also been reported. These tumors are typically 5 cm or less in size and are usually solitary and well circumscribed. Histologically, JG tumors are composed of sheets of polygonal or spindled tumor cells with central round regular nuclei with a complex vascular hemangiopericytic pattern that entraps normal renal tubules [3]. These tumors express renin, vimentin, CD34, CD117, and α-smooth muscle actin. Recurrence or metastasis has not been reported, although these tumors may be lethal if left untreated. Surgical excision is curative for JG tumors.

## Renomedullary Interstitial Cell Tumor

This is a common benign finding in adult autopsies and may be found incidentally in surgical resection specimens in patients >50 years of age [24]. This lesion has also been termed "medullary fibroma." Most patients are asymptomatic, although rare cases have been associated with hematuria and urinary tract infections. These lesions arise from the interstitial cells of the medulla and, as such, are typically immunoreactive for smooth muscle actin, COX-2, and PGE2. Microscopically, the tumor is composed of small stellate or polygonal cells in a background of loose faintly basophilic stroma reminiscent of that seen in renal medulla. At the periphery, renal medullary tubules often are entrapped in the matrix [3].

## Malignant Mesenchymal Neoplasms Involving the Kidney

Because of their usually larger size and invasive nature, malignant non-epithelial neoplasms are more frequently symptomatic with pain, a palpable mass, or hematuria being common presenting symptoms. On imaging, renal sarcomas are usually large, invasive tumors with areas of enhancement, necrosis, and occasionally calcifications [25].

Renal sarcomas are often large and locally invasive; therefore, radical nephrectomy is typically the primary treatment modality [25, 26]. The role of regional lymphadenectomy is widely debated for epithelial renal neoplasms, and there is no consensus regarding its use in malignant non-epithelial renal tumors. However, given that sarcomas may present with locoregional lymphadenopathy, a retroperitoneal lymphadenectomy may be of diagnostic and potentially therapeutic benefit. Complete surgical resection with no residual disease offers the best chance at cure [26]. These tumors may also be locally invasive, thereby requiring concomitant partial, or complete, resection of the involved structures (bowel, spleen, liver, psoas muscle, quadratus, ribs, vertebrae). Often the surgical team is comprised of multiple disciplines (urology, orthopedics, vascular and plastic surgery) and preoperative consultation and planning between surgeons is essential.

Malignant non-epithelial renal neoplasms are generally aggressive tumors with a poor prognosis. For renal sarcomas, the overall survival (OS) at 1, 3, and 5 years was 86.3, 40.7, and 14.5 %, respectively, according to one of the largest case series [26]. Other series report a relatively higher 5-year OS of 25 % [27]. Variables that appear to predict OS include complete surgical resection, tumor stage, and tumor grade [26, 27].

## Leiomyosarcoma

This is the most common renal sarcoma accounting for 50–60 % of cases [28, 29]. It may arise from the renal capsule, the renal parenchyma, smooth muscle fibers of the renal pelvis, or the main renal vein [6]. Histologically, it is composed of eosinophilic spindle cells with distinct smooth muscle features arranged in a fascicular, plexiform, or haphazard growth pattern (Fig. 10.5). The presence of necrosis, nuclear pleomorphism, and more than a rare mitotic figure helps in differentiating leiomyosarcomas from leiomyomas.

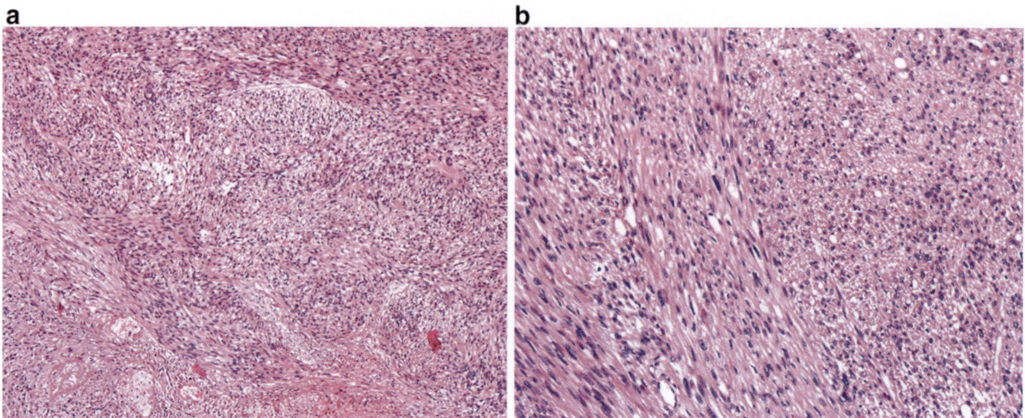

**Fig. 10.5** Leiomyosarcoma, exhibiting spindle cells with distinct smooth muscle features arranged in a fascicular or haphazard growth pattern. (**a**) Hematoxylin eosin, 4×. (**b**) Hematoxylin eosin, 20×

In the setting of unresectable leiomyosarcomas or for palliation, chemotherapy and radiation have been employed. Chemotherapy regimen includes cisplatin, adriamycin, etoposide, ifosfamide, and vincristine. Radiotherapy median dose is typically around 42Gy (range 30–60) [26, 30]. Renal lymphomas are managed with chemotherapy, and a common regimen is CHOP (cyclophosphamide, adriamycin, vincristine, prednisone) [31].

## Synovial Sarcoma

A characteristic feature of this mesenchymal neoplasm is the variable degree of epithelial differentiation that could be present. Histologically, synovial sarcoma displays monomorphic plump spindle cells with indistinct cell borders growing in short, intersecting fascicles or in solid sheets, often with prominent mitotic activity. At the molecular level, the tumor is characterized by a specific translocation t(X;18)(p11.2;q11). In contrast to soft tissue synovial sarcoma where the SYT-SSX1 gene fusion is more common than the alternative SYT-SSX2 form [32], the majority of renal synovial sarcomas have so far predominantly demonstrated the SYT-SSX2 gene fusion [33–35].

## Liposarcoma

Although retroperitoneal liposarcomas commonly occur in the perirenal area, primary liposarcomas of the kidney are very rare. Histologically, well-differentiated liposarcoma is composed of a relatively mature adipocytic proliferation, frequently with overt variation in cell size, focal cytologic atypia (Fig. 10.6), and consistent MDM2 (12q15) amplification [36]. This tumor is often associated with multiple recurrences, with about 10 % undergoing dedifferentiation. The latter most frequently resembles undifferentiated pleomorphic sarcoma or high-grade myxofibrosarcoma. Approximately 40 % of dedifferentiated liposarcomas recur locally and 15–20 % metastasize [36].

## Hematopoietic Tumors

Many lymphomas and leukemias can secondarily involve the kidney as part of systemic spread. In contrast, primary renal lymphoma is extremely rare. Some of these have been reported to develop in transplanted kidneys secondary to immunosuppression. Lymphomas can form discreet masses but secondary involvement more frequently appears as diffuse infiltration of the kidney parenchyma.

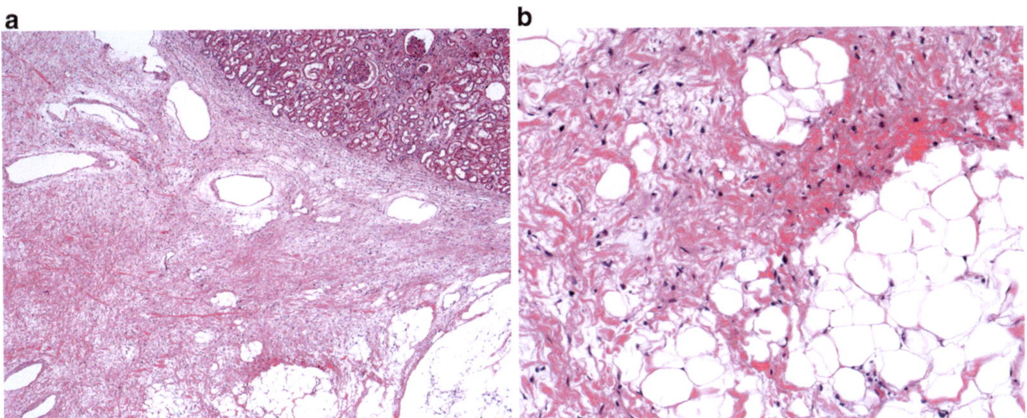

**Fig. 10.6** Well-differentiated liposarcoma, exhibiting a relatively mature adipocytic proliferation, frequently with overt variation in cell size and focal cytologic atypia. (**a**) Hematoxylin eosin, 4×. (**b**) Hematoxylin eosin, 20×

Patients with renal lymphoma and other hematopoietic neoplasms may present with "B" symptoms such as fevers, fatigue, and weight loss [31]. Renal lymphomas are often hypovascular and may appear as large infiltrative masses with nephromegaly [37]. In such situations, the absence of vena cava involvement is useful in the distinction from renal cell carcinoma [37]. Percutaneous renal biopsy should always be considered whenever there is a suspicion of lymphoma as this diagnosis will often change disease management compared to other renal tumors. Histological features of renal lymphoma and leukemia are described in Chap. 11. Survival for primary renal lymphoma ranges from 1 to 20 months based on case series [31].

## Neuroendocrine Tumors

These rarely occur in the kidney and include carcinoid tumor, neuroendocrine carcinoma, primitive neuroectodermal tumor, pheochromocytoma, and neuroblastoma. By definition, these tumors show morphological and immunohistochemical (synaptophysin and/or chromogranin expression) evidence of neuroendocrine differentiation. Of note, carcinoid tumor and neuroendocrine carcinoma also display evidence of epithelial differentiation. Primitive neuroectodermal tumor is an aggressive neoplasm, with the median OS in one series of 40 months and 5-year survival of 42 % [38]. Given

this aggressive behavior, this lesion is often treated with primary radical nephrectomy followed by chemotherapy and occasionally radiotherapy to the renal fossa [38]. Neuroendocrine tumors of the kidney are discussed in more detail in Chap. 9.

## References


1. Srigley JR, Delahunt B, Eble JN, et al. The International Society of Urological Pathology (ISUP) Vancouver classification of renal neoplasia. Am J Surg Pathol. 2013;37:1469–89.
2. Katabathina VS, Vikram R, Nagar AM, Tamboli P, Menias CO, Prasad SR. Mesenchymal neoplasms of the kidney in adults: imaging spectrum with radiologic-pathologic correlation. Radiographics. 2010;30: 1525–40.
3. Eble JN, Epstein JI, Sesterhenn IA, Sauter G. Pathology and genetics of tumours of the urinary system and male genital organs. 1st ed. Lyon: IARC; 2004.
4. Hajdu SI, Foote Jr FW. Angiomyolipoma of the kidney: report of 27 cases and review of the literature. J Urol. 1969;102:396–401.
5. Seyam RM, Bissada NK, Kattan SA, et al. Changing trends in presentation, diagnosis and management of renal angiomyolipoma: comparison of sporadic and tuberous sclerosis complex-associated forms. Urology. 2008;72:1077–82.
6. Prasad SR, Surabhi VR, Menias CO, Raut AA, Chintapalli KN. Benign renal neoplasms in adults: crosssectional imaging findings. AJR Am J Roentgenol. 2008;190:158–64.
7. Simpfendorfer C, Herts BR, Motta-Ramirez GA, et al. Angiomyolipoma with minimal fat on MDCT: can counts of negative-attenuation pixels aid diagnosis? AJR Am J Roentgenol. 2009;192:438–43.

8. Catalano OA, Samir AE, Sahani DV, Hahn PF. Pixel distribution analysis: can it be used to distinguish clear cell carcinomas from angiomyolipomas with minimal fat? Radiology. 2008;247:738–46.

9. Ro JY, Ayala AG, el-Naggar A, Grignon DJ, Hogan SF, Howard DR. Angiomyolipoma of kidney with lymph node involvement. DNA flow cytometric analysis. Arch Pathol Lab Med. 1990;114:65–7.

10. Eble JN. Angiomyolipoma of kidney. Semin Diagn Pathol. 1998;15:21–40.

11. Martignoni G, Pea M, Bonetti F, Brunelli M, Eble JN. Oncocytoma-like angiomyolipoma. A clinicopathologic and immunohistochemical study of 2 cases. Arch Pathol Lab Med. 2002;126:610–2.

12. Fine SW, Reuter VE, Epstein JI, Argani P. Angiomyolipoma with epithelial cysts (AMLEC): a distinct cystic variant of angiomyolipoma. Am J Surg Pathol. 2006;30:593–9.

13. Kilicaslan I, Gulluoglu MG, Dogan O, Uysal V. Intraglomerular microlesions in renal angiomyolipoma. Hum Pathol. 2000;31:1325–8.

14. Nese N, Martignoni G, Fletcher CD, et al. Pure epithelioid PEComas (so-called epithelioid angiomyolipoma) of the kidney: a clinicopathologic study of 41 cases: detailed assessment of morphology and risk stratification. Am J Surg Pathol. 2011;35:161–76.

15. Cho NH, Shim HS, Choi YD, Kim DS. Estrogen receptor is significantly associated with the epithelioid variants of renal angiomyolipoma: a clinicopathological and immunohistochemical study of 67 cases. Pathol Int. 2004;54:510–5.

16. Brimo F, Robinson B, Guo C, Zhou M, Latour M, Epstein JI. Renal epithelioid angiomyolipoma with atypia: a series of 40 cases with emphasis on clinicopathologic prognostic indicators of malignancy. Am J Surg Pathol. 2010;34:715–22.

17. Mohammed AY, Matthew L, Harmse JL, Lang S, Townell NH. Multiple leiomyoma of the renal capsule. Scand J Urol Nephrol. 1999;33:138–9.

18. Steiner M, Quinlan D, Goldman SM, et al. Leiomyoma of the kidney: presentation of 4 new cases and the role of computerized tomography. J Urol. 1990;143:994–8.

19. Tawfik OW, Moral LA, Richardson WP, Lee KR. Multicentric bilateral renal cell carcinomas and a vascular leiomyoma in a child. Pediatr Pathol. 1993;13:289–98.

20. Brown JG, Folpe AL, Rao P, et al. Primary vascular tumors and tumor-like lesions of the kidney: a clinicopathologic analysis of 25 cases. Am J Surg Pathol. 2010;34:942–9.

21. Kryvenko ON, Gupta NS, Meier FA, Lee MW, Epstein JI. Anastomosing hemangioma of the genitourinary system: eight cases in the kidney and ovary with immunohistochemical and ultrastructural analysis. Am J Clin Pathol. 2011;136:450–7.

22. Fine SW, McCarthy DM, Chan TY, Epstein JI, Argani P. Malignant solitary fibrous tumor of the kidney: report of a case and comprehensive review of the literature. Arch Pathol Lab Med. 2006;130:857–61.

23. Hirano D, Mashiko A, Murata Y, et al. A case of solitary fibrous tumor of the kidney: an immunohistochemical and ultrastructural study with a review of the literature. Med Mol Morphol. 2009;42:239–44.

24. Reis M, Faria V, Lindoro J, Adolfo A. The small cystic and noncystic noninflammatory renal nodules: a postmortem study. J Urol. 1988;140:721–4.

25. Srinivas V, Sogani PC, Hajdu SI, Whitmore Jr WF. Sarcomas of the kidney. J Urol. 1984;132:13–6.

26. Wang X, Xu R, Yan L, et al. Adult renal sarcoma: clinical features and survival in a series of patients treated at a high-volume institution. Urology. 2011;77:836–41.

27. Kendal WS. The comparative survival of renal leiomyosarcoma. Can J Urol. 2007;14:3435–42.

28. Grignon DJ, Ayala AG, Ro JY, el-Naggar A, Papadopoulos NJ. Primary sarcomas of the kidney. A clinicopathologic and DNA flow cytometric study of 17 cases. Cancer Am Cancer Soc. 1990;65:1611–8.

29. Vogelzang NJ, Fremgen AM, Guinan PD, Chmiel JS, Sylvester JL, Sener SF. Primary renal sarcoma in adults. A natural history and management study by the American Cancer Society, Illinois Division. Cancer Am Cancer Soc. 1993;71:804–10.

30. Deyrup AT, Montgomery E, Fisher C. Leiomyosarcoma of the kidney: a clinicopathologic study. Am J Surg Pathol. 2004;28:178–82.

31. Yasunaga Y, Hoshida Y, Hashimoto M, Miki T, Okuyama A, Aozasa K. Malignant lymphoma of the kidney. J Surg Oncol. 1997;64:207–11.

32. Ladanyi M, Antonescu CR, Leung DH, et al. Impact of SYT-SSX fusion type on the clinical behavior of synovial sarcoma: a multi-institutional retrospective study of 243 patients. Cancer Res. 2002;62: 135–40.

33. Argani P, Faria PA, Epstein JI, et al. Primary renal synovial sarcoma: molecular and morphologic delineation of an entity previously included among embryonal sarcomas of the kidney. Am J Surg Pathol. 2000;24:1087–96.

34. Kim DH, Sohn JH, Lee MC, et al. Primary synovial sarcoma of the kidney. Am J Surg Pathol. 2000;24:1097–104.

35. Koyama S, Morimitsu Y, Morokuma F, Hashimoto H. Primary synovial sarcoma of the kidney: report of a case confirmed by molecular detection of the SYT-SSX2 fusion transcripts. Pathol Int. 2001;51:385–91.

36. Fletcher CDM, World Health Organization, International Agency for Research on Cancer. WHO classification of tumours of soft tissue and bone. 4th ed. Lyon: IARC; 2013.

37. Ganeshan D, Iyer R, Devine C, Bhosale P, Paulson E. Imaging of primary and secondary renal lymphoma. AJR Am J Roentgenol. 2013;201:W712–9.

38. Thyavihally YB, Tongaonkar HB, Gupta S, et al. Primitive neuroectodermal tumor of the kidney: a single institute series of 16 patients. Urology. 2008;71:292–6.

# Pediatric Renal Neoplasms

**11**


Michael Yap, Mariah Zampieri Leivo,
Denise M. Malicki, Donna E. Hansel,
and George Chiang


Pediatric renal cancers are rare and constitute approximately 7 % of all childhood neoplasms [1]. Clinical findings are usually nonspecific, and asymptomatic patients are commonly seen. Tumors are frequently discovered incidentally, and precise diagnosis is quite challenging in both clinical and pathological scenario [2]. Oftentimes, these predominantly embryonal neoplasms mimic intra- and extrarenal and benign and malignant tumors that make appropriate patient management difficult. In this chapter, we will discuss key elements of the most common renal neoplasms in the pediatric population and provide guidance for accurate diagnosis and treatment.


M. Yap, M.D. • G. Chiang, M.D. (✉)
Division of Pediatric Urology, Rady Children's
Hospital, University of California at San Diego,
3020 Children's Way, San Diego, CA 92123, USA
e-mail: myap@rchsd.org; Gchiang@rchsd.org

M.Z. Leivo, M.D. • D.E. Hansel, M.D., Ph.D.
Department of Pathology, University of California at
San Diego, San Diego, CA, USA
e-mail: mleivo@ucsd.edu; dhansel@ucsd.edu

D.M. Malicki, M.D., Ph.D.
Department of Pathology, Rady Children's Hospital
San Diego, University of California at San Diego,
San Diego, CA, USA
e-mail: dmalicki@rchsd.org


## Malignant Pediatric Renal Tumors

## Wilms Tumor

### Introduction

Wilms tumor (WT), also named nephroblastoma, is the most common pediatric kidney tumor and represents about 92 % of all renal tumors in children younger than 5 years old. WT has an incidence of 1 in 10,000 newborns and approximately 500 cases are estimated annually in the USA [1–4]. WT has been tied to various syndromes involving deletion of the *WT1* gene. Syndromes associated with deletions of the *WT1* gene include WAGR syndrome, Denys-Drash syndrome, and Frasier syndrome. In WAGR syndrome, additional findings include aniridia, genitourinary abnormalities, and mental retardation. The risk of WT in these patients is 40–50 % [5, 6]. In Denys-Drash syndrome, additional findings include male pseudohermaphroditism and progressive renal failure. Approximately 50–90 % of these patients will develop WT [7, 8]. Frasier syndrome, which can present with undermasculanized genitalia in affected males, focal segmental glomerular sclerosis, and gonadoblastoma, is not typically associated with WT although several cases have been reported [9, 10]. Although the exact function of WT1 protein has not been identified, it may have a role in metanephric stem cell differentiation [11]. In




© Springer Science+Business Media New York 2016
D.E. Hansel et al. (eds.), *The Kidney*, DOI 10.1007/978-1-4939-3286-3_11

patients with isolated WT, evidence of *WT1* mutation exists in 5–10 % of cases. Alterations in the *WT2* gene are associated with Beckwith-Wiedemann syndrome, which consists of several abnormalities including macroglossia, macrosomia, hypoglycemia, visceromegaly, and omphalocele and carries an 8 % risk of WT [12].

## Clinical Presentation

Children with WT generally present with an asymptomatic abdominal mass, oftentimes discovered by a parent while bathing the child or by a relative who notices a protuberant abdomen. Associated signs and symptoms such as malaise, pain, and either microscopic or gross hematuria are found in approximately 25 % of children. Children presenting with a rapidly enlarging abdominal mass, anemia, hypertension, pain, and fever may have a subcapsular hemorrhage within the tumor [13]. Renal ultrasonography is usually the initial study for evaluation of suspected WT, followed by CT scan of the abdomen and pelvis. Intravenous tumor extension of WT occurs in about 11 % of cases with thrombus extending into the IVC in about 6 % of cases [4], for which evaluation can be performed by either Doppler ultrasonography, contrast-enhanced CT scans, or MRI. For evaluation of intracardiac tumor extension, echocardiogram may be helpful. Approximately 12 % of patients with WT will present with metastases. The most common site of metastasis in WT is the lung, and chest CT is the preferred imaging modality for evaluating this site [14, 15].

## Pathology

Grossly, WT appears well circumscribed and encapsulated with a uniform tan to gray cut surface (Fig. 11.1). Focal areas of necrosis, hemorrhage, and cystic change may be present, although they are more commonly seen following chemotherapy. Tumors with a firm consistency are usually associated with an abundant stromal component. Cystic masses are rare, and when large cysts are present, these lesions are characterized as cystic variants of Wilms tumor including cystic partially differentiated nephroblastoma and cystic nephroma [16, 17].

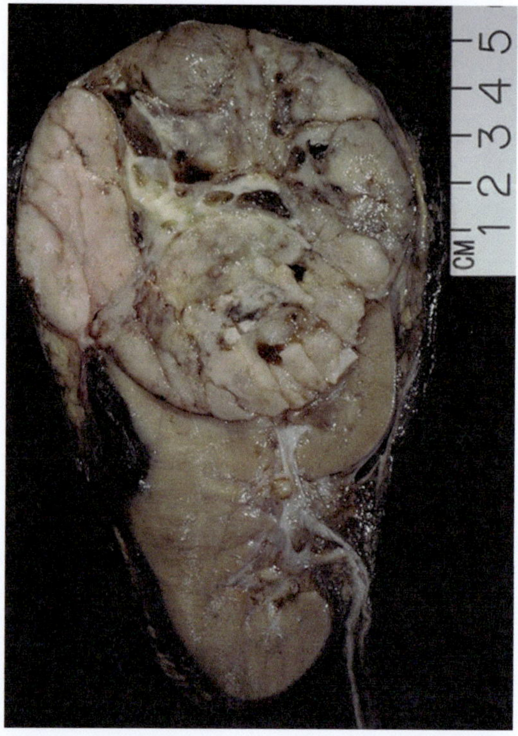

**Fig. 11.1** Wilms tumor

Histologically, WT most commonly shows three distinct components that consist of blastemal, epithelial, and stromal elements (Fig. 11.2a). Biphasic and monophasic patterns may also occur. The epithelial component is usually the most recognizable element in WT and can show a variety of differentiation patterns. Epithelial differentiation into tubular structures is the most common differentiation pattern and ranges from rudimentary, rosette-like tubular structures to mature tubules. Primitive glomeruli may also be seen (Fig. 11.2b). Heterologous differentiation may occur and include mucinous or squamous epithelial, or neural, and neuroendocrine differentiation. The blastemal component shows either a sheetlike or nested architectural pattern and typically consists of small crowded blue cells with minimal cytoplasm, overlapping oval nuclei, and coarse chromatin (Fig. 11.2c). Mitoses are frequently seen. In the setting of blastemal-predominant WT, the differential diagnosis includes other pediatric small round blue-cell tumors such as neuroblastoma, rhabdomyosar-

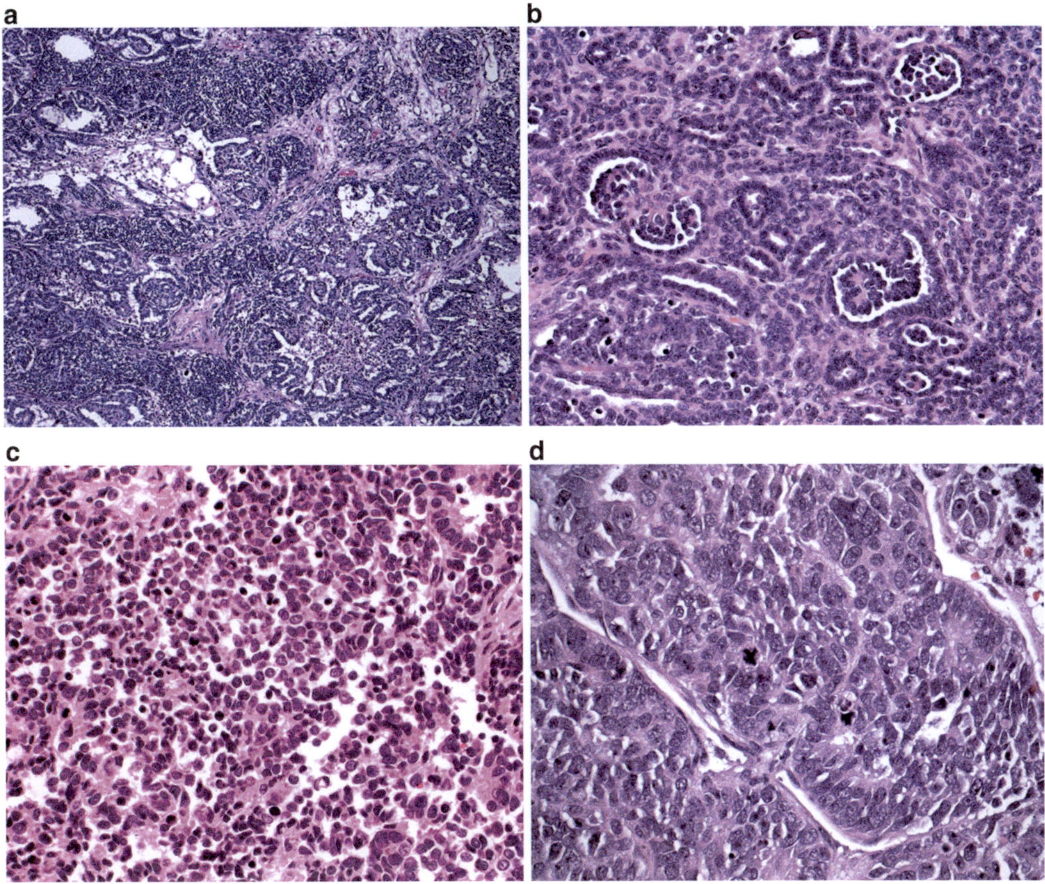

**Fig. 11.2** (**a**) Wilms tumor: blastemal, epithelial, and stromal elements. (**b**) Wilms tumor: primitive glomerular structures. (**c**) Wilms tumor: blastemal component. (**d**) Wilms tumor showing anaplasia with hyperchromatic and enlarged nuclei and mitotic figures

coma, primitive neuroectodermal tumor (PNET), and lymphoma. Preoperative chemotherapy has been associated with the presence of necrosis, fibrosis, and macrophage influx, as well as formation of mature skeletal muscle. The stromal component varies from lightly staining spindle cells occasionally to rhabdomyoblasts and cartilage or bone [18–20].

Anaplasia occurs in approximately 5 % of WT and may be seen in the epithelial, stromal, or blastemal elements. It is more common in older children, reaching a peak at approximately 5 years of age [20]. Anaplasia is defined as hyperchromatic, markedly enlarged nuclei, and the presence of multipolar or polypoid mitotic figures (Fig. 11.2d). Focal anaplasia is defined as one or a few limited foci of anaplastic cells within

a WT, with these anaplastic regions surrounded by areas without anaplasia or nuclear unrest approaching anaplasia. In contrast, diffuse anaplasia denotes a lesion that otherwise does not fit the "focal" definition and is associated with more aggressive behavior [21, 22].

Immunohistochemical analysis shows diffuse nuclear expression of WT1 in blastemal and epithelial cells, but not in stromal cells. In cases in which the stromal component is predominant, WT1 immunostain may not be a reliable indicator of the diagnosis [11, 23]. Epithelial elements can show cytokeratin immunoreactivity and blastemal cells may be positive for CD56 and negative for actin, myogenin, and MYOD1 [24–26].

Various genetic alterations may be associated with WT. These include deletion of the *WT1* gene at 11p13, alterations of the *WT2* gene at 11p15, p53 mutations, CTNNB1 gene mutations, and WTX mutations [27].

## Prognosis and Clinical Management

Management of WT has been advanced primarily by two large cooperative multinational trials: (1) the National Wilms Tumor Study Group (NWTSG), merged with three other groups to form the Children's Oncology Group (COG), and (2) the International Society of Pediatric Oncology (SIOP). SIOP and NWTSG differ in regard to risk stratification according to pathology. In SIOP, histological classification is divided into low-, intermediate-, and high-risk categories. Intermediate-risk tumors comprise 90 % of tumors and include epithelial-type WT, stromal-type WT, mixed-type WT, regressive-type WT and those with focal anaplasia. High-risk tumors, on the other hand, include blastemal-type WT and tumors with diffuse anaplasia. In NWTSG, histological classification is divided into two groups: favorable and unfavorable histology. Tumors with favorable histology include triphasic WT, epithelial-predominant WT, stromal-predominant WT, and blastemal-predominant WT. Tumors with unfavorable histology account for about 10 % of Wilms tumor and include tumors with either focal or diffuse anaplasia [15].

In SIOP and NWTSG, treatment protocols are based on stage and histology and involve various combinations of surgery, chemotherapy, and radiation. Whereas staging criteria are very similar between NWTSG and SIOP, there are fundamental differences between the two groups in regard to treatment of unilateral WT: primary surgery in NWTSG/COG versus initial or neoadjuvant chemotherapy in SIOP. In bilateral disease both NWTSG/COG and SIOP recommend preoperative chemotherapy. Radical nephrectomy is the mainstay of surgical therapy. Palpation of the renal vein before division is recommended to exclude the possibility of tumor thrombus. Intraoperative inspection of the liver and contralateral kidney is not required unless lesions were identified on preoperative imaging studies. Lymph node sampling is critically important, even in the setting of normal nodes on preoperative imaging. The role of partial nephrectomy has been suggested in cases of bilateral disease, as well as unilateral disease in the setting of syndromic conditions with increased risk of WT recurrence. Bilateral WT occurs in approximately 5 % of cases. Relapse occurs in about 15 % of children with favorable histology WT and 50 % of anaplastic histology WT. Most relapses occur early (within 2 years of diagnosis) and are found within the lungs (60 %) or abdomen (30 %). Currently survival is 90 % overall for children with Wilms tumor. Tumor histology and stage are the two most important prognostic factors [28, 29].

## Premalignant Neoplasms Associated with Wilms Tumor: Nephrogenic Rests and Nephroblastomatosis

### Introduction

Nephrogenic rests are clusters of residual embryonic metanephric cells, which normally disappear after 36 weeks of gestational age. The natural history of nephrogenic rests varies. Some regress and become sclerotic, while others have a hyperplastic overgrowth and may become neoplastic [30–32]. Nephrogenic rests can occur at any age but are most frequently found in infants [33]. It is estimated that they are present in about 1 % of unselected infants on postmortem biopsy [30]. Nephrogenic rests are classically divided into perilobar and intralobar types. Perilobar rests are much more common. They are usually found in subcapsular peripheral locations, are well demarcated, and often multiple. Intralobar rests, on the other hand, may be present anywhere within the kidney, often have a more irregular and intermixed margin, and are usually singular. Nephroblastomatosis is the presence of multiple or diffuse nephrogenic rests, and it can be perilobar or intralobar. Whereas perilobar nephroblastomatosis is found in association with synchronous bilateral WT, intralobar nephroblastomatosis is found in association with metachronous contralateral WT [33, 34].

## Clinical Presentation

Nephroblastomatosis (NB) is generally asymptomatic. It refers to the presence of multiple or diffuse nephrogenic rests. The clinical significance of nephrogenic rests is their association with WT. They are found in about 40 % of kidneys with unilateral WTs and almost 100 % of kidneys with bilateral WTs [30]. Its presence in the non-tumoral part of kidneys with WT may also increase the risk of subsequent relapse of WT after treatment [35]. Overall, less than 1 % of nephrogenic rests will progress to WT [32]. Both nephrogenic rests and NB have been associated with multiple syndromes, including Beckwith-Wiedemann syndrome, hemihypertrophy, Perlman syndrome, and trisomy 18 [30, 35].

On ultrasound, NB appears isoechoic or hypoechoic compared to the cortex, with small lesions being easily missed. On CT scan, the lesions are homogeneous and isodense on pre-contrast imaging, then become hypodense compared to the cortex on post-contrast imaging. Occasionally, regions of NB are so small they can be missed with CT as well [36]. On MRI, NB is isointense or slightly hypointense to the cortex on both T1-weighted and T2-weighted imaging. On gadolinium-enhanced T1-weighted images, the lesions remain homogeneously hypointense compared with the enhanced cortex. The major difference with NB and WT is the fact that the latter tends to show mixed echogenicity and heterogeneous structures on imaging [37]. An open biopsy that includes a portion of the lesion plus adjacent normal renal cortex can be helpful in distinguishing NB from WT. In WT, a pseudocapsule consisting of compressed renal parenchyma surrounds the tumor, while such a capsule does not exist with NB.

## Pathology

Perilobar rests are often multifocal and occur along the periphery of a renal lobe. The foci are well circumscribed and contain both blastemal and tubular elements with only scant stroma (Fig. 11.3a). In contrast, intralobar rests are randomly situated within the renal parenchyma, are poorly circumscribed, and show a prominent stromal component (Fig. 11.3b). Both subtypes can be

further subdivided into sclerosing (fibrotic background), obsolete (predominant fibrosis), dormant (small foci), and hyperplastic (large foci with abundant mitosis) subtypes. The distinction between hyperplastic RN and WT can be difficult, but may be more readily made if the border of the lesion is well sampled and surveyed for the presence of a pseudocapsule [30, 32].

Nephroblastomatosis is characterized by the presence of multifocal and diffuse nephrogenic rests lesions. Nephroblastomatosis can be subclassified as perilobar, intralobar, combined, or panlobar and can display all or any subclasses of nephrogenic rests patterns (dormant, hyperplastic, and neoplastic). Architecturally, nephroblastomatosis may be associated with a thick cortical outer layer of hyperplastic nephrogenic tissue [37, 38].

Similar to WT, NRs may contain alterations in the *WT1* and *WT2* genes. One model for the development of WT is the accumulation of one or more additional mutations within the NRs.

## Prognosis and Clinical Management

The treatment of NB remains controversial [30, 35]. It is a benign process, yet has a malignant potential [39]. Neither the National Wilms Tumor Study Group (NWTSG) nor the International Society of Pediatric Oncology (SIOP) provides formal guidance on how to treat NB or NRs in the absence of WT. As a consequence, patients with NB are treated in various ways, some with multiple chemotherapeutic regimens and some not at all [40]. The arguments in favor of chemotherapy for NB are (1) to treat undiagnosed WT within the NB lesion, (2) to decrease the number of target cells at risk for malignant transformation, and (3) to prevent damage to the normal renal cortex by compression from massive NB [30–32, 35]. The arguments against initial chemotherapy are (1) the risk of chemotherapy for treatment of a benign disease that may regress spontaneously, (2) the uncertainty that chemotherapy will prevent the development of WT, (3) the fear that chemotherapy will select for chemoresistant cells, and (4) the risk of NB regrowth after chemotherapy [38, 41]. There are sporadic case reports of spontaneous resolution of NB without

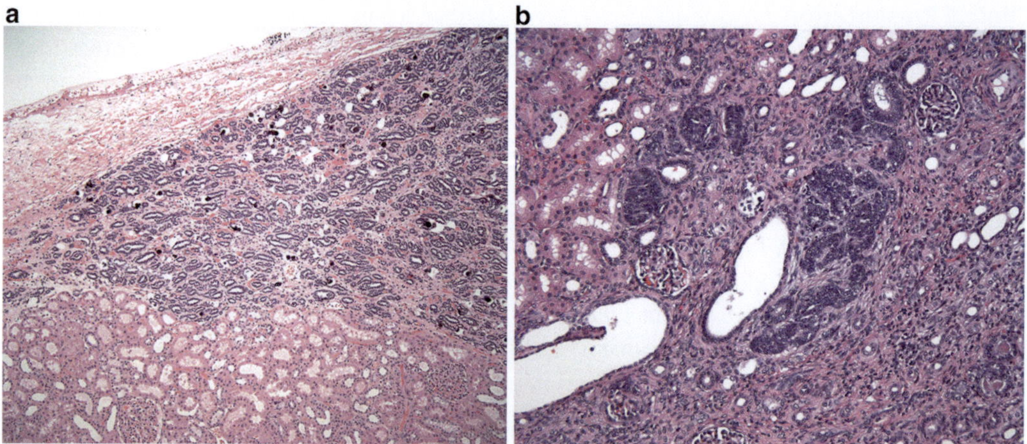

**Fig. 11.3** (**a**) Perilobar nephrogenic rests contain both blastemal and tubular elements with scant stroma. (**b**) Intralobar nephrogenic rests with prominent stromal component

treatment; however, the risk of developing WT persists even years after initial diagnosis.

## Clear Cell Sarcoma of the Kidney (CCSK)

### Introduction

Clear cell sarcoma of the kidney (CCSK) comprises approximately 5 % of all renal tumors in children. It is the second most common pediatric renal tumor after Wilms tumor [42–44]. The tumor presents at a mean age of about 36 months and rarely occurs in the first 6 months of life [44–59]. Recently a t(10;17)(q22;p13) translocation has been identified in CCSK, suggesting its possible role in tumorigenesis [60–62]. Gene expression profiles of CCSK suggest the cell of origin to be a renal mesenchymal cell with neural markers.

### Clinical Presentation

Presenting symptoms are similar to that of other pediatric renal tumors and include abdominal mass, abdominal and flank pain, and hematuria. Distributions by stages are 27 % for stage I, 33 % for stage II, 34 % for stage III, and 6 % for stage IV [42, 44, 45, 62–67]. Bilateral (stage V disease) has only been reported in a few case reports [44, 68, 69]. The most common sites of metastases are lymph nodes (60 %) and bone (13 %),

from which it derives the name "bone metastasizing renal tumor of childhood." Other metastatic sites include the brain, lung, liver, skin, and colon. CCSK is also able to invade the vena cava with extension into the right atrium. No specific syndromic or familial associations have been established [44, 45, 52, 66, 69, 70].

### Pathology

CCSK is typically a unifocal, well-circumscribed renal mass that is often large (mean diameter 11.3 cm). The cut surface shows a solid, homogeneous tan-gray appearance (Fig. 11.4a). Cystic structures, focal necrosis, and hemorrhage may be present [44].

Microscopically, CCSK shows a densely cellular proliferation of monotonous appearing cells with clear to mildly eosinophilic cytoplasm (Fig. 11.4b). Nuclei are round to oval, contain fine granular chromatin, and lack prominent nucleoli. Mitotic figures are frequent and may be atypical. Tumor cells invade into the adjacent renal parenchyma. The lesional background shows delicate branching vessels and occasional necrosis, which is an adverse prognostic indicator. Mucopolysaccharides may be present in the surrounding matrix. Several variants of CCSK have been described and include myxoid, sclerosing, epithelioid trabecular, palisading (Verocay body-like), spindle cell, and anaplastic forms [44, 48, 52, 71–73].

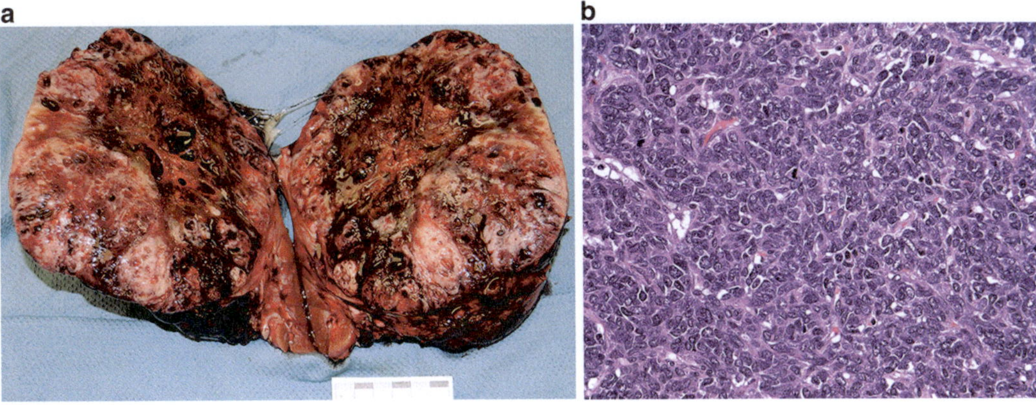

**Fig. 11.4** (**a**) Clear cell sarcoma of the kidney. (**b**) Clear cell sarcoma of the kidney showing dense populations of monotonous appearing cells

Immunohistochemical analysis shows the tumor cells to be positive for vimentin and bcl-2 and negative for cytokeratin, CD99, WT1, S100, and SNF5. No loss of INI1 occurs in this lesion [44, 74–76].

## Prognosis and Clinical Management

Current treatment strategies involve various combinations of surgery, chemotherapy, and radiation depending on stage. Although the optimal treatment for CCSK has not yet been established, with current intensive treatment schedules, 5-year relapse-free survival (RFS) now ranges from 75 to 85 % and 5-year overall survival (OS) from 85 to 90 % [44, 67, 73]. Younger children tend to have poorer outcomes (i.e., lower survival and higher recurrence rates) [67]. Relapses occur in 20–40 % of cases. Time interval to relapse is usually between 12 and 24 months, although late relapse up to 8 years after treatment has been reported [42, 44, 48, 52, 55, 64, 66, 67, 72, 77–81]. The most recent studies indicate that the brain has now surpassed bone as the most common site of CCSK recurrence [67, 77].

## Rhabdoid Tumor of the Kidney

### Introduction

Rhabdoid tumor of the kidney (RTK) is a highly aggressive malignant neoplasm, characterized by early metastases and a high mortality rate. It occurs primarily in the infant and newborn and is the second most common malignant tumor in the neonate [82]. Eighty percent of RTKs occur in patients under the age of 2 years and 60 % occur in patients under the age of 1 year [83]. After the age of 5 years, the diagnosis is unlikely [82–89]. The histologic origin of RTK remains obscure. RTK was named because microscopically it resembles rhabdomyosarcoma, although it does not show skeletal muscle markers either by staining or electron microscopy [18, 88].

### Clinical Presentation

The clinical presentation of children with RTK has not been well described. Gross hematuria can be seen in greater than 50 % of children with RTK and microscopic hematuria can be seen in nearly 75 % of patients. Hematuria as a presenting symptom suggests invasion of the renal pelvis by tumor [90–92]. RTK can also been diagnosed in utero by ultrasound and may present in the newborn as metastases to the skin or other sites [84, 86–88, 92–94]. Sites of metastasis include regional lymph nodes, the lungs, the liver, bone, and the brain [95]. Hypercalcemia has also been associated with RTK and is attributed to an increased serum PTH [96, 97]. Radiographically, RTK is indistinguishable from other malignant pediatric renal tumors. On CT, a prominent and eccentric crescent with attenuation of fluid—representing subcapsular renal hemorrhage or peripheral tumor necrosis adjacent to tumor lobules—may be seen in up to 71 % of cases; however, this finding is not specific to RTK [83].

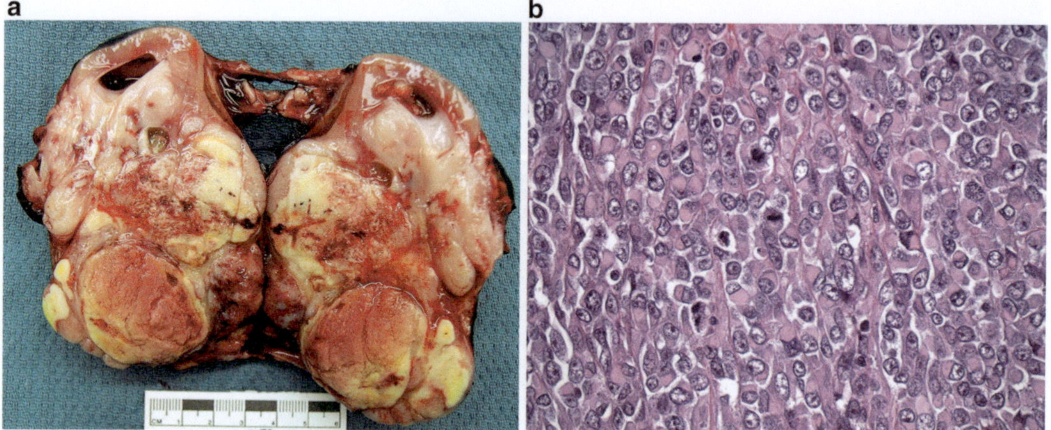

**Fig. 11.5** (**a**) Rhabdoid tumor of the kidney. (**b**) Rhabdoid tumor of the kidney: large polygonal cells with dense eosinophilic cytoplasmic inclusions and mitotic figures

## Pathology

On gross evaluation, RTK is a large, unencapsulated tumor that often overruns the kidney and extends into the perirenal tissue. The cut surface is often necrotic and hemorrhagic (Fig. 11.5a). Tumors can range up to 17 cm in size (mean 9.6 cm) [18, 82, 83, 86].

Histological evaluation shows sheets of loosely cohesive cells that extensively invade the surrounding renal parenchyma and perirenal tissue. Tumor cells are large and polygonal, often showing dense eosinophilic cytoplasmic inclusions that likely represent aggregates of intermediate filaments (Fig. 11.5b). Large, atypical vesicular nuclei are readily apparent, which contain clumped chromatin and prominent nucleoli [87–89, 98–101].

RTK often shows inactivation of the *HSNF5/INI1* tumor suppressor gene on 22q11.2, which can be demonstrated by negative nuclear immunohistochemical staining for INI1. Immunohistochemical stains for EMA/MUC1 and vimentin are often positive in this lesion [74, 88, 101].

## Prognosis and Clinical Management

Surgical excision is the mainstay of treatment, followed by adjuvant chemotherapy and/or radiotherapy. Prognosis associated with RTK is generally poor despite multimodal therapy [102].

## Desmoplastic Small round Cell Tumor of the Kidney

### Introduction

Desmoplastic small round cell tumor (DSRCT) is a rare, high-grade, malignant neoplasm usually seen in children, adolescents, and young adults, where it has an aggressive clinical course [103–107]. Recently a few cases involving the kidney have been reported in children (age 6–8 years of age) [108]. DSRCT is associated with a specific chromosomal translocation, t(11;22)(p13;q12), the identification of which is a requisite for diagnosis. The t(11;22)(p13;q12) translocation product is a chimeric transcript formed by fusion of the Ewing sarcoma gene (EWS) and the Wilms tumor gene (WT1), thought to be responsible for tumorigenesis [109].

### Clinical Presentation

Most of these tumors manifest as multinodular masses associated with the serosa of the abdominal cavity and usually minimal organ involvement. When these tumors involve the urogenital system, they are generally metastatic at the time of presentation and tend to have a poor prognosis [105, 110]. DSRCT specific to the kidney may present as an abdominal mass with associated symptoms that can include cramping, abdominal pain, weight loss, and constipation. It has been suggested that on imaging, these tumors may appear as hypovascular, well-circumscribed renal masses with associated punctate calcifications; however, the lack of these characteristics does not exclude the diagnosis [111].

## Pathology

On gross evaluation, DSRCT is often a solitary white-tan, nonencapsulated mass that can invade into the surrounding renal parenchyma and perirenal tissue. Necrosis and hemorrhage are common and tumor can range up to 13 cm in size [108, 112–114]. On microscopic assessment, nests of undifferentiated cells can be seen, occasionally associated with necrosis and calcification. The tumor cells display scant cytoplasm, and the nuclei are large and hyperchromatic. Mitotic figures are frequent. Very few pediatric cases of DSRCT have been reported in the literature; most describe an absence of desmoplasia, which makes DSRCT indistinguishable from other small round cell tumors [105, 108, 112, 114–117]. Molecular studies are essential for the diagnosis by identifying t(11;22)(p13;q12) translocation. Additionally, immunoreactivity for vimentin, desmin, cytokeratin, EMA, and WT-1 can also be seen [108, 111, 113].

## Prognosis and Clinical Management

Although there has been some reported success in achieving a response from multimodal chemotherapy, as well as surgery alone, there is no standard protocol for treatment of the disease and the mortality rate remains high [115, 118, 119].

## Anaplastic Sarcoma of the Kidney

### Introduction

Anaplastic sarcoma of the kidney (ASK) is a very rare renal pediatric tumor with just over 20 cases reported in the literature. ASK mainly occurs in children and adolescents younger than 15 years of age [120–122].

### Clinical Presentation

The most common presentation is a palpable abdominal mass and sometimes hematuria. Anaplastic Wilms tumor is the most important tumor in the differential [122].

## Pathology

On gross examination, ASK is a large, infiltrative lesion that shows frequent cystic change. Size ranges up to 21 cm (mean 12.7 cm) [122]. Histological review shows bundles of undifferentiated spindle cells that merge with small round primitive mesenchymal cells. The tumor background often shows myxoid change. Anaplastic foci that may demonstrate giant pleomorphic cells with enlarged irregular hyperchromatic nuclei can be seen throughout the tumor. Prominent areas of chondroid differentiation may be present, as well as small regions that contain osteoid with osteoclast-like giant cells [120–123].

## Prognosis and Clinical Management

Considering patients have been treated with various therapeutic protocols (nephrectomy, chemotherapy, and/or radiation), the overall outcome of ASK is reasonably good, with 75 % of patients in one series surviving after 8 years of follow-up [122].

## Indolent Renal Lesions and Malformations

## Congenital Mesoblastic Nephroma (CMN)

### Introduction

Congenital mesoblastic nephroma (CMN) is the most common renal tumor of young patients up to 3 months of age and accounts for 2–3 % of all pediatric renal tumors [124]. The median age at diagnosis is 30 days, with 90 % occurring within the first year of life and virtually none after the age of 3 years [125, 126]. Histologically, three variants are recognized. The classic type accounts for about 24 % of cases, the cellular type accounts for about 66 % of cases, and a mixed variant of both classic and cellular types comprises 10 % of cases. The cellular variant CMN is specific for a t(12;15)(p13;q25) translocation with resultant

ETV6-NTRK3 gene fusion transcript [127, 128]. Interestingly, this same translocation is shared by infantile fibrosarcoma (IFS), suggesting that cellular CMN represents intrarenal IFS [129].

## Clinical Presentation

CMN is usually detected prenatally by ultrasonography. In the infant, it most commonly presents as a palpable abdominal mass. On imaging, CMN is predominantly solid, but cystic or even calcified components may be identified [130]. Though CMN is largely a benign tumor, cases of metastases, especially of the cellular variant, have been reported. Reported sites of metastases include the brain, lung, liver, and heart.

## Pathology

On gross examination, CMN is often a unifocal mass that may replace a large portion of the kidney (Fig. 11.6a). The cut surface is gray to tan in color and shows a trabeculated, firm appearance. Cystic change, necrosis, and hemorrhage are occasionally present. Microscopically, CMN is comprised of fascicles of spindled cells with minimal atypia that often intercalate between adjacent renal elements (Fig. 11.6b). Mitotic figures are rare. A cellular variant of CMN has been described, which shows an increase in cellularity associated with a high mitotic rate, raising the differential diagnosis of infantile fibrosarcoma (Fig. 11.6c) [125, 126, 131, 132]. Both CMN and infantile fibrosarcoma have been reported to contain the t(12;15)(p13;q25) translocation, suggesting they may be potentially related entities [133].

The immunohistochemical profile of CMN shows the tumor cells to be frequently positive for vimentin, actin, and desmin and negative for CD34 [132, 134].

## Prognosis and Clinical Management

Complete surgical resection remains the most important prognostic criterion [131, 135]. Radical nephrectomy is preferable to partial nephrectomy in order to reduce the risk of local recurrence. Overall survival is greater than 95 % with a worse prognosis associated with older age, stage III disease, and the cellular variant [131]. Relapse occurs in only 5 % of patients and is

thought to be related to incomplete resection. Recurrences almost always develop within 12 months of surgery; thus, close surveillance is recommended during this period of time [136]. Cases that recur locally have been successfully treated with chemotherapy, with or without radiotherapy, with good outcomes [137].

## Metanephric Stromal Tumor

### Introduction

Metanephric stromal tumor (MST) is a benign pediatric tumor, most commonly seen in the first decade of life (mean age 2 years old). It is a rare renal pediatric neoplasm that is equally seen in both genders. MST was first described by Argani and Beckwith and was previously grouped as congenital mesoblastic nephroma (CMN). The distinction was clear given MST's benign behavior, which lacks the degree of microscopic infiltration seen in CMN [138–143].

### Clinical Presentation

Clinically, MST is often asymptomatic and presents itself as an incidental abdominal mass. Other symptoms, such as hypertension with hyperreninism, are seen when juxtaglomerular apparatus hyperplasia is involved and hematuria when the renal pelvis is involved. Radiologic findings are inconclusive, and diagnosis is made through pathologic analysis of excised tumor [138, 140, 142, 143].

### Pathology

MST is most commonly a solitary lesion in the renal medulla that shows a lobulated, tan to yellow appearance on cut surface. Small cysts may occasionally be present. Most MSTs are small to medium lesions, with an average approximate size of 4 cm [140]. On microscopy, bland stromal cells surround blood vessels and background renal parenchymal structures, giving an appearance of concentric rings (Fig. 11.7). A myxoid background may be present. Angiodysplasia may be present and is characterized by vessels showing epithelioid transformation of the medial smooth muscle. Heterologous

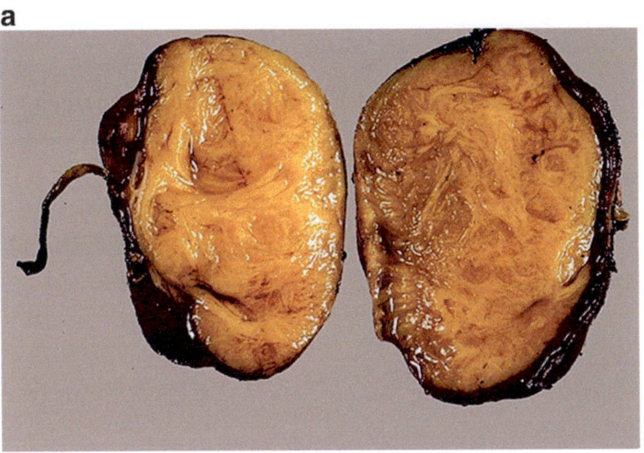

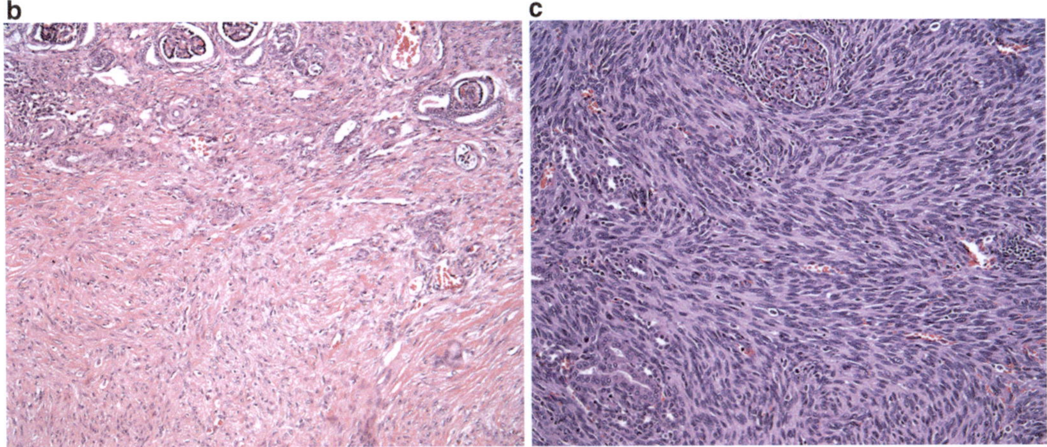

**Fig. 11.6** (**a**) Congenital mesoblastic nephroma. (**b**) Congenital mesoblastic nephroma, conventional pattern. (**c**) Congenital mesoblastic nephroma, cellular variant

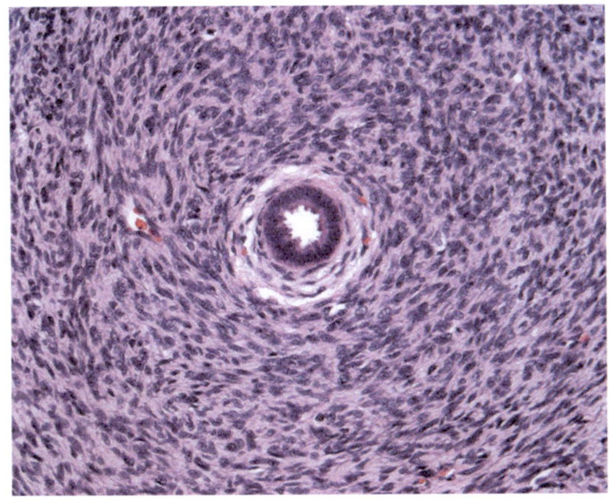

**Fig. 11.7** Metanephric stromal tumor

elements including glial tissue or cartilage may be present [140, 144].

The differential diagnosis of MST includes CMN and CCSK. In contrast to the deeply inter-digitating nature of CMN into the background renal parenchyma, MST is typically smaller with more focal regions of intercalation into the sur-rounding kidney. MST is occasionally more dif-ficult to distinguish at the cytological level from CCSK, although the more limited nature of MST lesions and the absence of the branching vascular pattern seen in CCSK can help in the distinction of these two entities. Immunohistochemical stains in MST show focal expression of CD34 (which is negative in CMN and CCSK) and absence of desmin, cytokeratin, and S100 immu-noreactivity [134, 138, 140–144].

## Prognosis and Clinical Management

In most cases, complete excision is both curative and diagnostic [138]. Once the diagnosis is established, no further adjuvant therapy is required. A single report of recurrence has been reported [139].

## Metanephric Adenofibroma

### Introduction

Metanephric adenofibroma (MAF), also called nephrogenic adenofibroma, is a rare biphasic tumor that combines the epithelial component of metanephric adenoma (MA) and stromal component of MST. Few cases have been reported in the literature with age ranging from 5 months to 36 years old (mean 6 years). It is more commonly seen in the male population (2:1). MAF can be morphologically similar to Wilms tumors (WT) and intralobar nephrogenic rests, and it has been considered a hyperdifferentiated version of these tumors [134, 144, 145].

### Clinical Presentation

The most common presenting symptom is hematuria. The radiologic appearance of MFA is nondiagnostic and indistinguishable from other solid pediatric renal tumors. Polycythemia is a peculiar incidental finding, which resolves after resection of the tumor [134, 145, 146].

### Pathology

MAF is localized to the renal medulla and is most commonly seen as a solitary lesion with a tan to yellow cut surface. Cystic change and nodularity have been reported. Average gross size is 3.85 cm [145]. Microscopically, there are a variable proportion of epithelial and stromal elements in MAF. The stromal element appears identical to that seen in MST, including the "onion skin" patterning, although is less likely to be associated with juxtaglomerular hyperplasia. The epithelial element shows unencapsulated groups of epithelial cells separated by bands of stroma. Numerous variants have been reported that overlap in appearance with more conventional metanephric adenoma. Immunohistochemical features of the stromal cells are similar to MST, with immunore-

activity to CD34 and absence of staining for desmin, muscle-specific actin, and cytokeratin. The epithelial component, however, is often immunoreactive for keratins and negative for AMACR [134, 144, 145].

## Prognosis and Clinical Management

Treatment is surgical excision with no reports of recurrence in the literature. MAF cases that may be associated with WT should receive adjuvant chemotherapy [144, 147, 148].

## Multicystic Dysplastic Kidney

### Introduction

Multicystic dysplastic kidney (MCDK) is a nonneoplastic lesion characterized by malformation of the kidney that manifests as variably sized cysts and frequently absence or diminishment of the vascular pedicle and ureter. Cysts may enlarge, remain stable in size, or involute [149–154]. The etiology of MCDKs remains unknown, but there are two leading theories. The obstruction theory proposes that the MCDK results from severe fetal obstructive hydronephrosis due to atresia of the renal pelvis or ureter [155]. The other theory suggests perturbation of the interaction between the ureteric bud and metanephric blastema [156, 157]. MCDK usually develops as a sporadic problem, although familial occurrence has been reported. The reported incidence of MCDK is estimated between 1 in 1000 and 1 in 4300 live births [158–161].

Vesicoureteral reflux (VUR), ureteropelvic junction (UPJ) obstruction, and megaureter of the contralateral kidney occur in children with MCDK more frequently than in the general population [152, 161–170]. VUR is the most frequent finding, with a reported incidence of up to 43 % in patients with MCDK. Therefore, VCUG is often recommended early in life. The majority of cases of VUR in these patients are asymptomatic, low grade, and self-limiting [152, 161–171]. The risk of hypertension among children with MCDK is similar to that seen in the general pediatric population [172–175]. While hypertension has been reported in association with retained

MCDKs, it is likely a result of damage to the contralateral functional solitary kidney rather than the MCDK itself [152, 159, 176]. Hypertension associated with MCDK may or may not resolve after nephrectomy of the MCDK [177–179]. There is a slight increased risk of Wilms tumor in patients with MCDK, with an incidence of 1 in 10,000 in the general population compared to 3 to 10 in 10,000 in children with MCDK in the USA. Approximately 16,000 MCDKs would have to be removed to prevent one Wilms tumor-related death and neither surveillance nor prophylactic nephrectomy seems warranted [180–184].

## Clinical Presentation

Most cases of MCDK are diagnosed on prenatal ultrasonography and less often because of a palpable abdominal mass. Most patients have neither symptoms nor a palpable abdominal mass [152]. The majority of cases of MCDK undergo spontaneous involution. Great variation in the prevalence of involution has been reported, ranging from 10 % at a mean of 33.5 months to 75 % at a mean of 16 months of observation [167, 179, 185–188]. Initially smaller MCDKs are more likely to involute and do so at an earlier age [189]. The contralateral kidney is often hypertrophic with compensatory growth.

## Pathology

On gross examination, the kidney may be diffusely involved by variably sized cysts and the pelvicalyceal system and ureter may be narrow and misshapen. On occasion, the process may be bilateral. On microscopy, immaturity and disorganization of the renal parenchyma are apparent. Epithelial structures are commonly present and include primitive ducts lined by cuboidal to columnar epithelium, cysts, and rudimentary glomerular elements (Fig. 11.8). Fibrous stroma may be present and can include the presence of heterologous cartilage [157].

## Prognosis and Clinical Management

Management involves observation and treatment of associated conditions. Indications for nephrectomy are restricted to large MCDKs that interfere with respiratory or intestinal function in the neonatal phase and those that contain solid components that grow on serial imaging [152]. Prognosis depends on whether involvement is unilateral or bilateral and on the presence and severity of associated anomalies. Bilaterality results in increased fetal loss or profound oligohydramnios with rapid respiratory death after birth [156]. Most patients with isolated unilateral MCDK, however, do not experience any problems or complications as a consequence of this congenital anomaly.

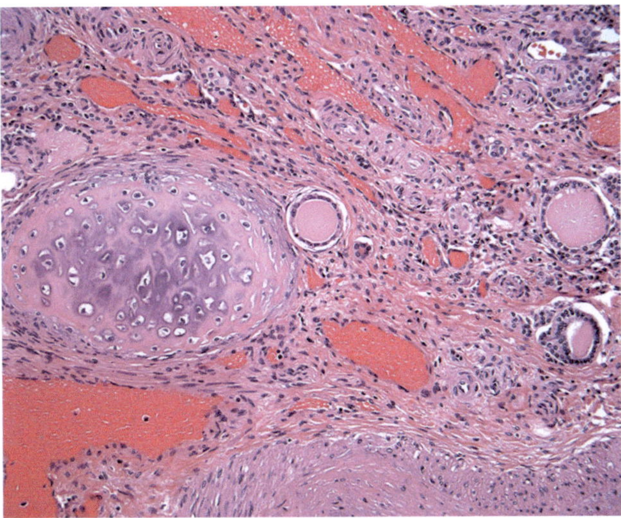

**Fig. 11.8** Multicystic dysplastic kidney

## Medullary Sponge Kidney

### Introduction
Medullary sponge kidney (MSK) results from a disruption of the ureteric bud-metanephric mesenchyme interface due to abnormalities in the glial cell line-derived neurotrophic factor (GDNF) or receptor tyrosine kinase (RET) genes [190, 191]. Defective acidification is the initial abnormality, which is followed by a sequence made up of defective bone mineralization, hypercalciuria, and stone formation. Patients may be in a negative calcium balance, which can cause hyperparathyroidism. Defective urinary concentrating ability and distal tubular acidosis can also be found which is a result of the functional abnormality of the terminal collecting ducts [192]. Exact prevalence is unknown although it is probably less than 0.5–1 %. It is much more frequent (12–20 %) in recurrent renal calcium stone formers [193].

### Clinical Presentation
MSK is generally diagnosed in young adulthood. Three different clinical profiles are recognized, all of which show the typical radiological feature of ectatic precalyceal papillary collecting ducts and nephrocalcinosis. The two most common include an indolent form rarely characterized by stones and diagnosed incidentally or with atypical signs and a much more prevalent form in which the patients manifest with many small stones that occasionally need urologic intervention. The third profile is a rare but severe condition dominated by intractable excruciating renal pain [194]. Urinary tract infection is considered to be the second most frequent clinical problem after renal stones in patients with MSK. Pyelonephritis can occur from urine stagnation in the dilated prepapillary tubule or by stones themselves. Recurrent infections can cause struvite stones, which may rarely lead to ESRD. Occasionally patients also discuss passing of sand in their urine. Diagnosis historically has been done via intravenous urogram to visualize tubular ectasia. With the increase in the use of CT and ultrasound, diagnosis is sometimes made erroneously based on multiple small stones which may or may not have the associated ectasia, which is specific for MSK [195].

### Pathology
On gross evaluation, the papillae in MSK are enlarged with rounded contours and blunted tips. The papillae may also show white and yellow plaques and variable numbers of stones. The classic histological triad for MSK consists of undifferentiated interstitial cells, multilayered hyperplastic epithelium of the medullary collecting ducts, and single-layered epithelium in dilated medullary collecting ducts. Small stones may be present in the latter structure. Immunohistochemical stains show expression of Runx2 in the nucleus of interstitial cells [193, 194, 196, 197].

### Prognosis and Clinical Management
Treatment with potassium citrate aids with the observed hypercalciuria and hypocitraturia [193]. A diet with high fluid intake, low salt, and low protein is also recommended for overall stone prevention, and thiazide diuretics are also used as an adjunct. Surgical intervention can be necessary as a result of infected or obstructing stones. Endourological approaches are available as well as complex reconstructions including autotransplantation with creation of a pyelovesicostomy to allow for stone passage [198].

## Reflux Nephropathy

### Introduction
Reflux nephropathy has been used to describe the renal abnormalities in patients diagnosed with vesicoureteral reflux (VUR). These lesions can include renal scarring, renal lesions, renal parenchymal abnormalities, dysplasia, and renal hypoplasia [199]. Several factors may contribute to reflux nephropathy including the severity of the VUR as well a possible genetic predisposition. VUR in itself is quite common with estimates at 1–2 % of all live births [200]. It is unknown how many of these children go on to have manifestations of reflux nephropathy. Familial clustering of VUR implies that genetic factors have an

important role in its pathogenesis, but no single major locus or gene for VUR has yet been identified and most researchers now acknowledge that VUR is genetically heterogeneous [201]. Since VUR is relatively common, there are a multitude of associated conditions along the CAKUT (congenital abnormalities of the kidney and urinary tract) spectrum. Many syndromes such as renal coloboma, Kallman, urofacial, de Lange, Bardet-Biedl, and Epstein syndrome can also be seen. The inheritance in these syndromes is usually autosomal dominant and multiple genes have been found to be disrupted including PAX2 [199, 200, 202–205].

## Clinical Presentation

In actuality, reflux nephropathy is a pathological entity that ideally would be documented histologically. However clinically it is diagnosed with recurrent urinary tract infections (UTIs) in the context of VUR and evidence of radiological abnormalities. A DMSA scan (dimercaptosuccinic acid renal scan) is the ideal imaging to confirm the presence of abnormalities although intravenous pyelography (IVP) has been used in the past. The differentiation between renal hypoplasia/dysplasia and reflux nephropathy can be difficult based on imaging alone, but the lack of UTIs is consistent with renal hypoplasia/dysplasia where the abnormality is in ureteral bud development.

Reflux nephropathy can cause long-term consequences of hypertension, loss of renal function, and even end-stage renal disease. Hypertension is thought to be mediated by the renin-angiotensin system with higher levels of serum renin. Eighteen percent of patients were noted to have hypertension after 15 years with initial findings of reflux nephropathy. Most patients become hypertensive between the ages of 15 and 30 [203]. In some studies hypertension can occur with any degree of renal damage [204]. Problems with hypertension can also manifest as preeclampsia during pregnancy. The incidence of preeclampsia was noted to be 24 % in women with bilateral renal scars versus 7 % with unilateral renal scarring [202]. The Italian Pediatric Registry of Renal Failure reported that 25 % of

patients with end-stage renal failure had a history of VUR [206].

## Pathology

Reflux nephropathy can be associated with inflammation and occasional colonization by bacterial organisms. The inflammatory response can cause local renal damage with deposition of collagen and destruction of the renal parenchyma over time. Histologically, the areas of damaged renal parenchyma show interstitial fibrosis, glomerulosclerosis, and dilated and atrophic tubules [199, 207].

## Prognosis and Clinical Management

The treatment of VUR continues to be controversial. The use of prophylactic antibiotics and surgical management can vary among providers. Ideally VUR will resolve after a period of observation. If it doesn't resolve, treatment can depend on the presence of scarring, the current grade of VUR, and parental or provider bias [208].

# Hematologic Malignancies Involving the Pediatric Kidney

## Renal Lymphoma and Leukemia

### Introduction

Primary renal lymphoma and leukemia are exceedingly rare in children [209, 210]. More often, renal involvement results from infiltration of the kidney by circulating malignant cells. Once within the kidneys, tumor infiltration is initially interstitial, with the nephrons, collecting ducts, and blood vessels acting as scaffolding for tumor growth. Further growth leads to destruction of the renal parenchyma scaffolding, resulting in an expansile growth pattern. Since only a fraction of these patients undergo CT imaging, the true incidence of renal leukemic involvement in children is unknown [211].

### Clinical Presentation

Renal lymphoma may present with renal failure, abdominal pain and abdominal mass, anemia, or hematuria [212–220]. On imaging, kidneys may appear unilaterally or bilaterally enlarged, as a single lesion, or as multiple mostly cortical lesions [221–223]. Regional lymph node involvement is common at presentation, as are metastases to the lungs, liver, choroid plexus, tonsils, and bone marrow [215, 220, 224–228]. Lymphoma infiltration may affect the kidney either primarily or secondarily [229, 230]. Secondary renal involvement as a part of systemic disease or contiguous infiltration from adjacent lymphoma is detected in only 3–8 % of all patients, most commonly through routine CT staging for lymphoma [222, 231–234]. In autopsy series, however, estimates of renal involvement in patients with known lymphoma range from 30 to 60 % [235].

Nephromegaly, hematuria, and renal dysfunction may be seen [209, 210, 224, 236–239]. However, renal leukemic involvement is usually an incidental finding. Unlike patients with lymphoma, children with leukemia do not generally require routine CT imaging for staging or follow-up. Instead, CT imaging in children with leukemia is typically utilized in the assessment of possible disease-related complications or for the evaluation of some other clinical problems. Renal leukemic involvement can present with a wide variety of contrast-enhanced CT imaging findings. The most common focal parenchymal abnormality is that of multiple bilateral renal low-attenuation masses. These may appear as small and large round low-attenuation masses, wedge-shaped and geographic low-attenuation masses, or ill-defined areas of low attenuation. Diagnosis involves core needle biopsy in association with hematologic findings [211].

## Pathology

Lymphomas and leukemias involving the kidney may appear as either a focal lesion or as diffuse involvement of the kidney on gross examination. The cut surface appears firm and pale, often with a homogeneous appearance. Necrosis, hemorrhage, cystic change, calcifications, and tumor thrombi can occur. Microscopically, abnormal lymphoid cells are present infiltrating between background renal elements [134]. These lymphoid cells may be present in sheets, which is often associated with diffuse renal enlargement, or as discrete nodules. Malignant lymphoid cells may also be primarily present within vascular spaces (intravascular lymphoma).

Immunohistochemical, flow, and molecular analyses can help to identify the lymphoid lineage of the neoplastic cells [134, 209, 211, 239].

## Prognosis and Clinical Management

The majority of cases of primary renal lymphoma in children have been treated with chemotherapy, although management with surgery, radiotherapy, and multimodal therapy has also been reported [212, 214, 218, 219, 240–244]. Treatment of secondary renal lymphoma is generally nonsurgical. Typically chemotherapy improves renal function [212, 214–216, 218–221]. The overall prognosis in these patients is poor due to its rapid dissemination with only a few long-term survivors reported in the literature [124, 240, 244–248]. Bilateral disease portends a worse outcome [219–221, 224, 227, 228, 240, 244].

There is no standardized recommendation for treatment of renal leukemia, but it usually involves chemotherapy and/or bone marrow transplant (BMT). Given the paucity of data, it is difficult to determine the prognosis with certainty [249–252].

## References


1. National Cancer Institute. Wilms tumor and other childhood kidney tumors treatment (PDQVR). http://www.cancer.gov/types/kidney/hp/wilms-treatment-pdq-section/_755. Accessed 14 June 2015.
2. Royer-Pokora B. Genetics of pediatric renal tumors. Pediatr Nephrol. 2013;28(1):13–23.
3. Ward E, DeSantis C, Robbins A, Kohler B, Jemal A. Childhood and adolescent cancer statistics, 2014. CA Cancer J Clin. 2014;64(2):83–103.
4. SEER Cancer Statistics Review Bethesda (MD). National Cancer Institute 1975–2010. http://seer.cancer.gov/archive/csr/1975_2010/. Accessed 12 June 2015.
5. Gronskov K, Olsen JH, Sand A, Pedersen W, Carlsen N, Bak Jylling AM, et al. Population-based risk estimates of Wilms tumor in sporadic aniridia. A comprehensive mutation screening procedure of PAX6

identifies 80% of mutations in aniridia. Hum Genet. 2001;109(1):11–8.

6. Muto R, Yamamori S, Ohashi H, Osawa M. Prediction by FISH analysis of the occurrence of Wilms tumor in aniridia patients. Am J Med Genet. 2002;108(4):285–9.

7. Huff V. Genotype/phenotype correlations in Wilms' tumor. Med Pediatr Oncol. 1996;27(5):408–14.

8. Royer-Pokora B, Beier M, Henzler M, Alam R, Schumacher V, Weirich A, et al. Twenty-four new cases of WT1 germline mutations and review of the literature: genotype/phenotype correlations for Wilms tumor development. Am J Med Genet A. 2004;127A(3):249–57.

9. Barbaux S, Niaudet P, Gubler MC, Grunfeld JP, Jaubert F, Kuttenn F, et al. Donor splice-site mutations in WT1 are responsible for Frasier syndrome. Nat Genet. 1997;17(4):467–70.

10. Koziell A, Charmandari E, Hindmarsh PC, Rees L, Scambler P, Brook CG. Frasier syndrome, part of the Denys Drash continuum or simply a WT1 gene associated disorder of intersex and nephropathy? Clin Endocrinol (Oxf). 2000;52(4):519–24.

11. Grubb GR, Yun K, Williams BR, Eccles MR, Reeve AE. Expression of WT1 protein in fetal kidneys and Wilms tumors. Lab Invest. 1994;71(4):472–9.

12. Tan TY, Amor DJ. Tumour surveillance in Beckwith-Wiedemann syndrome and hemihyperplasia: a critical review of the evidence and suggested guidelines for local practice. J Paediatr Child Health. 2006; 42(9):486–90.

13. Davidoff AM. Wilms tumor. Adv Pediatr. 2012; 59(1):247–67.

14. Shamberger RC, Ritchey ML, Haase GM, Bergemann TL, Loechelt-Yoshioka T, Breslow NE, et al. Intravascular extension of Wilms tumor. Ann Surg. 2001;234(1):116–21.

15. Sarin YK, Bhatnagar SN. Wilms' tumor-roadmaps of management. Indian J Pediatr. 2012;79(6):776–86.

16. Joshi VV, Beckwith JB. Multilocular cyst of the kidney (cystic nephroma) and cystic, partially differentiated nephroblastoma. Terminology and criteria for diagnosis. Cancer. 1989;64(2):466–79.

17. Blakely ML, Shamberger RC, Norkool P, Beckwith JB, Green DM, Ritchey ML, et al. Outcome of children with cystic partially differentiated nephroblastoma treated with or without chemotherapy. J Pediatr Surg. 2003;38(6):897–900.

18. Beckwith JB. Wilms' tumor and other renal tumors of childhood: a selective review from the National Wilms' Tumor Study Pathology Center. Hum Pathol. 1983;14(6):481–92.

19. Beckwith JB. National Wilms Tumor Study: an update for pathologists. Pediatr Dev Pathol. 1998;1(1):79–84.

20. Green DM, Beckwith JB, Breslow NE, Faria P, Moksness J, Finklestein JZ, et al. Treatment of children with stages II to IV anaplastic Wilms' tumor: a report from the National Wilms' Tumor Study Group. J Clin Oncol. 1994;12(10):2126–31.

21. Beckwith JB, Zuppan CE, Browning NG, Moksness J, Breslow NE. Histological analysis of aggressiveness and responsiveness in Wilms' tumor. Med Pediatr Oncol. 1996;27(5):422–8.

22. Faria P, Beckwith JB, Mishra K, Zuppan C, Weeks DA, Breslow N, et al. Focal versus diffuse anaplasia in Wilms tumor--new definitions with prognostic significance: a report from the National Wilms Tumor Study Group. Am J Surg Pathol. 1996;20(8):909–20.

23. Charles AK, Mall S, Watson J, Berry PJ. Expression of the Wilms' tumour gene WT1 in the developing human and in paediatric renal tumours: an immunohistochemical study. Mol Pathol. 1997;50(3): 138–44.

24. Magro G, Longo FR, Angelico G, Spadola S, Amore FF, Salvatorelli L. Immunohistochemistry as potential diagnostic pitfall in the most common solid tumors of children and adolescents. Acta Histochem. 2015;117(4–5):397–414.

25. Sehic D, Ciornei CD, Gisselsson D. Evaluation of CITED1, SIX1, and CD56 protein expression for identification of blastemal elements in Wilms tumor. Am J Clin Pathol. 2014;141(6):828–33.

26. Vasei M, Moch H, Mousavi A, Kajbafzadeh AM, Sauter G. Immunohistochemical profiling of Wilms tumor: a tissue microarray study. Appl Immunohistochem Mol Morphol. 2008;16(2): 128–34.

27. Huff V. Wilms' tumours: about tumour suppressor genes, an oncogene and a chameleon gene. Nat Rev Cancer. 2011;11(2):111–21.

28. Grundy P, Breslow N, Green DM, Sharples K, Evans A, D'Angio GJ. Prognostic factors for children with recurrent Wilms' tumor: results from the Second and Third National Wilms' Tumor Study. J Clin Oncol. 1989;7(5):638–47.

29. Pinkerton CR, Groot-Loonen JJ, Morris-Jones PH, Pritchard J. Response rates in relapsed Wilms' tumor. A need for new effective agents. Cancer. 1991;67(3):567–71.

30. Beckwith JB, Kiviat NB, Bonadio JF. Nephrogenic rests, nephroblastomatosis, and the pathogenesis of Wilms' tumor. Pediatr Pathol. 1990;10(1–2):1–36.

31. Beckwith JB. New developments in the pathology of Wilms tumor. Cancer Invest. 1997;15(2):153–62.

32. Beckwith JB. Nephrogenic rests and the pathogenesis of Wilms tumor: developmental and clinical considerations. Am J Med Genet. 1998;79(4):268–73.

33. Stabouli S, Printza N, Dotis J, Matis A, Koliouskas D, Gombakis N, et al. Perilobar nephroblastomatosis: natural history and management. Case Rep Pediatr. 2014;2014:756819.

34. Sebire NJ, Vujanic GM. Paediatric renal tumours: recent developments, new entities and pathological features. Histopathology. 2009;54(5):516–28.

35. Pizzo PA, Poplack DG. Principles and practice of pediatric oncology, vol. xiv. 5th ed. Philadelphia: Lippincott Williams & Wilkins; 2006. 1,780 pages.

36. Rohrschneider WK, Weirich A, Rieden K, Darge K, Troger J, Graf N. US, CT and MR imaging charac-

teristics of nephroblastomatosis. Pediatr Radiol. 1998;28(6):435–43.

37. Bergeron C, Iliescu C, Thiesse P, Bouvier R, Dijoud F, Ranchere-Vince D, et al. Does nephroblastomatosis influence the natural history and relapse rate in Wilms' tumour? A single centre experience over 11 years. Eur J Cancer. 2001;37(3):385–91.

38. Perlman EJ, Faria P, Soares A, Hoffer F, Sredni S, Ritchey M, et al. Hyperplastic perilobar nephroblastomatosis: long-term survival of 52 patients. Pediatr Blood Cancer. 2006;46(2):203–21.

39. Stone MM, Beaver BL, Sun CC, Hill JL. The nephroblastomatosis complex and its relationship to Wilms' tumor. J Pediatr Surg. 1990;25(9):933–7. discussion 7–8.

40. Coppes M, Ritchey M. Commentary: managing nephroblastomatosis. Med Pediatr Oncol. 2000;35: 433.

41. Prasil P, Laberge JM, Bond M, Bernstein M, Pippi-Salle JL, Bernard C, et al. Management decisions in children with nephroblastomatosis. Med Pediatr Oncol. 2000;35(4):429–32. discussion 33.

42. Sotelo-Avila C, Gonzalez-Crussi F, Sadowinski S, Gooch 3rd WM, Pena R. Clear cell sarcoma of the kidney: a clinicopathologic study of 21 patients with long-term follow-up evaluation. Hum Pathol. 1985;16(12):1219–30.

43. Huang CC, Cutcliffe C, Coffin C, Sorensen PH, Beckwith JB, Perlman EJ, et al. Classification of malignant pediatric renal tumors by gene expression. Pediatr Blood Cancer. 2006;46(7):728–38.

44. Argani P, Perlman EJ, Breslow NE, Browning NG, Green DM, D'Angio GJ, et al. Clear cell sarcoma of the kidney: a review of 351 cases from the National Wilms Tumor Study Group Pathology Center. Am J Surg Pathol. 2000;24(1):4–18.

45. Seibel NL, Li S, Breslow NE, Beckwith JB, Green DM, Haase GM, et al. Effect of duration of treatment on treatment outcome for patients with clear-cell sarcoma of the kidney: a report from the National Wilms' Tumor Study Group. J Clin Oncol. 2004;22(3):468–73.

46. Green DM, Breslow NE, Beckwith JB, Moksness J, Finklestein JZ, D'Angio GJ. Treatment of children with clear-cell sarcoma of the kidney: a report from the National Wilms' Tumor Study Group. J Clin Oncol. 1994;12(10):2132–7.

47. Hung NA. Congenital "clear cell sarcoma of the kidney". Virchows Arch. 2005;446(5):566–8.

48. Amin MB, de Peralta-Venturina MN, Ro JY, El-Naggar A, Mackay B, Ordonez N, et al. Clear cell sarcoma of kidney in an adolescent and in young adults: a report of four cases with ultrastructural, immunohistochemical, and DNA flow cytometric analysis. Am J Surg Pathol. 1999;23(12):1455–63.

49. Kural AR, Onal B, Ozkara H, Cakarir C, Ayan I, Agaoglu FY. Adult clear cell sarcoma of the kidney: a case report. BMC Urol. 2006;6:11.

50. Rosso D, Ghignone GP, Bernardi D, Zitella A, Casetta G, De Zan A, et al. Clear cell sarcoma of the kidney with invasion of the inferior vena cava. Urol Int. 2003;70(3):251–2.

51. Bhayani SB, Liapis H, Kibel AS. Adult clear cell sarcoma of the kidney with atrial tumor thrombus. J Urol. 2001;165(3):896–7.

52. Oda H, Shiga J, Machinami R. Clear cell sarcoma of kidney. Two cases in adults. Cancer. 1993;71(7): 2286–91.

53. Mishra VK, Krishnani N, Bhandari M. Clear cell sarcoma of kidney in an adult. Br J Urol. 1993; 72(1):118.

54. Toyoda Y, Yamashita C, Sugimoto T, Yoshida M, Okada M. Clear cell sarcoma of kidney with tumor extension into the right atrium. J Cardiovasc Surg (Torino). 1998;39(4):489–91.

55. Adnani A, Latib R, Bouklata S, Ajana A, Hammani L, Imani F. Clear cell sarcoma of the kidney in an adult: a case report. J Radiol. 2006;87(2 Pt 1): 136–8.

56. Suzuki H, Honzumi M, Itoh Y, Umehara N, Moriyama S, Funada M. Clear-cell sarcoma of the kidney seen in a 3-day-old newborn. Z Kinderchir. 1983;38(6):422–4.

57. Newbould MJ, Kelsey AM. Clear cell sarcoma of the kidney in a 4-month-old infant: a case report. Med Pediatr Oncol. 1993;21(7):525–8.

58. Mazzoleni S, Vecchiato L, Alaggio R, Cecchetto G, Zorzi C, Carli M. Clear cell sarcoma of the kidney in a newborn. Med Pediatr Oncol. 2003;41(2):153–5.

59. Benchekroun A, Ghadouane M, Zannoud M, Alami M, Amhajji R, Faik M. Clear cell sarcoma of the kidney in an adult. A case report. Ann Urol (Paris). 2002;36(1):33–5.

60. Punnett HH, Halligan GE, Zaeri N, Karmazin N. Translocation 10;17 in clear cell sarcoma of the kidney. A first report. Cancer Genet Cytogenet. 1989;41(1):123–8.

61. Rakheja D, Weinberg AG, Tomlinson GE, Partridge K, Schneider NR. Translocation (10;17)(q22;p13): a recurring translocation in clear cell sarcoma of kidney. Cancer Genet Cytogenet. 2004;154(2):175–9.

62. Brownlee NA, Perkins LA, Stewart W, Jackle B, Pettenati MJ, Koty PP, et al. Recurring translocation (10;17) and deletion (14q) in clear cell sarcoma of the kidney. Arch Pathol Lab Med. 2007;131(3): 446–51.

63. Kalapurakal JA, Perlman EJ, Seibel NL, Ritchey M, Dome JS, Grundy PE. Outcomes of patients with revised stage I clear cell sarcoma of kidney treated in National Wilms Tumor Studies 1–5. Int J Radiat Oncol Biol Phys. 2013;85(2):428–31.

64. Morgan E, Kidd JM. Undifferentiated sarcoma of the kidney: a tumor of childhood with histopathologic and clinical characteristics distinct from Wilms' tumor. Cancer. 1978;42(4):1916–21.

65. Cheah PL, Looi LM. Implications of p53 protein expression in clear cell sarcoma of the kidney. Pathology. 1996;28(3):229–31.

66. El Kababri M, Khattab M, El Khorassani M, Hessissen L, Kili A, Nachef MN, et al. Clear cell sar-

coma of the kidney. A study of 13 cases. Arch Pediatr. 2004;11(7):794–9.

67. Furtwangler R, Gooskens SL, van Tinteren H, de Kraker J, Schleiermacher G, Bergeron C, et al. Clear cell sarcomas of the kidney registered on International Society of Pediatric Oncology (SIOP) 93–01 and SIOP 2001 protocols: a report of the SIOP Renal Tumour Study Group. Eur J Cancer. 2013;49(16):3497–506.

68. Manchanda V, Mohta A, Khurana N, Gupta CR, Neogi S. Bilateral clear cell sarcoma of the kidney. J Pediatr Surg. 2010;45(9):1927–30.

69. Parikh SH, Chintagumpala M, Hicks MJ, Trautwein LM, Blaney S, Minifee P, et al. Clear cell sarcoma of the kidney: an unusual presentation and review of the literature. J Pediatr Hematol Oncol. 1998; 20(2):165–8.

70. Iyer VK, Kapila K, Verma K. Fine needle aspiration cytology of clear cell sarcoma of the kidney with spindle cell pattern. Cytopathology. 2003;14(3): 160–4.

71. Haas JE, Bonadio JF, Beckwith JB. Clear cell sarcoma of the kidney with emphasis on ultrastructural studies. Cancer. 1984;54(12):2978–87.

72. Kusumakumary P, Chellam VG, Rojymon J, Hariharan S, Krishnan NM. Late recurrence of clear cell sarcoma of the kidney. Med Pediatr Oncol. 1997;28(5):355–7.

73. Gooskens SL, Furtwangler R, Vujanic GM, Dome JS, Graf N, van den Heuvel-Eibrink MM. Clear cell sarcoma of the kidney: a review. Eur J Cancer. 2012;48(14):2219–26.

74. Hoot AC, Russo P, Judkins AR, Perlman EJ, Biegel JA. Immunohistochemical analysis of hSNF5/INI1 distinguishes renal and extra-renal malignant rhabdoid tumors from other pediatric soft tissue tumors. Am J Surg Pathol. 2004;28(11):1485–91.

75. Rubin BP, Fletcher JA, Renshaw AA. Clear cell sarcoma of soft parts: report of a case primary in the kidney with cytogenetic confirmation. Am J Surg Pathol. 1999;23(5):589–94.

76. Shao L, Hill DA, Perlman EJ. Expression of WT-1, Bcl-2, and CD34 by primary renal spindle cell tumors in children. Pediatr Dev Pathol. 2004;7(6): 577–82.

77. Seibel N, Sun J, Anderson J. Outcome of clear cell sarcoma of the kidney (CCSK) treated on the National Wilms Tumor Study-5 (NWTS). J Clin Oncol. 2006;24(abstr 9000).

78. Hsueh C, Wang H, Gonzalez-Crussi F, Lin JN, Hung IJ, Yang CP, et al. Infrequent p53 gene mutations and lack of p53 protein expression in clear cell sarcoma of the kidney: immunohistochemical study and mutation analysis of p53 in renal tumors of unfavorable prognosis. Mod Pathol. 2002;15(6):606–10.

79. Park DY, Kim YM, Chi JG. Intracranial metastasis from clear cell sarcoma of the kidney--a case report. J Korean Med Sci. 1997;12(5):473–6.

80. Yumura-Yagi K, Inoue M, Wakabayashi R, Mabuchi S, Nakayama M, Yoneda A, et al. Successful double autografts for patients with relapsed clear cell sarcoma of the kidney. Bone Marrow Transplant. 1998;22(4):381–3.

81. Wood Jr DP, Kay R, Norris D. Renal sarcomas of childhood. Urology. 1990;36(1):73–8.

82. Isaacs Jr H. Fetal and neonatal rhabdoid tumor. J Pediatr Surg. 2010;45(3):619–26.

83. Agrons GA, Kingsman KD, Wagner BJ, Sotelo-Avila C. Rhabdoid tumor of the kidney in children: a comparative study of 21 cases. AJR Am J Roentgenol. 1997;168(2):447–51.

84. Isaacs H. Tumors in pathology of the fetus and infants. 4th ed. St Louis, MO: Mosby Year Book; 1996. p. 1242–339.

85. Isaacs H. Tumors of the fetus and newborn, vol. xii. Philadelphia: W.B. Saunders; 1997. 384 pages.

86. Isaacs Jr H. Perinatal (congenital and neonatal) neoplasms: a report of 110 cases. Pediatr Pathol. 1985;3(2–4):165–216.

87. Vujanic GM, Sandstedt B, Harms D, Boccon-Gibod L, Delemarre JF. Rhabdoid tumour of the kidney: a clinicopathological study of 22 patients from the International Society of Paediatric Oncology (SIOP) nephroblastoma file. Histopathology. 1996;28(4):333–40.

88. Weeks DA, Beckwith JB, Mierau GW, Luckey DW. Rhabdoid tumor of kidney. A report of 111 cases from the National Wilms' Tumor Study Pathology Center. Am J Surg Pathol. 1989;13(6):439–58.

89. Marsden HB, Lawler W. Primary renal tumours in the first year of life. A population based review. Virchows Arch A Pathol Anat Histopathol. 1983;399(1):1–9.

90. Arey JB. Abdominal masses in infants and children. Pediatr Clin North Am. 1963;10:665–91.

91. Boles Jr ET. Tumors of the abdomen in children. Pediatr Clin North Am. 1962;9:467–84.

92. Chung CJ, Cammoun D, Munden M. Rhabdoid tumor of the kidney presenting as an abdominal mass in a newborn. Pediatr Radiol. 1990;20(7): 562–3.

93. Fuchs IB, Henrich W, Kalache KD, Lippek F, Dudenhausen JW. Prenatal sonographic features of a rhabdoid tumor of the kidney. Ultrasound Obstet Gynecol. 2004;23(4):407–10.

94. Luo CC, Lin JN, Jaing TH, Yang CP, Hsueh C. Malignant rhabdoid tumour of the kidney occurring simultaneously with a brain tumour: a report of two cases and review of the literature. Eur J Pediatr. 2002;161(6):340–2.

95. Bonnin JM, Rubinstein LJ, Palmer NF, Beckwith JB. The association of embryonal tumors originating in the kidney and in the brain. A report of seven cases. Cancer. 1984;54(10):2137–46.

96. Mayes LC, Kasselberg AG, Roloff JS, Lukens JN. Hypercalcemia associated with immunoreactive parathyroid hormone in a malignant rhabdoid tumor of the kidney (rhabdoid Wilms' tumor). Cancer. 1984;54(5):882–4.

97. Papadakis V, Vlachopapadopoulou EA, Levine L. Rhabdoid tumor of the kidney with humoral hypercalcemia and parathyroid hormone-related protein production. Med Pediatr Oncol. 1995;24(2):133–6.

98. Haas JE, Palmer NF, Weinberg AG, Beckwith JB. Ultrastructure of malignant rhabdoid tumor of the kidney. A distinctive renal tumor of children. Hum Pathol. 1981;12(7):646–57.

99. Parham DM, Weeks DA, Beckwith JB. The clinicopathologic spectrum of putative extrarenal rhabdoid tumors. An analysis of 42 cases studied with immunohistochemistry or electron microscopy. Am J Surg Pathol. 1994;18(10):1010–29.

100. Weeks DA, Beckwith JB, Mierau GW, Zuppan CW. Renal neoplasms mimicking rhabdoid tumor of kidney. A report from the National Wilms' Tumor Study Pathology Center. Am J Surg Pathol. 1991;15(11):1042–54.

101. Wick MR, Ritter JH, Dehner LP. Malignant rhabdoid tumors: a clinicopathologic review and conceptual discussion. Semin Diagn Pathol. 1995;12(3):233–48.

102. Malkan AD, Loh A, Bahrami A, Navid F, Coleman J, Green DM, et al. An approach to renal masses in pediatrics. Pediatrics. 2015;135(1):142–58.

103. Baltogiannis N, Mavridis G, Keramidas D. Intraabdominal desmoplastic small round cell tumour: report of two cases in paediatric patients. Eur J Pediatr Surg. 2002;12(5):333–6.

104. Crapanzano JP, Cardillo M, Lin O, Zakowski MF. Cytology of desmoplastic small round cell tumor. Cancer. 2002;96(1):21–31.

105. Furman J, Murphy WM, Wajsman Z, Berry 3rd AD. Urogenital involvement by desmoplastic small round-cell tumor. J Urol. 1997;158(4):1506–9.

106. Kim JH, Goo HW, Yoon CH. Intra-abdominal desmoplastic small round-cell tumour: multiphase CT findings in two children. Pediatr Radiol. 2003;33(6):418–21.

107. Pickhardt PJ, Fisher AJ, Balfe DM, Dehner LP, Huettner PC. Desmoplastic small round cell tumor of the abdomen: radiologic-histopathologic correlation. Radiology. 1999;210(3):633–8.

108. Wang LL, Perlman EJ, Vujanic GM, Zuppan C, Brundler MA, Cheung CR, et al. Desmoplastic small round cell tumor of the kidney in childhood. Am J Surg Pathol. 2007;31(4):576–84.

109. Liu J, Nau MM, Yeh JC, Allegra CJ, Chu E, Wright JJ. Molecular heterogeneity and function of EWS-WT1 fusion transcripts in desmoplastic small round cell tumors. Clin Cancer Res. 2000;6(9):3522–9.

110. Carroll JC, Klauber GT, Kretschmar CS, Ucci A, Cendron M. Urological aspects of intra-abdominal desmoplastic small round cell tumor of childhood: a preliminary report. J Urol. 1994;151(1):172–3.

111. Egloff AM, Lee EY, Dillon JE, Callahan MJ. Desmoplastic small round cell tumor of the kidney in a pediatric patient: sonographic and multiphase CT findings. AJR Am J Roentgenol. 2005;185(5):1347–9.

112. Gerald WL, Miller HK, Battifora H, Miettinen M, Silva EG, Rosai J. Intra-abdominal desmoplastic small round-cell tumor. Report of 19 cases of a distinctive type of high-grade polyphenotypic malignancy affecting young individuals. Am J Surg Pathol. 1991;15(6):499–513.

113. Ordonez NG. Desmoplastic small round cell tumor: II: an ultrastructural and immunohistochemical study with emphasis on new immunohistochemical markers. Am J Surg Pathol. 1998;22(11):1314–27.

114. Raney B, Anderson J, Arndt C, Crist W, Maurer H, Qualman S, et al. Primary renal sarcomas in the Intergroup Rhabdomyosarcoma Study Group (IRSG) experience, 1972–2005: a report from the Children's Oncology Group. Pediatr Blood Cancer. 2008;51(3):339–43.

115. Lae ME, Roche PC, Jin L, Lloyd RV, Nascimento AG. Desmoplastic small round cell tumor: a clinicopathologic, immunohistochemical, and molecular study of 32 tumors. Am J Surg Pathol. 2002;26(7):823–35.

116. Ordonez NG. Desmoplastic small round cell tumor: I: a histopathologic study of 39 cases with emphasis on unusual histological patterns. Am J Surg Pathol. 1998;22(11):1303–13.

117. Rao P, Tamboli P, Fillman EP, Meis JM. Primary intra-renal desmoplastic small round cell tumor: expanding the histologic spectrum, with special emphasis on the differential diagnostic considerations. Pathol Res Pract. 2014;210(12):1130–3.

118. Eaton SH, Cendron MA. Primary desmoplastic small round cell tumor of the kidney in a 7-year-old girl. J Pediatr Urol. 2006;2(1):52–4.

119. Gil A, Gomez Portilla A, Brun EA, Sugarbaker PH. Clinical perspective on desmoplastic small round-cell tumor. Oncology. 2004;67(3–4):231–42.

120. Gomi K, Hamanoue S, Tanaka M, Matsumoto M, Kitagawa N, Niwa T, et al. Anaplastic sarcoma of the kidney with chromosomal abnormality: first report on cytogenetic findings. Hum Pathol. 2010;41(10):1495–9.

121. Labanaris A, Zugor V, Smiszek R, Nutzel R, Kuhn R. Anaplastic sarcoma of the kidney. Scientific World Journal. 2009;9:97–101.

122. Vujanic GM, Kelsey A, Perlman EJ, Sandstedt B, Beckwith JB. Anaplastic sarcoma of the kidney: a clinicopathologic study of 20 cases of a new entity with polyphenotypic features. Am J Surg Pathol. 2007;31(10):1459–68.

123. Watanabe N, Omagari D, Yamada T, Nemoto N, Furuya T, Sugito K, et al. Anaplastic sarcoma of the kidney: case report and literature review. Pediatr Int. 2013;55(5):e129–32.

124. van den Heuvel-Eibrink MM, Grundy P, Graf N, Pritchard-Jones K, Bergeron C, Patte C, et al. Characteristics and survival of 750 children diag-

nosed with a renal tumor in the first seven months of life: a collaborative study by the SIOP/GPOH/SFOP, NWTSG, and UKCCSG Wilms tumor study groups. Pediatr Blood Cancer. 2008;50(6):1130–4.

125. Bolande RP. Congenital mesoblastic nephroma of infancy. Perspect Pediatr Pathol. 1973;1:227–50.

126. Pettinato G, Manivel JC, Wick MR, Dehner LP. Classical and cellular (atypical) congenital mesoblastic nephroma: a clinicopathologic, ultrastructural, immunohistochemical, and flow cytometric study. Hum Pathol. 1989;20(7):682–90.

127. Knezevich SR, McFadden DE, Tao W, Lim JF, Sorensen PH. A novel ETV6-NTRK3 gene fusion in congenital fibrosarcoma. Nat Genet. 1998;18(2): 184–7.

128. Murphy WM, Grignon DJ, Perlman EJ, Armed Forces Institute of Pathology (U.S.), Universities Associated for Research and Education in Pathology. Tumors of the kidney, bladder, and related urinary structures, vol. xii. Washington, DC: Armed Forces Institute of Pathology; 2004. 394 pages.

129. Knezevich SR, Garnett MJ, Pysher TJ, Beckwith JB, Grundy PE, Sorensen PH. ETV6-NTRK3 gene fusions and trisomy 11 establish a histogenetic link between mesoblastic nephroma and congenital fibrosarcoma. Cancer Res. 1998;58(22):5046–8.

130. Matsumura M, Nishi T, Sasaki Y, Yamada R, Yamamoto H, Ohhama Y, et al. Prenatal diagnosis and treatment strategy for congenital mesoblastic nephroma. J Pediatr Surg. 1993;28(12):1607–9.

131. Gormley TS, Skoog SJ, Jones RV, Maybee D. Cellular congenital mesoblastic nephroma: what are the options. J Urol. 1989;142(2 Pt 2):479–83. discussion 89.

132. Nadasdy T, Roth J, Johnson DL, Bane BL, Weinberg A, Verani R, et al. Congenital mesoblastic nephroma: an immunohistochemical and lectin study. Hum Pathol. 1993;24(4):413–9.

133. Rubin BP, Chen CJ, Morgan TW, Xiao S, Grier HE, Kozakewich HP, et al. Congenital mesoblastic nephroma t(12;15) is associated with ETV6-NTRK3 gene fusion: cytogenetic and molecular relationship to congenital (infantile) fibrosarcoma. Am J Pathol. 1998;153(5):1451–8.

134. Eble JN. WHO classification. France: Lyon; 2004.

135. Furtwaengler R, Reinhard H, Leuschner I, Schenk JP, Goebel U, Claviez A, et al. Mesoblastic nephroma—a report from the Gesellschaft fur Padiatrische Onkologie und Hamatologie (GPOH). Cancer. 2006;106(10):2275–83.

136. Beckwith JB. Letter to editor. Pediatr Pathol. 1993;13:886–7.

137. Gruver AM, Hansel DE, Luthringer DJ, MacLennan GT. Congenital mesoblastic nephroma. J Urol. 2010;183(3):1188–9.

138. Argani P, Beckwith JB. Metanephric stromal tumor: report of 31 cases of a distinctive pediatric renal neoplasm. Am J Surg Pathol. 2000;24(7):917–26.

139. De Pasquale MD, Diomedi-Camassei F, Serra A, Boldrini R, Inserra A, Caione P, et al. Recurrent metanephric stromal tumor in an infant. Urology. 2011;78(6):1411–3.

140. Kacar A, Azili MN, Cihan BS, Demir HA, Tiryaki HT, Argani P. Metanephric stromal tumor: a challenging diagnostic entity in children. J Pediatr Surg. 2011;46(12):e7–10.

141. Lorenzo AJ, Timmons C, Weinberg A, Megison SM, Snodgrass WT. Metanephric stromal tumor with urothelial extension. J Urol. 2003;169(3):1095–7.

142. Palese MA, Ferrer F, Perlman E, Gearhart JP. Metanephric stromal tumor: a rare benign pediatric renal mass. Urology. 2001;58(3):462.

143. Rajalakshmi V, Chandran P, Selvambigai, Ganesh J. Metanephric stromal tumor: a novel pediatric renal neoplasm. Indian J Pathol Microbiol. 2009;52(3): 389–91.

144. Argani P. Metanephric neoplasms: the hyperdifferentiated, benign end of the Wilms tumor spectrum? Clin Lab Med. 2005;25(2):379–92.

145. Arroyo MR, Green DM, Perlman EJ, Beckwith JB, Argani P. The spectrum of metanephric adenofibroma and related lesions: clinicopathologic study of 25 cases from the National Wilms Tumor Study Group Pathology Center. Am J Surg Pathol. 2001; 25(4):433–44.

146. Comerci SC, Levin TL, Ruzal-Shapiro C, Berdon WE, Beckwith JB, Hibshoosh H, et al. Benign adenomatous kidney neoplasms in children with polycythemia: imaging findings. Radiology. 1996;198(1):265–8.

147. Bigg SW, Bari WA. Nephrogenic adenofibroma: an unusual renal tumor. J Urol. 1997;157(5):1835–6.

148. Guzman E, Turc-Carel C, Soler C, Pierre C, Chevallier P, Michiels JF. Nephrogenic adenofibroma in a young child. Pathol Res Pract. 2000;196(12):853–6.

149. Avni EF, Thoua Y, Lalmand B, Didier F, Droulle P, Schulman CC. Multicystic dysplastic kidney: natural history from in utero diagnosis and postnatal follow-up. J Urol. 1987;138(6):1420–4.

150. Felson B, Cussen LJ. The hydronephrotic type of unilateral congenital multicystic disease of the kidney. Semin Roentgenol. 1975;10(2):113–23.

151. Hashimoto BE, Filly RA, Callen PW. Multicystic dysplastic kidney in utero: changing appearance on US. Radiology. 1986;159(1):107–9.

152. Kuwertz-Broeking E, Brinkmann OA, Von Lengerke HJ, Sciuk J, Fruend S, Bulla M, et al. Unilateral multicystic dysplastic kidney: experience in children. BJU Int. 2004;93(3):388–92.

153. Mesrobian HG, Rushton HG, Bulas D. Unilateral renal agenesis may result from in utero regression of multicystic renal dysplasia. J Urol. 1993;150 (2 Pt 2):793–4.

154. Pedicelli G, Jequier S, Bowen AD, Boisvert J. Multicystic dysplastic kidneys: spontaneous regression demonstrated with US. Radiology. 1986; 161(1):23–6.

155. Osathanondh V, Potter EL. Pathogenesis of polycystic kidneys. Historical survey. Arch Pathol. 1964;77:459–65.

156. Kleiner B, Filly RA, Mack L, Callen PW. Multicystic dysplastic kidney: observations of contralateral disease in the fetal population. Radiology. 1986; 161(1):27–9.

157. Matsell DG, Bennett T, Goodyer P, Goodyer C, Han VK. The pathogenesis of multicystic dysplastic kidney disease: insights from the study of fetal kidneys. Lab Invest. 1996;74(5):883–93.

158. Gordon AC, Thomas DF, Arthur RJ, Irving HC. Multicystic dysplastic kidney: is nephrectomy still appropriate? J Urol. 1988;140(5 Pt 2):1231–4.

159. James CA, Watson AR, Twining P, Rance CH. Antenatally detected urinary tract abnormalities: changing incidence and management. Eur J Pediatr. 1998;157(6):508–11.

160. Kalyoussef E, Hwang J, Prasad V, Barone J. Segmental multicystic dysplastic kidney in children. Urology. 2006;68(5):1121e9–11.

161. Menster M, Mahan J, Koff S. Multicystic dysplastic kidney. Pediatr Nephrol. 1994;8(1):113–5.

162. Al-Khaldi N, Watson AR, Zuccollo J, Twining P, Rose DH. Outcome of antenatally detected cystic dysplastic kidney disease. Arch Dis Child. 1994;70(6):520–2.

163. Atiyeh B, Husmann D, Baum M. Contralateral renal abnormalities in multicystic-dysplastic kidney disease. J Pediatr. 1992;121(1):65–7.

164. Flack CE, Bellinger MF. The multicystic dysplastic kidney and contralateral vesicoureteral reflux: protection of the solitary kidney. J Urol. 1993;150(6):1873–4.

165. John U, Rudnik-Schoneborn S, Zerres K, Misselwitz J. Kidney growth and renal function in unilateral multicystic dysplastic kidney disease. Pediatr Nephrol. 1998;12(7):567–71.

166. Karmazyn B, Zerin JM. Lower urinary tract abnormalities in children with multicystic dysplastic kidney. Radiology. 1997;203(1):223–6.

167. Oliveira EA, Diniz JS, Vilasboas AS, Rabelo EA, Silva JM, Filgueiras MT. Multicystic dysplastic kidney detected by fetal sonography: conservative management and follow-up. Pediatr Surg Int. 2001;17(1):54–7.

168. Rudnik-Schoneborn S, John U, Deget F, Ehrich JH, Misselwitz J, Zerres K. Clinical features of unilateral multicystic renal dysplasia in children. Eur J Pediatr. 1998;157(8):666–72.

169. Selzman AA, Elder JS. Contralateral vesicoureteral reflux in children with a multicystic kidney. J Urol. 1995;153(4):1252–4.

170. Zerin JM, Leiser J. The impact of vesicoureteral reflux on contralateral renal length in infants with multicystic dysplastic kidney. Pediatr Radiol. 1998;28(9):683–6.

171. Ismaili K, Avni FE, Alexander M, Schulman C, Collier F, Hall M. Routine voiding cystourethrography is of no value in neonates with unilateral multicystic dysplastic kidney. J Pediatr. 2005;146(6): 759–63.

172. Narchi H. Risk of hypertension with multicystic kidney disease: a systematic review. Arch Dis Child. 2005;90(9):921–4.

173. Okada T, Yoshida H, Matsunaga T, Kouchi K, Ohtsuka Y, Saitou T, et al. Multicystic dysplastic kidney detected by prenatal ultrasonography: natural history and conservative management. Pediatr Surg Int. 2003;19(3):207–10.

174. Tiryaki S, Alkac AY, Serdaroglu E, Bak M, Avanoglu A, Ulman I. Involution of multicystic dysplastic kidney: is it predictable? J Pediatr Urol. 2013;9(3): 344–7.

175. Weinstein A, Goodman TR, Iragorri S. Simple multicystic dysplastic kidney disease: end points for subspecialty follow-up. Pediatr Nephrol. 2008;23(1):111–6.

176. Webb NJ, Lewis MA, Bruce J, Gough DC, Ladusans EJ, Thomson AP, et al. Unilateral multicystic dysplastic kidney: the case for nephrectomy. Arch Dis Child. 1997;76(1):31–4.

177. Husmann DA. Renal dysplasia: the risks and consequences of leaving dysplastic tissue in situ. Urology. 1998;52(4):533–6.

178. Snodgrass WT. Hypertension associated with multicystic dysplastic kidney in children. J Urol. 2000;164(2):472–3. discussion 3–4.

179. Sukthankar S, Watson AR. Unilateral multicystic dysplastic kidney disease: defining the natural history. Anglia Paediatric Nephrourology Group. Acta Paediatr. 2000;89(7):811–3.

180. Psooy K. Multicystic dysplastic kidney in the neonate: the role of the urologist. Can Urol Assoc J. 2010;4(2):95–7.

181. Perez LM, Naidu SI, Joseph DB. Outcome and cost analysis of operative versus nonoperative management of neonatal multicystic dysplastic kidneys. J Urol. 1998;160(3 Pt 2):1207–11. discussion 16.

182. Onal B, Kogan BA. Natural history of patients with multicystic dysplastic kidney-what followup is needed? J Urol. 2006;176(4 Pt 1):1607–11.

183. Narchi H. Risk of Wilms' tumour with multicystic kidney disease: a systematic review. Arch Dis Child. 2005;90(2):147–9.

184. Beckwith J. Ask the expert. Pediatr Nephrol. 1992;6:511.

185. Orejas G, Malaga S, Santos F, Rey C, Lopez MV, Merten A. Multicystic dysplastic kidney: absence of complications in patients treated conservatively. Child Nephrol Urol. 1992;12(1):35–9.

186. Strife JL, Souza AS, Kirks DR, Strife CF, Gelfand MJ, Wacksman J. Multicystic dysplastic kidney in children: US follow-up. Radiology. 1993;186(3): 785–8.

187. Vinocur L, Slovis TL, Perlmutter AD, Watts Jr FB, Chang CH. Follow-up studies of multicystic dysplastic kidneys. Radiology. 1988;167(2):311–5.

188. Wacksman J, Phipps L. Report of the multicystic kidney registry: preliminary findings. J Urol. 1993;150(6):1870–2.

189. Hayes WN, Watson AR, Trent & Anglia MCDK Study Group. Unilateral multicystic dysplastic kidney: does initial size matter? Pediatr Nephrol. 2012;27(8):1335–40.

190. Diouf B, Ka EH, Calender A, Giraud S, Diop TM. Association of medullary sponge kidney disease and multiple endocrine neoplasia type IIA due to RET gene mutation: is there a causal relationship? Nephrol Dial Transplant. 2000;15(12):2062–3.

191. Torregrossa R, Anglani F, Fabris A, Gozzini A, Tanini A, Del Prete D, et al. Identification of GDNF gene sequence variations in patients with medullary sponge kidney disease. Clin J Am Soc Nephrol. 2010;5(7):1205–10.

192. Higashihara E, Nutahara K, Tago K, Ueno A, Niijima T. Medullary sponge kidney and renal acidification defect. Kidney Int. 1984;25(2):453–9.

193. Fabris A, Lupo A, Bernich P, Abaterusso C, Marchionna N, Nouvenne A, et al. Long-term treatment with potassium citrate and renal stones in medullary sponge kidney. Clin J Am Soc Nephrol. 2010;5(9):1663–8.

194. Gambaro G, Danza FM, Fabris A. Medullary sponge kidney. Curr Opin Nephrol Hypertens. 2013;22(4):421–6.

195. Chu HY, Yan MT, Lin SH. Recurrent pyelonephritis as a sign of 'sponge kidney'. Cleve Clin J Med. 2009;76(8):479–80.

196. Evan AP, Worcester EM, Williams Jr JC, Sommer AJ, Lingeman JE, Phillips CL, et al. Biopsy proven medullary sponge kidney: clinical findings, histopathology, and role of osteogenesis in stone and plaque formation. Anat Rec (Hoboken). 2015;298(5):865–77.

197. Geavlete P, Nita G, Alexandrescu E, Geavlete B. The impact of modern endourological techniques in the treatment of a century old disease--medullary sponge kidney with associated nephrolithiasis. J Med Life. 2013;6(4):482–5.

198. Flechner SM, Noble M, Tiong HY, Coffman KL, Wee A. Renal autotransplantation and modified pyelovesicostomy for intractable metabolic stone disease. J Urol. 2011;186(5):1910–5.

199. Cendron M. Reflux nephropathy. J Pediatr Urol. 2008;4(6):414–21.

200. Kaefer M, Curran M, Treves ST, Bauer S, Hendren WH, Peters CA, et al. Sibling vesicoureteral reflux in multiple gestation births. Pediatrics. 2000;105 (4 Pt 1):800–4.

201. Puri P, Gosemann JH, Darlow J, Barton DE. Genetics of vesicoureteral reflux. Nat Rev Urol. 2011;8(10): 539–52.

202. El-Khatib M, Packham DK, Becker GJ, Kincaid-Smith P. Pregnancy-related complications in women with reflux nephropathy. Clin Nephrol. 1994;41(1):50–5.

203. Goonasekera CD, Shah V, Wade AM, Barratt TM, Dillon MJ. 15-year follow-up of renin and blood pressure in reflux nephropathy. Lancet. 1996; 347(9002):640–3.

204. Kohler JR, Tencer J, Thysell H, Forsberg L, Hellstrom M. Long-term effects of reflux nephropathy on blood pressure and renal function in adults. Nephron Clin Pract. 2003;93(1):C35–46.

205. Ransley PG, Risdon RA. Renal papillary morphology and intrarenal reflux in the young pig. Urol Res. 1975;3(3):105–9.

206. Ardissino G, Avolio L, Dacco V, Testa S, Marra G, Vigano S, et al. Long-term outcome of vesicoureteral reflux associated chronic renal failure in children. Data from the ItalKid Project. J Urol. 2004;172(1):305–10.

207. Mattoo TK. Vesicoureteral reflux and reflux nephropathy. Adv Chronic Kidney Dis. 2011;18(5):348–54.

208. Lee OT, Durbin-Johnson B, Kurzrock EA. Physician preference is a major factor in management of vesicoureteral reflux. Pediatr Nephrol. 2015;30(1):131–8.

209. Boueva A, Bouvier R. Precursor B-cell lymphoblastic leukemia as a cause of a bilateral nephromegaly. Pediatr Nephrol. 2005;20(5):679–82.

210. Pradeep R, Madhumathi DS, Lakshmidevi V, Premalata CS, Appaji L, Patil SA, et al. Bilateral nephromegaly simulating wilms tumor: a rare initial manifestation of acute lymphoblastic leukemia. J Pediatr Hematol Oncol. 2008;30(6):471–3.

211. Hilmes MA, Dillman JR, Mody RJ, Strouse PJ. Pediatric renal leukemia: spectrum of CT imaging findings. Pediatr Radiol. 2008;38(4):424–30.

212. Camitta BM, Casper JT, Kun LE, Lauer SJ, Starshak RJ, Oechler HW. Isolated bilateral T-cell renal lymphoblastic lymphoma. Am J Pediatr Hematol Oncol. 1986;8(1):8–12.

213. Choi JH, Choi GB, Shim KN, Sung SH, Han WS, Baek SY. Bilateral primary renal non-Hodgkin's lymphoma presenting with acute renal failure: successful treatment with systemic chemotherapy. Acta Haematol. 1997;97(4):231–5.

214. Dobkin SF, Brem AS, Caldamone AA. Primary renal lymphoma. J Urol. 1991;146(6):1588–90.

215. Hain RD, Harvey E, Poon AO, Weitzman S. Acute tumour lysis syndrome with no evidence of tumour load. Pediatr Nephrol. 1994;8(5):537–9.

216. Jaffe N, Tefft M. Unsuspected lymphosarcoma of the kidneys diagnosed as bilateral Wilms tumor. J Urol. 1973;110(5):593–5.

217. Lowe LH, Isuani BH, Heller RM, Stein SM, Johnson JE, Navarro OM, et al. Pediatric renal masses: Wilms tumor and beyond. Radiographics. 2000;20(6): 1585–603.

218. McGuire PM, Merritt CR, Ducos RS. Ultrasonography of primary renal lymphoma in a child. J Ultrasound Med. 1996;15(6):479–81.

219. Sieniawska M, Bialasik D, Jedrzejowski A, Sopylo B, Maldyk J. Bilateral primary renal Burkitt lym-

phoma in a child presenting with acute renal failure. Nephrol Dial Transplant. 1997;12(7):1490–2.

220. Tisnado J, Amendola MA, Beachley MC, Urizar R. Renal lymphoma, angiographic findings in a child. Rev Interam Radiol. 1980;5(2):55–8.

221. Brouland JP, Meeus F, Rossert J, Hernigou A, Gentric D, Jacquot C, et al. Primary bilateral B-cell renal lymphoma: a case report and review of the literature. Am J Kidney Dis. 1994;24(4):586–9.

222. Chepuri NB, Strouse PJ, Yanik GA. CT of renal lymphoma in children. AJR Am J Roentgenol. 2003;180(2):429–31.

223. Cruz Villalon F, Escribano Fernandez J, Ramirez Garcia T. The hypoechoic halo: a finding in renal lymphoma. J Clin Ultrasound. 1995;23(6):379–81.

224. Gilboa N, Lum GM, Urizar RE. Early renal involvement in acute lymphoblastic leukemia and non-Hodgkin's lymphoma in children. J Urol. 1983;129(2):364–7.

225. Hugosson C, Mahr MA, Sabbah R. Primary unilateral renal lymphoblastic lymphoma. Pediatr Radiol. 1997;27(1):23–5.

226. Laxer RM, de Chadarevian JP, Anderson RJ, Kaplan BS. Malignant lymphoma presenting with nonoliguric renal failure. Clin Pediatr (Phila). 1983;22(12): 819–21.

227. Malbrain ML, Lambrecht GL, Daelemans R, Lins RL, Hermans P, Zachee P. Acute renal failure due to bilateral lymphomatous infiltrates. Primary extranodal non-Hodgkin's lymphoma (p-EN-NHL) of the kidneys: does it really exist? Clin Nephrol. 1994; 42(3):163–9.

228. Neuhauser TS, Lancaster K, Haws R, Drehner D, Gulley ML, Lichy JH, et al. Rapidly progressive T cell lymphoma presenting as acute renal failure: case report and review of the literature. Pediatr Pathol Lab Med. 1997;17(3):449–60.

229. Kanfer A, Vandewalle A, Morel-Maroger L, Feintuch MJ, Sraer JD, Roland J. Acute renal insufficiency due to lymphomatous infiltration of the kidneys: report of six cases. Cancer. 1976;38(6): 2588–92.

230. Srinivasa NS, McGovern CH, Solez K, Poppema S, Halloran PF. Progressive renal failure due to renal invasion and parenchymal destruction by adult T-cell lymphoma. Am J Kidney Dis. 1990;16(1): 70–2.

231. Cohan RH, Dunnick NR, Leder RA, Baker ME. Computed tomography of renal lymphoma. J Comput Assist Tomogr. 1990;14(6):933–8.

232. Heiken JP, Gold RP, Schnur MJ, King DL, Bashist B, Glazer HS. Computed tomography of renal lymphoma with ultrasound correlation. J Comput Assist Tomogr. 1983;7(2):245–50.

233. Ng YY, Healy JC, Vincent JM, Kingston JE, Armstrong P, Reznek RH. The radiology of non-Hodgkin's lymphoma in childhood: a review of 80 cases. Clin Radiol. 1994;49(9):594–600.

234. Reznek RH, Mootoosamy I, Webb JA, Richards MA. CT in renal and perirenal lymphoma: a further look. Clin Radiol. 1990;42(4):233–8.

235. Richmond J, Sherman RS, Diamond HD, Craver LF. Renal lesions associated with malignant lymphomas. Am J Med. 1962;32:184–207.

236. Basker M, Scott JX, Ross B, Kirubakaran C. Renal enlargement as primary presentation of acute lymphoblastic leukaemia. Indian J Cancer. 2002; 39(4):154–6.

237. Frei 3rd E, Fritz RD, Price E, Moore EW, Thomas LB. Renal and hepatic enlargement in acute leukemia. Cancer. 1963;16:1089–92.

238. Hayek M, Srinivasan A. Acute lymphoblastic leukemia presenting with lactic acidosis and renal tubular dysfunction. J Pediatr Hematol Oncol. 2003; 25(6):488–90.

239. Sato A, Imaizumi M, Chikaoka S, Niizuma H, Hoshi Y, Takeyama J, et al. Acute renal failure due to leukemic cell infiltration followed by relapse at multiple extramedullary sites in a child with acute lymphoblastic leukemia. Leuk Lymphoma. 2004; 45(4):825–8.

240. Arranz Arija JA, Carrion JR, Garcia FR, Tejedor A, Perez-Manga G, Tardio J, et al. Primary renal lymphoma: report of 3 cases and review of the literature. Am J Nephrol. 1994;14(2):148–53.

241. Kutluk MT, Buyukpamukcu M, Gogus S, Sarialioglu F, Akhan O, Besbas N. Renal lymphoma. An unusual presentation in a child. Turk J Pediatr. 1989; 31(1):71–7.

242. Levine C, Vrlenich L. Renal lymphoma in ataxia-telangiectasia: CT contribution. J Comput Assist Tomogr. 1989;13(3):537–9.

243. Vujanic GM, Webb D, Kelsey A. B-cell non-Hodgkin's lymphoma presenting as a primary renal tumour in a child. Med Pediatr Oncol. 1995; 25(5):423–6.

244. Yasunaga Y, Hoshida Y, Hashimoto M, Miki T, Okuyama A, Aozasa K. Malignant lymphoma of the kidney. J Surg Oncol. 1997;64(3):207–11.

245. Ferry JA, Harris NL, Papanicolaou N, Young RH. Lymphoma of the kidney. A report of 11 cases. Am J Surg Pathol. 1995;19(2):134–44.

246. Harris GJ, Lager DJ. Primary renal lymphoma. J Surg Oncol. 1991;46(4):273–7.

247. Kandel LB, McCullough DL, Harrison LH, Woodruff RD, Ahl Jr ET, Munitz HA. Primary renal lymphoma. Does it exist? Cancer. 1987;60(3):386–91.

248. Okuno SH, Hoyer JD, Ristow K, Witzig TE. Primary renal non-Hodgkin's lymphoma. An unusual extranodal site. Cancer. 1995;75(9):2258–61.

249. Gaynon PS, Qu RP, Chappell RJ, Willoughby ML, Tubergen DG, Steinherz PG, et al. Survival after relapse in childhood acute lymphoblastic leukemia: impact of site and time to first relapse--the Children's Cancer Group Experience. Cancer. 1998;82(7): 1387–95.

250. Jones DP, Stapleton FB, Kalwinsky D, McKay CP, Kellie SJ, Pui CH. Renal dysfunction and hyperuricemia at presentation and relapse of acute lymphoblastic leukemia. Med Pediatr Oncol. 1990;18(4): 283–6.

251. Kebaili K, Manel AM, Chapelon C, Taylor P, Philippe N, Bertrand Y. Renal enlargement as presentation of isolated renal relapse in childhood leukemia. J Pediatr Hematol Oncol. 2000;22(5): 454–6.

252. Rivera G, Murphy SB, Aur RJ, Verzosa MS, Dahl GV, Mauer AM. Recurrent childhood lymphocytic leukemia: clinical and cytokinetic studies of cytosine arabinoside and methotrexate for maintenance of second hematologic remission. Cancer. 1978; 42(6):2521–8.

# Glomerular Disease

**12**

Edward R. Gould and Anna Marie Burgner

## Renal Anatomy

The kidneys receive approximately 25 % of the cardiac output. This blood is delivered via the renal arteries, which very rapidly divide into segmental arteries, lobar arteries, interlobar arteries, and finally the arcuate arteries before delivering blood to individual nephrons. The parenchyma of the kidney can be divided into the outer renal cortex—which houses approximately one to two million glomeruli per kidney—and the inner renal medulla, which is imperative in urinary concentration and water conservation.

The renal medulla can be appreciated macroscopically as the renal pyramids. These pyramids orient the final collecting ducts of the individual nephron subunits toward the renal calyces which then drain into the renal pelvis and into the lower genitourinary system.

## The Nephron

The basic functional unit of the kidney is the nephron. These can be divided into two subtypes: the cortical nephrons, which have relatively short loops of Henle, and the juxtamedullary nephrons, which have long loops of Henle that dive to the deepest parts of the medulla. The latter play a significant role in renal concentrating capacity.

Individual nephrons can be divided into several individual segments, each with unique transport and functional characteristics and susceptibility to injury. These include the glomerulus, proximal tubule, loop of Henle, distal convoluted tubule, the connecting segment, and finally the collecting duct, which delivers the tubular filtrate to the renal calyx [1, 2].

## The Glomerulus

All serum filtration is performed in the glomerulus. The glomerulus consists of an afferent arteriole which branches into the glomerular tuft before coalescing back into a single efferent arteriole. The glomerular tuft is a delicate bouquet of capillaries that is composed of a specialized fenestrated endothelium, which is surrounded by a basement membrane and a layer of epithelial cells that are unique to the glomerulus called podocytes. The tuft is supported by the mesangium, which is made up of cells and matrix. The

E.R. Gould, M.D. (✉) • A.M. Burgner, M.D.
Division of Nephrology, Department of Medicine,
Vanderbilt University Medical Center,
2213 Garland Avenue, S3223 MCN,
Nashville, TN 37232, USA
e-mail: edward.r.gould@vanderbilt.edu; anna.
burgner@vanderbilt.edu

© Springer Science+Business Media New York 2016
D.E. Hansel et al. (eds.), *The Kidney*, DOI 10.1007/978-1-4939-3286-3_12

mesangial cells provide mechanical structure to the glomerular capillaries and may have other nutritive or hormonal roles.

The glomerular filtration apparatus is highly specialized and creates a size and charge barrier that allows blood filtration to occur. The barrier is composed of three layers. The endothelium of the glomerular capillary tuft is considered the first layer. It is one of the few capillary beds in the body that is fenestrated, with pores that measure approximately 70–100 nm across [3]. Given that platelets are approximately five- to tenfold larger that those pores, this layer provides an important barrier to cellular elements found in the blood.

Deep to the basal side of the fenestrated epithelium lies the glomerular basement membrane. The basement membrane is the fusion product of the endothelial basement membrane and the basement membrane from the podocyte [3]. Morphologically, it is composed of three layers: the lamina rara interna adjacent to the endothelial cell, a dense inner layer called the lamina densa, and the lamina rara externa adjacent to the podocyte. The composition of the basement membrane is also unique from other basement membranes, being composed primarily of type IV collagen. The meshwork of collagen fibers provides the superstructure of the basement membrane and generates smaller pores than those found in the fenestrated endothelium. These collagen fibers are then further modified with the addition of specific proteins that help maintain adhesion to the overlying cellular products and, more importantly, modify the barrier to limit the passage of charged particles [4].

On the urinary side of the glomerular tuft, deep to the basement membrane lies the podocyte. This is a highly specialized epithelial cell type that provides the final specificity to the filtration of blood. The podocytes spread out over the basement membrane in interdigitated foot processes that abut the membrane itself. In between these foot processes, several protein products coalesce into the slit diaphragm. This is believed to primarily add to the charge selectivity of the filtration barrier. This is highlighted in states of disease, namely, focal segmental glomerulosclerosis and minimal change disease, wherein the podocytes lose their structure and the foot processes lose cohesion, the result being the loss of charge selectivity and large protein losses in the urine; this will be further discussed later [3, 4].

## The Proximal Tubule

The glomerulus is surrounded by Bowman's capsule, which collects the glomerular filtrate and shuttles it toward the tubule. The normal adult human filters approximately 160–170 L of ultrafiltrate daily. Most of this is reabsorbed through the length of the nephron, with the proximal tubule doing much of this work. In addition to reabsorption of valuable water and important solutes, it is also the site responsible for secretion of drugs, secretion of acids, as well as having some important metabolic activities [5].

The proximal tubule reabsorbs nearly all of the amino acids, glucose, and bicarbonate that are filtered through the glomerulus each day. This is largely through secondary active transport, with a favorable electrochemical gradient established by the Na-K ATPase found on the basal membrane driving sodium reclamation along with other solutes of interest. Since total body water is largely dependent on sodium balance, the reclamation of sodium also facilitates substantial resorption of water from the tubular ultrafiltrate, with approximately 66 % of the filtered water volume being recovered in this segment [5].

The proximal tubule also houses specialized active transporters for secretion of proteins and molecules that would otherwise not be adequately secreted into urine; the most common example of this is the secretion of pharmaceuticals into the urine through organic anion transporters. It is also the site for some of the renal metabolic functions such as vitamin D activation.

## The Loop of Henle

The tubular filtrate not reabsorbed in the proximal tubule enters the loop of Henle. This segment can be divided into its descending limb, the thin ascending limb, and the thick ascending limb, each with a specific role. This segment is largely focused on managing water balance. Much of this function is through the establishment of the medullary concentration gradient against which water can be reclaimed later in the nephron at the level of the collecting duct.

The loop is best described by beginning distally at the thick ascending limb (TAL). The TAL is considered to be water impermeable—that is, there are no aquaporins found in the TAL and the tight junctions limit paracellular movement of water. Here, the Na-K-2Cl transporter facilitates sodium reclamation from the tubular lumen into the medullary interstitium and begins the process of countercurrent exchange. Again, the reclamation of sodium here is considered a secondarily active process, with subsequent water reabsorption from the descending limb driven by the local increases in interstitial osmolarity. Because of the hairpin design of this segment, the local increases in sodium concentration at the beginning of the descending limb lead to water reclamation as the descending limb moves further into the interstitium, increasing the osmolarity of both the tubular and interstitial compartments down the length of the segment. In times of water avidity (dehydration, hypotension, etc.), this apparatus works maximally and can generate a medullary osmolarity of ~1200 mOsms which facilitates maximal water reclamation in the collecting duct.

It is important to appreciate the specialized arrangement of blood flow through this region as well. The efferent arteriole for a given glomerulus leads to the vasa recta for *that same glomerulus.* So the juxtamedullary glomeruli with long loops of Henle have vasa recta that follow them into the papillary medulla. Branching anastomoses in these vasa recta prevent high blood flows in the area and therefore prevent high blood flow at the deepest layers of the medulla, thereby preventing medullary washout, which impairs the nephron's concentrating ability.

## Distal Convoluted Tubule and Connecting Segment

The remaining tubular filtrate then moves to the convoluted tubule. This is the home of the Na-Cl cotransporter. This site is responsible for approximately 5 % of the sodium reclamation in the kidney. This reabsorption is also by secondarily active transport with the favorable gradient being established by the basal Na-K ATPase. It is also one of the primary sites for calcium reabsorption from the urinary filtrate, an important factor in the generation of nephrolithiasis, considered elsewhere.

## Collecting Duct

The distal-most tubular segment is responsible for final refinement of the tubular filtrate. Only about 5 % of the total filtered sodium and water enter the collecting duct. The cortical segment of the collecting duct houses two cell types, each with a specific role. The principal cell modulates potassium secretion via an aldosterone-sensitive pathway. The intercalated cell facilitates hydrogen secretion and therefore influences a patients' acid–base status.

The principal cell houses apical epithelial sodium channels (ENaC), which are aldosterone sensitive. In times of high aldosterone output—in general, periods of intravascular volume depletion—aldosterone both increases nuclear transcription of ENaC and facilitates the intracellular movement of preformed ENaC to the apical surface of the principal cell. This then allows sodium to move down its concentration gradient into the principal cell where it can be recovered through the Na-K ATPase. Concurrently, apical potassium channels allow for potassium secretion into the tubular filtrate in order to maintain electroneutrality.

The more distal collecting duct houses more of these cell types but becomes increasingly sensitive to circulating antidiuretic hormone (ADH). This circulating hormone increases the insertion of apical aquaporin 4 channels, which in times of volume depletion dramatically increase water recovery in this segment against a very favorable osmotic gradient that was established by countercurrent exchange in the loop of Henle. In that setting, urinary osmolarity will be very high, approaching 1200 mOsms, reflecting the water reclamation in this region.

The renal pelvis, ureters, and bladder are largely impermeable to water and solutes, though

**Table 12.1** Indications and contraindications to renal biopsy

|  | Contraindications | |
|---|---|---|
| Indications | Relative | Absolute |
| Nephrotic syndrome | Severe azotemia | Uncooperative patient |
| Routinely in adults | Renal anatomic abnormalities | Uncontrollable hypertension |
| If atypical for MCD in children | Antiplatelet therapy or anticoagulation | Uncontrollable bleeding diathesis |
| Nephritic syndrome | Solitary native kidney | |
| Systemic disease with renal insufficiency | Skin infection over the biopsy site | |
| Unexplained CKD | Active kidney infection | |
| Familial renal disease | Pregnancy | |
| Renal transplant dysfunction | | |

*MCD* minimal change disease, *CKD* chronic kidney disease

in low flow states, some water and urea reclamation can occur. In animal models, this has been shown to change the urinary composition by approximately 7–15 % [6].

## Renal Biopsy

The processing of renal tissue for pathologic review is somewhat different than typical tissue preparation that may be used for other biopsy samples. The nature of the diseases that can be detected through pathologic evaluation demands that optimal preparative technique be used. Proper handling at the time of biopsy facilitates light microscopy, immunofluorescence evaluation, electron microscopy (EM), and—where necessary—immunohistochemical staining.

Tissue adequacy has historically been a limiting factor in renal biopsy, though with newer technologies and safer sampling techniques, that issue has become less prevalent [7]. In order to make an accurate diagnosis of native renal disease, a minimum of 10 glomeruli are required, though to ensure a 95 % sensitivity for more focal lesions, 20–25 glomeruli are recommended [8].

Presently, the standard of care for outpatients who need renal tissue sampling for diagnosis of their underlying renal disease is the percutaneous renal biopsy. There are both relative and absolute contraindications to this procedure that would preclude percutaneous sampling, and in those

instances CT-guided renal biopsy, laparoscopic or open renal biopsy, or transvenous renal biopsy can be considered (Table 12.1) [8].

## Percutaneous Kidney Biopsy

The percutaneous renal biopsy has been adopted as the principal technique for sampling renal parenchyma. When doing percutaneous biopsy, most renal pathologists agree that at least two core samples are necessary for adequate sampling and to avoid missed diagnoses. Where available, it is also useful to hand tissue directly to a trained technician at the time of biopsy for review under either a dissection or light microscope to evaluate for tissue adequacy based on the number of observed glomeruli [9].

This procedure is typically done with the patient awake and in the prone position. CT or ultrasound is used to locate the desired target—typically the lower pole of either kidney. The patient is given instructions on breath holding and regional anesthetics are used to numb the patient from the skin to the renal capsule. Since renal parenchyma lacks sensory innervation, there is no need to anesthetize deeper renal tissues. A biopsy needle is passed through the anesthetized tract and core samples taken with the patient instructed to hold their breath during period when the biopsy will be taken. Typically precautions are taken following the procedure to decrease the risk of bleeding and provide time for hemostasis to occur. Patients are maintained in the supine position with frequent vital sign monitoring for the ensuing 8–24 h. Urine collections are also preserved for physician review to ensure that gross hematuria, if present initially, improves during that same period.

A number of clinical studies have tried to address the exact amount of time that a patient should be observed for complications following the procedure. Early literature on the topic suggested that most complications would be noted by 12 h, thus perhaps eliminating the need for overnight hospitalization [10]. More recent data suggests that it may take longer to recognize complications, with one observational study noting that while 46 % of complications were noted before 4 h and 67 % by 8 h, 89 % could be identified by 24 h [11]. Presently, consensus recommendation is to observe patients in the inpatient setting for 24 h post procedure.

## Open Kidney Biopsy

Laparoscopic and open biopsies have been shown to be largely safe and well tolerated. In the largest case series of 934 patients, a modified laparoscopic approach with general anesthesia had 100 % tissue adequacy for diagnosis, no major complications, and only one minor complication related to anesthesia [12].

However, given the invasive nature of the procedure, the risks of general anesthesia on a population basis, and the prolonged recovery time, open biopsy is typically only used in patients who have either an absolute or relative contraindication that precludes percutaneous biopsy [13].

## Transvenous Kidney Biopsy

The transvenous—transjugular or transfemoral—approach is a procedural technique first described by Mal in France in 1990 [14]. Various reasons have been cited as prompting this choice of procedure, including need for other organ biopsies (heart, liver), bleeding dia-

theses, and uncontrolled hypertension, among others. Since that time a number of studies have been published reviewing the adequacy of this technique as well as their complication rates [13, 15]. Studies have reported adequate parenchymal sampling, with rates ranging from 73 to 97 %. In the published literature, no patient has died or required dialysis after these procedures [13]. Comparison to the other available biopsy options is difficult because of inherent selection bias. At present, the use of this technique largely depends on local availability and patient-specific factors that would preclude percutaneous biopsy.

## Tissue Fixation and Preparation

The fixatives used for preserving the tissue vary by microscopy modality. It is important that the proceduralist be familiar with the handling preferences of their renal pathology lab in order to ensure appropriate handling once collected. Here we will discuss the handling of the percutaneous biopsy, given its prevalent use in parenchymal sampling.

The core samples taken by percutaneous biopsy are typically divided into portions destined for the varying histologic uses. Samples are taken from both the cortical end of the tissue and the medullary end for use in electron microscopy. The remaining tissue from each tissue core is divided for use with immunofluorescence of light microscopy.

## Light Microscopy

Most pathology laboratories prefer light samples to be collected and stored in 10 % aqueous formaldehyde solution (formalin). Formalin is safe and readily disposed of and preserves morphologic features for review. It also allows for additional tissue processing using immunohistochemical techniques or molecular studies to be used if necessary. Alternative solutions include Bouin's, Duboscq-Brazil, Zenker's, or 4 % paraformaldehyde fixatives, each with varying uses [9].

Slide preparation also varies according to pathology laboratory, but typically includes sectioning of the preserved tissue into 2 μm slices and serial staining with hematoxylin and eosin (H&E) stain, periodic acid-Schiff reaction (PAS), silver stain, or trichrome stain [9].

## Electron Microscopy

Tissue fixation for EM requires fixation in either 2–3 % glutaraldehyde or 1–4 % paraformaldehyde. This provides the greatest degree of structural preservation. It is occasionally necessary to reprocess samples stored in either the frozen section or the paraffin-embedded section if glomeruli are not available on the EM processed sections. This can lead to cellular artifact, but generally is considered acceptable for review of the GBM for both structural integrity and for immune deposition [9].

## Immunofluorescence or Immunoperoxidase

Some pathology laboratories have gone to immunoperoxidase (IP) staining for review of immune deposition due to relative ease of processing. However, most renal pathologists agree that dark field imaging with IF is the preferred modality to identify immune deposition in pathology samples. The processing of these materials is laboratory dependent, though formalin fixation is typically adequate with freezing and subsequent sectioning used to label the immune complexes [9].

## Glomerular Syndromes and Mechanisms of Injury

Medical renal disease affects the kidneys in a variety of ways and can manifest clinically as any number of clinical syndromes. Each of the individual classes of renal disease has their own hallmarks; here, however, we will be focusing diseases primarily affecting the glomerulus.

The glomerular diseases manifest according to the pattern of underlying injury, which we will briefly review, before discussing specific clinical syndromes.

## Structural Patterns of Injury

As discussed previously, the glomerular tuft houses the filtration apparatus that generates the tubular ultrafiltrate and is composed of three layers: the fenestrated endothelium, the glomerular basement membrane, and the podocytes. Each of these layers can suffer injury and the nature of that injury correlates closely with the observed clinical syndrome.

Immune conditions or vasculitis conditions that affect the endothelium lead directly to a robust inflammatory cascade that typically leads to endothelial proliferation and filtration barrier disruption. That disruption can be detected clinically as the nephritic syndrome with loss of both protein and cellular elements (typically red blood cells) into the urinary space with concomitant changes in filtration efficacy as detected by changes in the glomerular filtration rate (GFR).

Conditions that affect the glomerular basement membrane include both congenital and acquired conditions. The congenital disorders tend to be more indolent with adaptive changes in the associated glomerular cell types and long latency to diagnosis. These include disease like thin basement membrane disease and Alport's disease. The acquired types can lead directly to disruption of the GBM and has implications for both the size and charge selectivity of the filtration barrier. These acquired conditions, like anti-GBM disease, typically lead to robust immune activation and consequences similar to those seen with endothelial diseases.

The podocytopathies are a family of disease that classically disrupt the cellular architecture of the podocyte leading to breakdown of the interdigitated foot processes with associated loss of charge selectivity. That loss of charge specificity leads to robust proteinuria, but relatively limited, if any, hematuria.

Each of these will be discussed in more detail below.

## Nephritic Syndromes

The nephritic syndrome is a collection of signs and symptoms that denote underlying glomerular injury, the hallmark of which is the presence of both proteinuria and hematuria in the urine. The classic nomenclature is used to describe a limited amount of protein, with any amount of glomerular hematuria. This contrasts with the nephrotic syndrome, which denotes a disease wherein there is significant proteinuria and no hematuria. Some providers also discuss the nephritic/nephrotic syndrome where there are significant hematuria and nephrotic-range proteinuria, though this is better described as an advanced nephritic syndrome, given that the underlying mechanism of injury, as discussed above, mandates endothelial injury in order to facilitate the observed hematuria.

## Rapidly Progressive Glomerulonephritis

The most striking examples of the nephritic syndrome are the crescentic glomerulopathies, which frequently present as rapidly progressive glomerulonephritis (RPGN). RPGN does not refer to a single disease process; rather, it describes a clinical syndrome of rapidly progressive acute renal failure associated with hematuria and proteinuria, which is typically caused by advanced histologic injury to the glomerular tuft.

## Clinical Presentation

Clinically, this collection of diseases share certain features, namely, the presence of a nephritic sediment with red blood cells either in red cell casts or with dysmorphic characteristics, some amount of proteinuria, and rapid loss of renal function. Renal failure with oliguria, severe azotemia, and hypertension are the hallmark of the initial presentation and typically lead to progression to ESRD within 3 months of diagnosis if left untreated [16]. Patients may also have evidence of hypertension—owing to disrupted sodium regulation and possibly renin-mediated mechanisms—and edema. There are of course more distant or systemic effects that can be seen as well, though these are generally a characteristic of the underlying disease. An example would be

the pulmonary hemorrhage seen in anti-GBM disease (Goodpasture's disease) [17].

The number of disease conditions that are known to cause RPGN is limited. Each has a specific pathogenic mechanism by which it leads to glomerular capillary injury and disruption, outlined separately, but they can be organized according to their pattern of injury. The first and most straightforward is anti-GBM disease, the second group being a far more heterogeneous array of disease wherein immune complexes in the glomerular capillary tuft lead to local injury, and the last being the pauci-immune vasculitides wherein no immune depositions can be detected, but pathogenic antineutrophil cytoplasmic antibodies (ANCA) lead to notable inflammatory activation which can be observed histologically. The latter is the most common form of crescentic glomerulonephritis, accounting for approximately 60–80 % of all cases [16].

## Pathogenesis

While the underlying pathogenesis of the specific disease entities is reviewed below, their progression to an RPGN is typical and includes necrotizing inflammation which leads to GBM disruption and leakage of serum proteins including fibrin and fibronectin into the urinary space which generates a robust activation of both the visceral and parietal epithelial layers in Bowman's space. In turn, these cells dedifferentiate and proliferate and lead to the formation of the prototypical crescent (Fig. 12.1) [16].

The crescents themselves are a histologic signal of injury; the association of this pattern of injury with the clinical manifestations of the RPGNs has led to these terms being considered near synonymous [18].

## Treatment

Despite their differences, the initial treatment of these diseases is similar, largely because of the incredibly high risk of irreversible renal injury and risk of other morbidities and mortality [19].

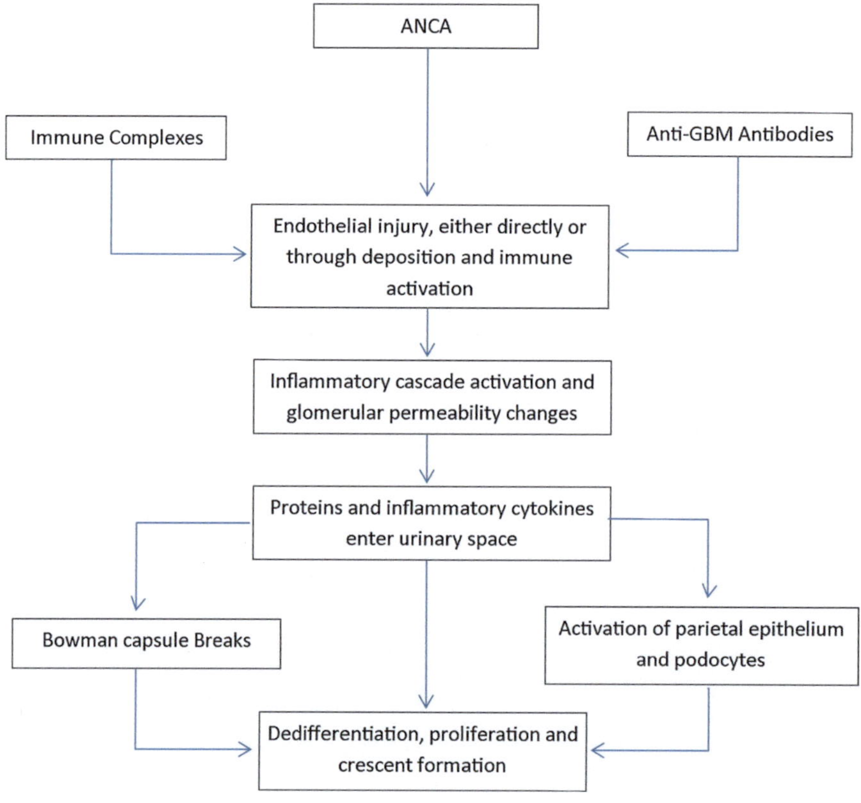


**Fig. 12.1** Pathogenesis of crescent formation

Typically the treatment of any of these diseases is divided into induction and maintenance phases. Induction therapy is often initiated in advance of definitive diagnosis. Sometimes this is with serologic evidence, but often, even that is not yet available. The cornerstones of treatment have been steroid therapy and plasma exchange for nearly 40 years [20]. Recent meta-analysis on the topic has shown that the use of adjunct plasma exchange can reduce the rate of progression to ESRD in these patients, noting that ESRD rates are reduced at both 3 and 12 months [21]. Pulse glucocorticoid therapy is also typically started at the time of clinical presentation. While subject to varying patterns of administration, typically 500–1000 mg of methylprednisolone is given over 2–3 days as initial therapy to help calm the inflammatory cascades active in the tuft. Lastly the use of immunosuppression therapy is used to reign in the production of the injurious autoantibodies. The classical treatment for RPGN has been oral or intravenous cyclophosphamide (CYC) administered according to a variety of protocols either as continuous oral therapy or as pulse intravenous therapy [21]. With the advent of newer immunosuppressive therapies, the treatments used in practice have increased, though the details of their selection are outside the scope of this publication.

## Anti-glomerular Basement Membrane Disease

Typically this disease presents as a pulmonary renal syndrome with acute onset of both lower respiratory complaints and changes in urinary character [17, 19]; however, more subtle cases can be seen. Because of its tendency to rapidly progress, it should be considered in all cases of acute pulmonary renal disease, and coordination with a nephrologist is recommended for urgent initiation of plasmapheresis if needed in the setting of diffuse alveolar hemorrhage [21, 22].

## Pathogenesis

The GBM is formed through the fusion of the endothelial and podocyte basement membranes. The normal GBM is a tight meshwork of collagen fibers, with alpha 3, alpha 4, and alpha 5 subtypes of type IV collagen fibers forming hexamers that then crosslink through their non-collagenous (NC1) domains. In patients with anti-GBM disease, immunoglobulin G (IgG) can be identified on immunofluorescence overlying all of the glomerular basement membrane, and the causative antibodies have been found to be directed against those NC1 domains of alpha 3 or alpha 5 type IV collagen [23].

Recent work has demonstrated that the disease is one of quaternary conformational change—the specific cause of which is unknown, though it has been linked to smoking, viral infections, and solvent exposure—which leads to molecular conformational shifting and exposure of the normally sheltered NC1 domains with subsequent autoantibody formation. Those autoantibodies then bind to the NC1 domains and lead complement fixation and to a type II hypersensitivity reaction with robust inflammatory recruitment and consequent local injury [22, 23].

This disease manifests as the nephritic syndrome due to the ongoing glomerular injury, and patients have pulmonary symptoms as well given that the alpha-3 subunit is also expressed in the alveoli of the lungs. This can lead to a very dramatic clinical presentation of the disease with diffuse pulmonary hemorrhage as the initial presenting symptom. Prior to the use of the above-described therapies, anti-GBM disease was nearly universally fatal, though with the use of modern treatments, the 5-year survival now exceeds 80 % [22].

## Pathology

Anti-GBM disease has characteristics on light microscopy that are typical for RPGN, typically with areas of GBM destruction with nearby fibrinoid necrosis. In early disease, there may not be evidence of crescent formation on the biopsy sample, though in more advanced cases, lymphoplasmacytic infiltration and endocapillary proliferation may become apparent. Immunofluorescence is diagnostic with smooth GBM staining for IgG and c3. IgG is usually more positive than c3 staining. Electron microscopy reveals the absence of immune deposits and can highlight the broken GBM with associated fibrin tactoids notable in areas of discrete necrosis.

## Management

The challenges present in diagnosing this disease combined with its rarity make this a challenging disease on which to do randomized clinical trials. However, given that it is understood to be an immune-mediated disease, immunosuppressive therapies are considered necessary as part of its treatment. If diagnosed during its fulminant phase, plasmapheresis is often indicated. At the same time, induction is achieved, as described above for all of the RPGNs, classically done with CYC and high-dose glucocorticoid therapy [16, 19, 22]. The introduction of anti-CD20 monoclonal antibody (rituximab) therapies has been used as well in small patient cohorts, the largest a series of eight patients who had received steroids and CYC as well as plasmapheresis. All were started on rituximab within 2 months of diagnosis. At approximately 2 years follow-up, patient and renal survival were 100 and 75 %, respectively [24].

The prognosis for patients affected by anti-GBM disease is largely dependent on the promptness of the diagnosis and initiation of effective treatment. While historically the disease was considered fatal [25], the above therapies have led to a 5-year survival rate in excess of 80 %, and only about a third of patients require long-term dialysis [22].

**Table 12.2** Features of ANCA-associated vasculitides

| | Renal limited disease | Microscopic polyangiitis | Granulomatosis with polyangiitis | Eosinophilic granulomatosis with polyangiitis (Churg-Strauss syndrome) |
|---|---|---|---|---|
| Frequency of renal involvement | 100 | 90 | 80 | 45 |
| Frequency of ANCA positivity | 80 | 90 | 95 | 70 |
| MPO | 60 | 50 | 25 | 60 |
| PR3 | 40 | 50 | 75 | 40 |
| Extrarenal manifestations | None | Musculoskeletal complaints, pulmonary | Pulmonary, sinus, head, and neck | Pulmonary, neurologic, allergy symptoms |

*ANCA* antineutrophil cytoplasmic antibody, *MPO* myeloperoxidase, *PR3* proteinase 3

## Pauci-immune Glomerular Disease

Accounting for just over half of all diagnosed RPGN syndromes and sometimes recognized in more indolent circumstances, this group of diseases is characterized by necrotizing changes on biopsy in the absence of immune deposits [19]. This group of diseases includes granulomatosis with polyangiitis (GPA), eosinophilic granulomatosis with polyangiitis (EGPA, formerly Churg-Strauss syndrome), and microscopic polyangiitis (MPA). The bulk of these patients have circulating ANCA. Clinically they present in a variety of different ways, each of which is typically associated with a collection of extrarenal manifestations that can suggest which disease is causative, though it does require tissue biopsy to establish the definitive diagnosis. The varying extrarenal characteristics, as well as the frequency of specific ANCA subtypes with those diseases, are summarized in Table 12.2. These diseases do occasionally present with less fulminant disease. So-called early systemic disease is defined as serologic positivity, but with sCr below 1.7 mg/dL and no critical extrarenal organ dysfunction [26]. This distinction has implications for treatment.

## Pathogenesis

The association of ANCA and necrotizing glomerular disease was first recognized by Davies in 1982 [27]; subsequent work has gone on to support a pathogenic mechanism for these autoantibodies. There are two identified culpable antibody subtypes, the anti-myeloperoxidase (MPO) subtype and the anti-proteinase 3 subtype (PR-3). These antigens are typically sequestered into neutrophilic granules and are exposed only during periods of inflammatory activation [17, 19]. Directly linking this antibody activity to the disease, however, has been proven difficult. Renal biopsies of affected patients are rife with activated neutrophils, and indeed, the number of activated neutrophils seen on biopsy has been correlated with the degree of renal insufficiency [28], but they do not have observable immune complexes attributable to ANCA, hence the name "pauci-immune." Additional evidence for a pathogenic role of ANCA has grown with ANCA being elutable from affected kidney tissue, and in the case of anti-MPO antibodies, necrotizing glomerulonephritis can be induced with infusion of ANCA [29]. Interestingly, anti-LAMP 2 (antibodies directed against lysosomal membrane protein-2) have been shown to be present in upward of 80 % of all active ANCA-associated vasculitides (AAV) [30, 31]. While the understanding of the disease is improving, there are many aspects of the pathogenesis that remain to be understood.

## Pathology

The ANCA-associated vasculitides have similar histologic appearances. Common among all of them are segmental glomerular necrosis with

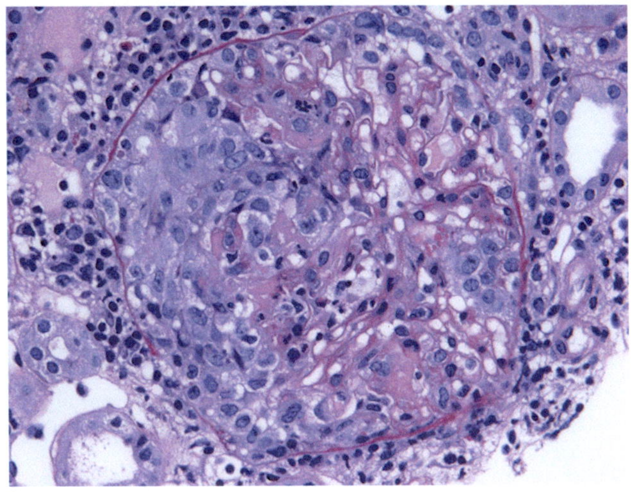

**Fig. 12.2** A cellular crescent with fibrinoid necrosis is noted on the left side of this glomerulus in a patient with pauci-immune (ANCA-associated) glomerulonephritis (PAS)

crescent formation (Fig. 12.2) and the absence of either immunofluorescence findings or changes by electron microscopy. In GPA and microscopic polyangiitis, there is typically evidence of an active interstitial nephritis with or without larger vessel involvement. In EGPA there may or may not be an eosinophilic predominance in the interstitial infiltrate, and this does not have bearing on the pathologic diagnosis. The granulomatous changes seen in GPA are more typically identified in lung biopsy than in renal biopsy, and often the diagnostic distinction between these diseases (GPA/MPA/EGPA) is made clinically.

## Management

Again, the induction therapy for this disease has included treatment as described for an RPGN with cyclophosphamide as the core of the induction immunosuppressive regimen since the 1970s. Typically, maintenance therapy is necessary due to high rates of relapse and has historically been accomplished with azathioprine. Recent studies have also set out to explore the utility of B cell-depleting agents like rituximab both as an alternative induction agent and a maintenance therapy.

In situations where patients may present with less threatening disease, so-called early systemic AAV, several studies have shown non-inferiority of methotrexate (MTX) as an induction agent. In one randomized controlled trial patients with confirmed ANCA positivity, sCr <1.7 mg/dL and no evidence of critical organ dysfunction were randomized to receive either oral cyclophosphamide or oral MTX for 12 months. There were similar rates of remission at 18-month follow-up, though the time to remission was longer in the MTX patients, particularly those with more extensive disease [26].

Cyclophosphamide is the historical gold standard for induction therapy. Oral or intravenous (IV) administration of CYC has also been extensively studied [32–34]. Indeed similar response rates were seen in patients receiving either oral or IV CYC, though the cumulative dose of those patients receiving IV therapy was less. Given that the complication profile of CYC is largely directed by its cumulative dose, there may be some long-term benefit to limiting the absolute amount of CYC administered. However, long-term follow-up of patients previously enrolled in the largest of these trials has failed to show a difference in treatment-related adverse events. It did, however, show a higher relapse rate among patients receiving the IV therapy, though this ultimately was not reflected in differences in the overall patient morbidity or mortality at just over 4 years [35].

Rituximab has also been used for both induction and maintenance in these patients as well with high efficacy. Two large, well-conducted trials have evaluated the use of rituximab for induc-

**Table 12.3** Overview of the treatment of AAV according to EULAR recommendations

| Disease stage | Treatment | Study/level of evidence, grade of recommendation |
|---|---|---|
| *Induction of remission* | | |
| Early systemic | Methotrexate 15 mg/week (oral/parenteral), increase to 20–25 mg/week, folic acid+GC | NORAM (level 1B, grade B) |
| Generalized | Cyclophosphamide IV/oral+GC | CYCLOPS (level 1A/1B, grade A) |
| | duration: 3–6 months (oral) or 6–9 pulses (IV) | RAVE (level 1B) |
| | Rituximab 4×375 mg/m$^2$ in weekly intervals | |
| Severe (creatinine >500 µmol/L) | Standard therapy+plasma exchange | MEPEX (level 1B, grade A) |
| | Rituximab 4×375 mg/m$^2$ in weekly intervals (as substitute for cyclophosphamide) | RITUXVAS (level 1B) |
| Concomitant glucocorticoids (GC) | Prednisolone/prednisone 1 mg/kg/day oral taper to 15 mg/day or less within 3 months | (level 3, grade C) |
| *Maintenance of remission* | | |
| Maintenance options | Azathioprine 2 mg/kg/day oral+low-dose GC | CYCAZAREM (level 1B, grade A) |
| | Methotrexate 20–25 mg/week+low-dose GC | WEGENT (level1B, grade B/A) |
| | Leflunomide 20 mg/day oral+low–dose GC | LEM (level 1B, grade B) |
| | Duration: at least 18 months | |
| Concomitant GC | Prednisolone/prednisone less than 10 mg/day | |
| *Refractory, relapsing and persistent disease* | | |
| Options for refractory disease | IVIG 2 g/kg IV for 5 days | |
| | Rituximab IV | |
| | Infliximab 3–5 mg/kg IV 1–2 months | |
| | MMF 2 g/day oral | |
| | 15-deoxyspergualin 0.5 mg/kg/day SUBQ until nadir; then stop until leucocyte recovery (six cycles) | |
| | Anti-thymocyte globulin 2.5 mg/kg/day IV for 10 days (adjusted to lymphocyte count) | |

New trials have been incorporated into the overview and are presented in gray letters

Adapted with permission from Elsevier: Holle and Gross [39]

tion therapy with similar efficacy [36, 37]. Follow-up trials have gone on to show non-inferiority for maintenance therapy with rituximab as well [38]. The current treatment recommendations for AAV are summarized in Table 12.3.

## Immune Complex Deposit Mediated Disease

This heterogeneous group of diseases is often consequent to ongoing immune activation with accumulation of immune elements in the glomerular tuft. Those immune complexes may form in circulation and deposit in the glomerular basement membrane, or they may be circulating antibodies which preferentially favor deposition in the glomerular tuft with in situ complex formation with circulating antigens.

These diseases can manifest as RPGN pictures depending on the variable amount of immune activation and tissue injury associated with that activation. They stem from a variety of underlying clinical illnesses ranging from the autoimmune condition systemic lupus erythematosus (SLE) to the mixed cryoglobulinemic conditions commonly associated with chronic viral infections like hepatitis C and Epstein-Barr virus. Here we will review the most common immune complex diseases and their pathology.

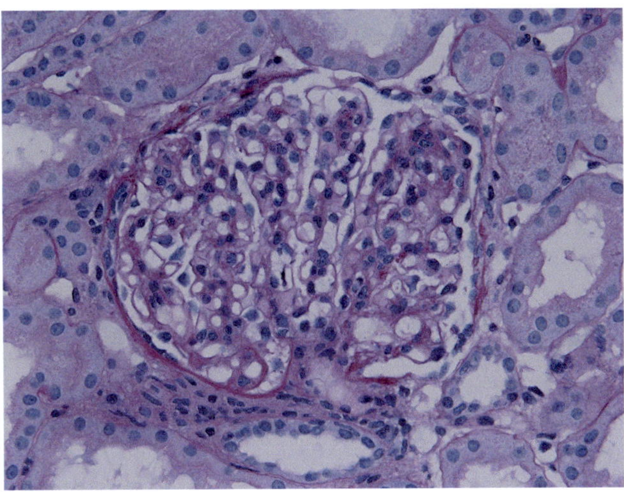

**Fig. 12.3** There is segmental mesangial hypercellularity, which should be assessed in regions removed from the vascular pole, in this glomerulus from a patient with IgA nephropathy (PAS)

## IgA Nephropathy

IgA nephropathy is the most common primary glomerulonephritis globally. First described in 1968 by Berger, it is also commonly referred to as Berger's disease. Clinically it most commonly presents as hematuria with or without overt proteinuria. It has a male predominance that ranges from 2:1 in Japan up to 6:1 in Europe and the United States [40]. It has long been considered a relatively indolent disease, but has recently been recognized to frequently lead to progressive CKD and ESRD and may present as a RPGN [40, 41].

### Pathophysiology

Recent advances in the understanding of IgA nephropathy have led to a deeper understanding of the complex genetic and environmental interplay that are important in the development of this disease. Clinically, patients who manifest gross hematuria would note that hematuria would closely follow episodes of respiratory or gastrointestinal illness. Given that IgA is an important component of mucosal defense, this led to the hypothesis that it was primarily an overproduction of immunoglobulin with glomerular trapping that led to disease manifestations. While this may be true, we now recognize that aberrant *O*-galactosylation—a genetic phenomenon—in the hinge region of the immunoglobulin predisposes patients to the disease.

There are two subclasses of IgA: IgA1 and IgA2. Glomerular disease seems to be exclusively the consequence of IgA1, which houses a hinge region that IgA2 does not. This hinge region is heavily galactosylated. These carbohydrate modifications in patients with IgA nephropathy lack terminal galactose, which is considered to be the principal defect in the pathogenesis of this disease [42]. While IgA1 is dominantly in the mucosal tissues, some can be found in circulation. The galactosylation aberrancy is thought to lead either to easier trapping in the mesangium with in situ complex formation or to immune complex formation in circulation. These immune complexes lead to local inflammation and injury to the surrounding tuft [42].

### Pathology

The most common finding by renal biopsy worldwide, IgA nephropathy is characterized by mesangial deposits of IgA that are readily apparent by immunofluorescence. As its name suggests, IgA is typically the dominant immunoglobulin identified by immunofluorescence, though it can be codominate with IgG. The deposits are readily apparent by electron microscopy in the mesangium—and occasionally at subendothelial deposits. Light microscopy varies and often correlates with the clinical findings observed (Fig. 12.3). It can range from normal histology to isolated mesangial proliferation and, in very severe cases, can have focal or diffuse endocapillary proliferation with or without necrosis and crescent formation.

## Management

Despite an expanding understanding of the pathogenesis of this disease, no specific disease-targeted therapy yet exists. In most cases management of this disease is conservative with emphasis on blood pressure and proteinuria management with renin-angiotensin-aldosterone system (RAAS) blockade. There have been a variety of treatments that have been considered but which have failed to show improvement in randomized studies (tonsillectomy, fish oil, immunosuppression therapy, etc.). If, despite conservative treatment for 4–6 months, proteinuria continues in excess of 1 g/day and the patient has preserved renal function, a course of high-dose oral steroids is often completed [43]. Patients that present with a crescentic RPGN are treated similar to other RPGNs with steroids and CYC.

## Postinfectious Glomerulonephritis

Infection remains a common cause acute proliferative glomerulonephritis. Recognized and described first in the eighteenth century, the association between acute infection and subsequent renal manifestations is well known. In contrast to the renal manifestations that accompany IgA nephropathy, which are synpharyngitic, postinfectious glomerulonephritis (PIGN) typically presents 2–4 weeks after infection, earlier following upper respiratory tract infection, later after skin infections. Classically the patient is young with a recent infection with group A *Streptococcus pyogenes*, and they present with edema, oliguria, and hematuria. They have declining renal function and an active urinary sediment with dysmorphic red cells, red cell casts, and white cells in their urine. Evidence of complement activity is also an important clue to the diagnosis with low serum complement levels. The natural history is widely variable with some patients requiring renal replacement therapy and others recovering renal function relatively rapidly.

## Pathogenesis

Multiple offending organisms have been implicated in the pathogenesis of acute PIGN. The most common among them is a streptococcal infection. Specific streptococcal Lancefield M types have been associated with PIGN and have been termed the "nephritogenic" strains. In patients who have disease that follows a typical upper respiratory or tonsillitis, types 1, 2, 4, and 12 have been implicated. In patients whose disease follows a skin infection, types 47, 49, and 57 have been shown to be associated [44]. That is not to suggest that *Streptococcus* is the only culpable organism, as *Staphylococcus* and many others have also been associated [45]. The antigenic organism forms circulating immune complexes that are then deposited between the GBM and the podocyte ("subepithelial") of the glomerulus. This leads to complement activation either through the alternative or lectin pathways and the proinflammatory milieu recruits additional immune cells to the area [44]. This robust activation leads to the endocapillary proliferation.

## Pathology

Light microscopy is highly suggestive of postinfectious glomerulonephritis with diffuse endocapillary proliferation and infiltration with numerous polymorphonuclear cells (Fig. 12.4). Typically there are chunky subepithelial deposits, "humps" that can be seen along the capillary loops by electron microscopy, and these correlate with strong IgG and c3 staining by immunofluorescence. It is important to recognize that they will remain the longest in areas where the capillary loop meets the mesangium and these areas should be thoroughly investigated by electron microscopy if this diagnosis is suspected.

## Management

Thankfully, in most children and young adults, the disease is self-limited. It can be more prolonged and have longer-lasting renal consequences in the elderly. This may be in part due to less renal reserve or perhaps due to a waning immune system unable to clear the immune mediators trapped in the glomerulus. In cases where there is pronounced activity on biopsy or where dialysis is

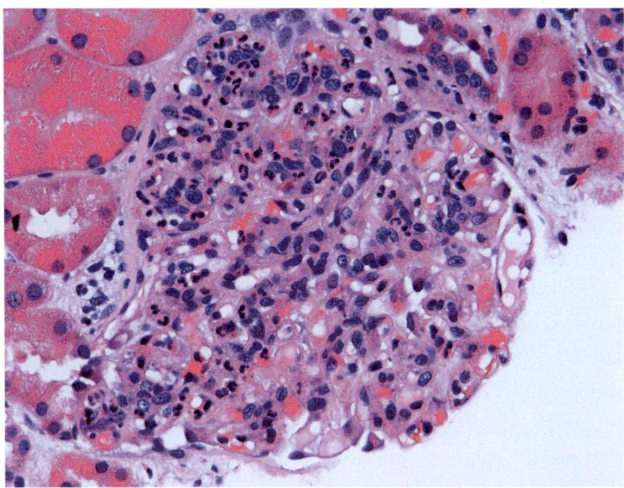

**Fig. 12.4** Numerous neutrophils are present in the glomerular capillaries which are characteristic of postinfectious glomerulonephritis (H&E)

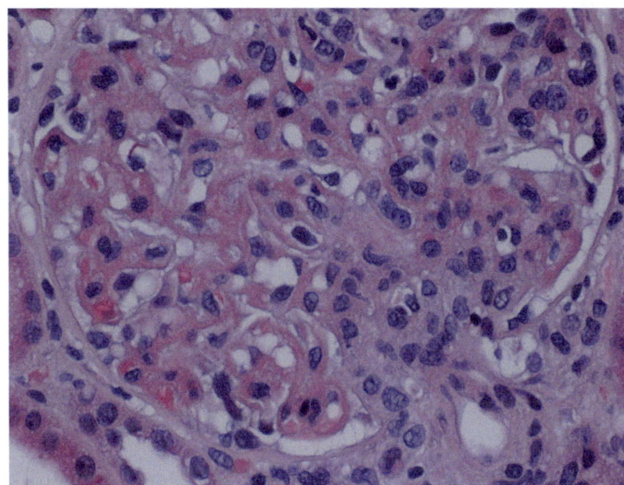

**Fig. 12.5** This glomerulus from a lupus patient contains prominent immune complex deposition in the form of "wire-loop" deposits at the 4 and 6 o'clock aspects of this glomerulus, which is a feature of activity (H&E)

required, corticosteroids and sometimes immunosuppressants are used, though it is important to be sure the infection that led to the insult is cleared.

## Lupus Nephritis

Systemic lupus erythematosus (SLE) is a multi-organ autoimmune disease that has a number of implicated autoantibodies recognized to cause the disease. Those antibodies include antinuclear antibodies (ANAs), anti double-stranded DNA antibodies (anti-ds DNA), anti-histone antibodies, and anti-ribonucleoprotein antibodies (anti-

RNP). The diagnosis is made clinically based on a variety of clinical, laboratory, and pathologic characteristics (Fig. 12.5). One of the end-organ injuries that can result from SLE is lupus nephritis, a varied disease entity with clinical manifestations that differ both between patients and across time.

Unfortunately there is no hallmark clinical presentation of lupus nephritis. It ranges from subnephrotic range proteinuria, to nephrotic syndrome, to the RPGN syndrome according to how the immune deposits culpable in the disease align within the glomerulus. Treatment is variable depending on the type of lupus nephritis.

## Nephrotic Syndrome

The nephrotic syndrome is characterized by ≥3.5 g proteinuria per day, edema, and hypercholesterolemia. In this disease state, the primary defect driving the proteinuria—which may be secondary to a systemic disease process—is the loss of charge discrimination at the level of the glomerular filtration barrier.

As this charge barrier breaks down, small proteins, typically albumin, begin to move from the capillary into the urinary space where they are minimally reabsorbed, leading to microalbuminuria. This decline in serum colloid also leads to increased hepatic synthetic function, an increase that is thought to help rectify the hypoalbuminemia, but as an unintended side effect also leads to hypercholesterolemia as the hepatic apparatus also generates cholesterol.

The physiologic underpinning of edema development is felt to have both an "underfill" and "overfill" component. The "underfill" hypothesis describes the loss of albumin and decrease in intravascular oncotic pressure as being central to edema formation. It describes the loss of plasma proteins into the urine and the consequent decrease in intravascular oncotic pressure. This change in intravascular oncotic pressure leads to changes in the starling equilibrium such that there is a net ultrafiltration from the capillary to peripheral tissues. Early in the disease, lymphatic drainage is able to accommodate this increase in extravascular fluid, thus preventing tissue swelling, but as that system becomes saturated, edema develops.

Despite being a simple explanation, it is worth noting that experimental evidence has shown that there is a concurrent decrease in both intravascular and interstitial proteins. Classic literature on the topic has, in fact, shown that the difference in osmotic pressure between the intravascular and extravascular spaces is relatively constant across a wide array of serum albumins [46–48].

The "overfill" hypothesis explains the sodium avidity in these patients and helps to explain the process by which intravascular volume expansion occurs. Increased sodium retention in this hypothesis occurs at the level of the collecting duct via ENaC. Activation of ENaC appears to

occur secondary to the filtration of proteinases into the urine that activate the channel and lead to sodium retention [49].

In addition to the classical features of the nephrotic syndrome, these patients are also at increased risk of both arterial and venous thrombosis, particularly renal vein thrombosis, due to loss of innate anticoagulant elements in the urine leading to an aberrant coagulation cascade [50]. They also are at increased risk of infection due to nonspecific loss of immunoglobulins in advanced nephrosis [51].

# The Podocytopathies: Minimal Change Disease and Focal Segmental Glomerulosclerosis

The podocyte is the glomerular tuft cell with a complex array of microtubular arrays that create interdigitated foot processes along the GBM that are interconnected at the slit diaphragm. As noted previously, this structure is necessary to impose the final charge selectivity to the GBM. In recent years the importance of this cell has become increasingly apparent and, indeed, has realized a wealth of new insights, thanks to reliable mouse models allowing new investigation. Minimal change disease and focal segmental glomerulosclerosis (FSGS) are the two most common podocytopathies and we will review them here.

## Minimal Change Disease

Minimal change disease is a major cause of nephrotic syndrome in children, with onset typically in childhood, after the first year of life with a peak incidence between 24 and 36 months of life. The disease seems to have a strong male predilection in children as well. In children between 85 and 95 % of cases of the nephrotic syndrome are due to minimal change disease. That frequency falls as children become adolescence, accounting for only 50 % in that age group. It can occur in adults, but other diseases, like focal segmental glomerulosclerosis, begin to also occur at higher frequencies.

**Table 12.4**  Secondary causes of minimal change disease

| Drugs | Malignancy | Infection |
|---|---|---|
| NSAIDs | Hodgkin's disease | Tuberculosis |
| Lithium | Non-Hodgkin's lymphoma | HIV |
| Gold | Leukemia | Ehrlichiosis |
| Antimicrobials | RCC | Syphilis |
| Methimazole | Bronchogenic carcinoma | |
| Penicillamine | Colon CA | |
| Tamoxifen | Pancreatic CA | |

The classic presentation, especially in the above-described age group, is significant proteinuria with advancing edema. In most patients, proteinuria and its associated edema are the dominant presenting complaints, often described as having arisen over a very short period of time. The incidences of associated hematuria, hypertension, or declining GFR are relatively uncommon. While any one of these abnormalities can be seen in approximately 15 % of patients with MCD, the presence of more than one should prompt consideration of another disease process. Its frequency in younger patients often leads to presumptive treatment with high-dose corticosteroids by the treating physician without a kidney biopsy. In adults, given the significantly lower pretest probability and the risks of inadequately treating other causes of the nephrotic syndrome, a biopsy is generally pursued before initiating therapy.

In adults, not only is the disease less frequently the cause of nephrotic syndrome, it is also less frequently considered idiopathic. There are a number of other drugs and primary or systemic disease that can manifest as minimal change disease in the kidney. A list of these is reviewed in Table 12.4.

## Pathophysiology

The specific inciting factor in MCD is not known. In some inherited forms, specific defects have been identified in proteins that are integral for slit diaphragm function. In cases that are not inherited, it has been proposed that there is a circulating T cell-secreted factor that may be culpable [52]. While no such circulating factor has yet been positively identified, early work suggested a significant role for T regulatory ($T_{reg}$) cells, and indeed, studies have gone on to show that supplementing MCD patients with $T_{reg}$ cells reduces proteinuria in mouse models [53]. Additional work has evaluated specific cellular markers, though these studies have thus far failed to provide a definitive answer.

Regardless of the specific inciting stimulus, the result is loss of cytoskeletal architecture of the podocyte. This decay leads to foot process effacement and disordered slit diaphragm proteins, without which protein efflux across the glomerular basement membrane is unimpeded. This disorganization is not visible at the level of the light microscope and, as such, was named "minimal change."

## Pathology

As the name suggests, minimal change disease has a normal histologic appearance when reviewed by light microscopy (Fig. 12.6). Notably absent, especially if distinguishing between MCD and FSGS, are areas of focal sclerosis within glomerular tuft. Indeed, immunofluorescence also lacks positivity attributable to the condition. Electron microscopy, however, shows diffuse foot process effacement. If patients have been previously treated, the effacement can be incomplete.

## Management

The mainstay of therapy is glucocorticoids. This treatment is highly efficacious leading to complete remission approaches 90 %. Indeed, even in adults, most patients will have a response to therapy, with approximately 80 % responding to treatment [54]. In two controlled studies in adults that evaluated the use of corticosteroids, significant

**Fig. 12.6** This glomerulus appears normal by light microscopy and electron microscopy (not shown) revealed diffuse podocyte foot process effacement consistent with minimal change disease (Jones methenamine silver)

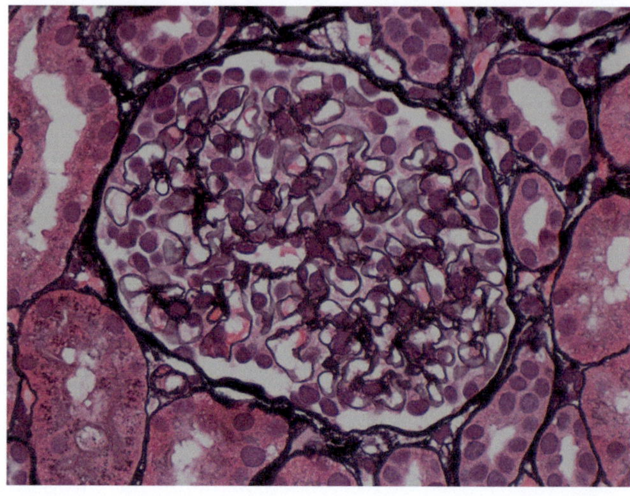

**Table 12.5** Secondary causes of FSGS

| Genetic mutations | Viral associations | Medications | Others |
|---|---|---|---|
| Podocin | HIV | Pamidronate | Obesity |
| α-Actinin 4 | Parvovirus B19 | Heroin | Sickle cell disease |
| | | Interferon alpha | Reflux nephropathy |
| | | Lithium | Renal agenesis |
| | | | Cholesterol atheroemboli |

response rates were achieved at 2 months with complete resolution of proteinuria, though long-term follow-up showed similar rates of remission, suggesting that many patients will experience a spontaneous remission in time [55, 56].

In large part there continues to be debate regarding dosing frequency (daily versus alternate day dosing), though there may be some benefit, particularly in children, for preserving activity of the adrenal axis during growth periods [56, 57]. Oral dosing has been thought to be superior to intravenous dosing forms, largely because of the ease of use and evidence that trends toward higher rates of remission at 3 months. In children, current recommendations are for 6 months of therapy at a minimum given higher rates of relapse with shorter course [58]. In adults it is less certain, though current recommendations are for trials of at least 16 weeks prior to declaring the treatment a failure.

## Focal Segmental Glomerulosclerosis

Similar to MCD, FSGS is a disease primarily of the podocyte. Its clinical presentation is similar, though it affects adolescents and adults more frequently than MCD. Unlike MCD, if left untreated it will progress to end-stage renal disease (ESRD). It is considered the most common cause of nephrotic syndrome among African Americans and, in some studies, the most common cause in all races.

Like MCD, it has both idiopathic forms wherein no underlying or associated disease can be identified as well as many different secondary forms, shown in Table 12.5. Many of these seen in patients seem to be related to the development first of hyperfiltration and associated glomerular hypertrophy. While the specific mechanism of how hyperfiltration causes slerosis remains uncertain, it may be related to slow podocyte loss or insufficiency in those circumstances.

**Table 12.6** FSGS subtypes and disease associations

| Subtype | Histologic pattern | Disease associations |
| --- | --- | --- |
| NOS, classical | Segmental sclerosis without features of subtype | |
| Collapsing | Glomerular tuft collapse with corrugated zGBM and podocyte proliferation | HIV, parvovirus, TB, hemophagocytic syndrome |
| Cellular | Endocapillary proliferation without evidence of collapsing or tip lesion | |
| Perihilar | Perihilar sclerosis and hyalinosis involving more than half of affected glomeruli | Nephron loss (HTNive disease, other causes CKD) |
| Tip variant | Glomerulosclerosis involving only the tubular pole of the glomerular tuft | |

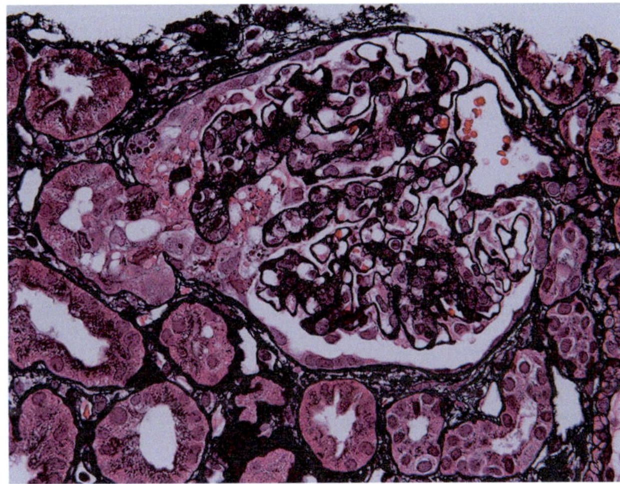

**Fig. 12.7** The glomerular capillaries at the tip of this glomerulus demonstrate prominence of the visceral epithelial cells (podocytes), which also contain numerous protein reabsorption droplets, and there are some intracapillary foam cells. These findings are characteristic of the tip variant of focal segmental glomerulosclerosis (Jones methenamine silver)

## Pathophysiology

Like many diseases, inherited forms of the disease allowed researchers to hone in on various key proteins in the podocyte that trigger FSGS. For example, mutations in the nephrin gene identified in congenital Finnish-type nephrotic syndrome have allowed researchers to appreciate the importance of slit diaphragm maintenance in podocyte health. However, many mouse models have identified other mutations both in proteins directly related to the slit diaphragm and in trafficking proteins. Whatever the error, there seems to be an association with progressive podocyte loss, podocyte effacement, and progressive sclerosis of portions of any given glomerular tuft.

And while the recognition of these congenital variants show that defects in the slit diaphragm are sufficient to cause disease, they are unlikely to explain idiopathic FSGS. Indeed, it has also been suggested that the different histologic variants of FSGS may be related to different pathophysiologic mechanisms. These are summarized in Table 12.6.

## Pathology

Focal segmental glomerulosclerosis has a number of histologic subtypes that have important prognostic features for the patient (Fig. 12.7). The primary features are areas of sclerosis within the glomerular tuft (focal) that are apparent by light microscopy and associated foot process effacement of the podocytes that involve some but not all of the glomeruli (focal). As noted previously, this diagnosis is largely dependent on sample size given that even a single glomeruli with segmental sclerosis can distinguish between MCD and FSGS. Immunofluorescence may reveal IgM and c3 deposition in the sclerotic segment.

The subtypes of FSGS can also be distinguished on their histology and are summarized in Table 12.6.

## Management

Although the clinical course in FSGS varies between patients, the natural history is one of progressive glomerular sclerosis and loss. Unlike MCD, if left untreated, only 5–10 % of patients will experience a spontaneous remission in proteinuria. In early studies of the disease, only 10–30 % of patients treated with corticosteroids (or other early immunosuppressive regimens like azathioprine, chlorambucil, etc.) achieved a remission. Later observational studies suggested that while the response was not as robust as that seen in MCD, immunosuppressants did have an impact [59].

Presently, the standard of care in FSGS is to consider a trial of corticosteroids, with consideration of cyclosporine or cyclophosphamide if contraindicated to steroids or failure of corticosteroids (defined as lack of partial remission after 16 weeks of therapy). Mycophenolic acid has also been used, but is considered third-line therapy.

If the disease is known or presumed to be secondary, treatment and optimization of the underlying disease are recommended. In both idiopathic and secondary FSGS ongoing management of other risk factors for loss of renal function should be pursued (blood pressure management, RAAS blockade, etc.).

## Membranous Nephropathy

Membranous nephropathy (MN) is a disease of IgG immune deposition between the GBM and the podocyte with reaction at the level of the podocyte leading to foot process effacement. Typically affecting men more than women (2:1) with a median age of onset in the mid-1950s, the disease often presents as isolated proteinuria that is incidentally detected. However, the disease can lead to profound protein losses in the urine with overt nephrotic syndrome manifestations.

Several genetic associations have been made with patients expressing HLA-DR3 having a threefold risk of the disease [60]. Other HLA subtypes have similarly been associated with increased disease risk, including HLA-DQA1 which seems to track with MN quite closely [61]. These risk factors may suggest a tendency toward autoantibody formation in these groups, although, until only the last decade, the specific antigens were largely unknown, with most cases of MN being dubbed idiopathic.

Patients with the disease have variable clinical courses with up to a third of patients exhibiting a spontaneous remission, even in the face of substantial of proteinuria. The remaining patients will have persistent proteinuria, with either preserved renal function or with progressive chronic kidney disease as a result with approximately 0.5 % of current US ESRD patients being dialysis-dependent from MN [62].

## Pathophysiology

The pathology in the disease has long suggested in situ formation of immune complexes with resultant structural changes in the GBM. Those structural changes lead to loss of integrity of the overlying podocytes with effacement. While elusive up until the last decade, recent work has identified several target autoantigens including the best-described example, the M-type phospholipase $A_2$ receptor (PLA$_2$R) as a target for autoantibody formation. PLA$_2$R is a member of the mannose receptor family that is expressed as a transmembrane protein in the basolateral aspect of the podocyte [63]. Circulating autoantibodies against this protein likely migrate across the GBM and react with the membrane-bound PLA$_2$R protein.

There are a number of secondary causes of membranous nephropathy as well that range from viral infections to malignancies. While some of these may lead to autoantibody formation against proteins intrinsic to the podocyte, others are thought to lead to the formation of antigens that get trapped at the level of the podocyte [62]. Cationic antigens of the right size can easily traverse the GBM and then be targeted by autoanti-

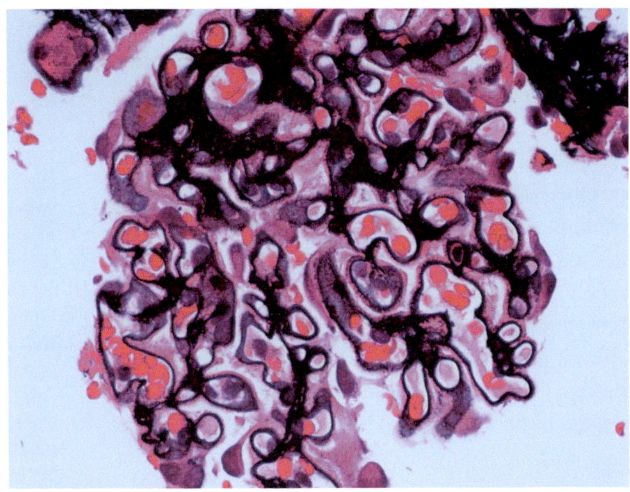

**Fig. 12.8** Subepithelial "spike" formation is frequently observed along the capillaries due to membranous nephropathy

bodies. This is exemplified in mouse models of MN where the animal is immunized with cationized bovine serum albumin (cBSA) [62]. Planted antigens are thought to explain class V lupus nephritis and hepatitis B-associated MN [64, 65].

## Pathology

MN is diagnosed by finding subepithelial and intramembranous immune deposits that can typically be seen (Fig. 12.8). The immune deposits give the GBM a rarefacted appearance on light microscopy—especially on silver stain, which stains for GBM—that can show the absence of immune deposit staining which appear as "holes." These can be seen early in the disease in tangential sections of GBM. As the disease progresses and the matrix reaction progresses, light microscopy can reveal "spikes" of basement membrane that reach outward toward the overlying podocytes. Immunofluorescence shows staining of the immunoglobulins present as a granular pattern along the length of the GBM. Most typically this is IgG, though other immunoglobulins can be appreciated in some cases and may bespeak a secondary cause of the disease.

## Management

As noted previously, many cases of MN will spontaneously resolve if left untreated. Early trials evaluating prednisone, chlorambucil, or cyclophosphamide as therapy were mixed with some showing benefits in remission and renal survival and others showing no difference with increased adverse events from immunosuppressive therapy [66–68]. In the 1980s 140 cases of biopsy proven MN were reviewed and their clinical courses noted. Most of them, 83 % were nephrotic at the time of diagnosis. At last follow-up available, 57 % of the untreated group had achieved full remission. Indeed, at 10 years there was no statistical difference in either renal survival or mortality between the two groups [69]. All of these early randomized trials were limited by their follow-up, noting no difference over the short term. As time passed, though longer-term follow-up of treated cohorts became available, it became apparent that in patients who had a high likelihood of progression, the use of an immunosuppression regimen was beneficial [70, 71].

Presently, most nephrologists attempt to stratify patients with MN according to their risk of progression, with low-risk patients (subnephrotic proteinuria with normal renal function) being treated conservatively and high-risk patients receiving immunosuppression. First-line therapy is cytotoxic therapy with cyclophosphamide or chlorambucil and glucocorticoids for 6 months of therapy. Calcineurin inhibitors have also been shown to be efficacious, but are considered to be second-line therapy.

## References


1. Salvatore SP et al. Nonneoplastic renal cortical scarring at tumor nephrectomy predicts decline in kidney function. Arch Pathol Lab Med. 2013;137(4): 531–40.
2. Bijol V et al. Evaluation of the nonneoplastic pathology in tumor nephrectomy specimens: predicting the risk of progressive renal failure. Am J Surg Pathol. 2006;30(5):575–84.
3. Pollak MR et al. The glomerulus: the sphere of influence. Clin J Am Soc Nephrol. 2014;9(8):1461–9.
4. Rose BD, Post TW. Clinical physiology of acid–base and electrolyte disorders. 5th ed. New York: McGraw-Hill; 2001.
5. Curthoys NP, Moe OW. Proximal tubule function and response to acidosis. Clin J Am Soc Nephrol. 2014;9(9):1627–38.
6. Levinsky NG, Davidson DG, Berliner RW. Changes in urine concentration during prolonged administration of vasopressin and water. Am J Physiol. 1959;196(2):451–6.
7. Whittier WL. Complications of the percutaneous kidney biopsy. Adv Chronic Kidney Dis. 2012;19(3): 179–87.
8. Laurin L-P, Alain B, Dube M, Leblanc M. Percutaneous renal biopsy. In: Mubarak M, Kazi JI, editors. Topics in renal biopsy and pathology. Rijeka: InTech; 2012.
9. Walker PD. The renal biopsy. Arch Pathol Lab Med. 2009;133(2):181–8.
10. Jones B et al. Reduced duration of bed rest after percutaneous renal biopsy. Clin Nephrol. 1991;35(1): 44–5.
11. Whittier WL, Korbet SM. Timing of complications in percutaneous renal biopsy. J Am Soc Nephrol. 2004;15(1):142–7.
12. Nomoto Y et al. Modified open renal biopsy: results in 934 patients. Nephron. 1987;45(3):224–8.
13. Whittier WL, Korbet SM. Renal biopsy: update. Curr Opin Nephrol Hypertens. 2004;13(6):661–5.
14. Mal F et al. Transjugular renal biopsy. Lancet. 1990;335(8704):1512–3.
15. Navuluri R, Ahmed O. Complications of transjugular biopsies. Semin Intervent Radiol. 2015;32(1): 42–8.
16. Moroni G, Ponticelli C. Rapidly progressive crescentic glomerulonephritis: early treatment is a must. Autoimmun Rev. 2014;13(7):723–9.
17. Lee RW, D'Cruz DP. Pulmonary renal vasculitis syndromes. Autoimmun Rev. 2010;9(10):657–60.
18. Jennette JC. Rapidly progressive crescentic glomerulonephritis. Kidney Int. 2003;63(3):1164–77.
19. Kambham N. Crescentic Glomerulonephritis: an update on Pauci-immune and Anti-GBM diseases. Adv Anat Pathol. 2012;19(2):111–24.
20. Chen X, Chen N. Plasma exchange in the treatment of rapidly progressive glomerulonephritis. Contrib Nephrol. 2013;181:240–7.
21. Walters G, Willis NS, Craig JC. Interventions for renal vasculitis in adults. Cochrane Database Syst Rev. 2008;3, CD003232.
22. Greco A et al. Goodpasture's syndrome: a clinical update. Autoimmun Rev. 2015;14(3):246–53.
23. Pedchenko V et al. Molecular architecture of the Goodpasture autoantigen in anti-GBM nephritis. N Engl J Med. 2010;363(4):343–54.
24. Touzot M et al. Rituximab in anti-GBM disease: a retrospective study of 8 patients. J Autoimmun. 2015;60:74–9.
25. Benoit FL et al. Goodpasture's syndrome: a clinicopathologic entity. Am J Med. 1964;37:424–44.
26. De Groot K et al. Randomized trial of cyclophosphamide versus methotrexate for induction of remission in early systemic antineutrophil cytoplasmic antibody-associated vasculitis. Arthritis Rheum. 2005;52(8):2461–9.
27. Davies DJ et al. Segmental necrotising glomerulonephritis with antineutrophil antibody: possible arbovirus aetiology? Br Med J. 1982;285(6342):606.
28. Brouwer E et al. Neutrophil activation in vitro and in vivo in Wegener's granulomatosis. Kidney Int. 1994;45(4):1120–31.
29. Xiao H et al. The role of neutrophils in the induction of glomerulonephritis by anti-myeloperoxidase antibodies. Am J Pathol. 2005;167(1):39–45.
30. Kain R, Rees AJ. What is the evidence for antibodies to LAMP-2 in the pathogenesis of ANCA associated small vessel vasculitis? Curr Opin Rheumatol. 2013;25(1):26–34.
31. Peschel A et al. Autoantibodies to hLAMP-2 in ANCA-negative pauci-immune focal necrotizing GN. J Am Soc Nephrol. 2014;25(3):455–63.
32. de Groot K, Adu D, Savage CO. The value of pulse cyclophosphamide in ANCA-associated vasculitis: meta-analysis and critical review. Nephrol Dial Transplant. 2001;16(10):2018–27.
33. Adu D et al. Controlled trial of pulse versus continuous prednisolone and cyclophosphamide in the treatment of systemic vasculitis. QJM. 1997;90(6):401–9.
34. Guillevin L et al. A prospective, multicenter, randomized trial comparing steroids and pulse cyclophospha-

mide versus steroids and oral cyclophosphamide in the treatment of generalized Wegener's granulomatosis. Arthritis Rheum. 1997;40(12):2187–98.

35. Harper L et al. Pulse versus daily oral cyclophosphamide for induction of remission in ANCA-associated vasculitis: long-term follow-up. Ann Rheum Dis. 2012;71(6):955–60.

36. Jones RB et al. Rituximab versus cyclophosphamide in ANCA-associated renal vasculitis. N Engl J Med. 2010;363(3):211–20.

37. Stone JH et al. Rituximab versus cyclophosphamide for ANCA-associated vasculitis. N Engl J Med. 2010;363(3):221–32.

38. Specks U et al. Efficacy of remission-induction regimens for ANCA-associated vasculitis. N Engl J Med. 2013;369(5):417–27.

39. Holle JU, Gross WL. Treatment of ANCA-associated vasculitides (AAV). Autoimmun Rev. 2013;12(4): 483–6.

40. Donadio JV, Grande JP. IgA nephropathy. N Engl J Med. 2002;347(10):738–48.

41. Yu HH, Chiang BL. Diagnosis and classification of IgA nephropathy. Autoimmun Rev. 2014;13(4–5): 556–9.

42. Wyatt RJ, Julian BA. IgA nephropathy. N Engl J Med. 2013;368(25):2402–14.

43. Lv J et al. Corticosteroid therapy in IgA nephropathy. J Am Soc Nephrol. 2012;23(6):1108–16.

44. Rodriguez-Iturbe B. Postinfectious glomerulonephritis. Am J Kidney Dis. 2000;35(1):XLVI–VIII.

45. Nasr SH, Radhakrishnan J, D'Agati VD. Bacterial infection-related glomerulonephritis in adults. Kidney Int. 2013;83(5):792–803.

46. Joles JA et al. Colloid osmotic pressure in young analbuminemic rats. Am J Physiol. 1989;257(1 Pt 2): F23–8.

47. Fiorotto M, Coward WA. Pathogenesis of oedema in protein-energy malnutrition: the significance of plasma colloid osmotic pressure. Br J Nutr. 1979;42(1):21–31.

48. Siddall EC, Radhakrishnan J. The pathophysiology of edema formation in the nephrotic syndrome. Kidney Int. 2012;82(6):635–42.

49. Bockenhauer D. Over- or underfill: not all nephrotic states are created equal. Pediatr Nephrol. 2013;28(8): 1153–6.

50. Llach F. Hypercoagulability, renal vein thrombosis, and other thrombotic complications of nephrotic syndrome. Kidney Int. 1985;28(3):429–39.

51. Orth SR, Ritz E. The nephrotic syndrome. N Engl J Med. 1998;338(17):1202–11.

52. Shalhoub RJ. Pathogenesis of lipoid nephrosis: a disorder of T-cell function. Lancet. 1974;2(7880): 556–60.

53. Le Berre L et al. Induction of T regulatory cells attenuates idiopathic nephrotic syndrome. J Am Soc Nephrol. 2009;20(1):57–67.

54. Hogan J, Radhakrishnan J. The treatment of minimal change disease in adults. J Am Soc Nephrol. 2013;24(5):702–11.

55. Black DA, Rose G, Brewer DB. Controlled trial of prednisone in adult patients with the nephrotic syndrome. Br Med J. 1970;3(5720):421–6.

56. Coggins CH. Adult minimal change nephropathy: experience of the collaborative study of glomerular disease. Trans Am Clin Climatol Assoc. 1986;97: 18–26.

57. Lange K, Wasserman E, Slobody LB. Prolonged intermittent steroid therapy for nephrosis in children and adults. J Am Med Assoc. 1958;168(4):377–81.

58. Palmer SC, Nand K, Strippoli GF. Interventions for minimal change disease in adults with nephrotic syndrome. Cochrane Database Syst Rev. 2008;1, CD001537.

59. Pei Y et al. Evidence suggesting under-treatment in adults with idiopathic focal segmental glomerulosclerosis. Regional Glomerulonephritis Registry Study. Am J Med. 1987;82(5):938–44.

60. Couser WG, Nangaku M. Cellular and molecular biology of membranous nephropathy. J Nephrol. 2006;19(6):699–705.

61. Stanescu HC et al. Risk HLA-DQA1 and PLA(2)R1 alleles in idiopathic membranous nephropathy. N Engl J Med. 2011;364(7):616–26.

62. Beck Jr LH, Salant GJ. Membranous nephropathy: from models to man. J Clin Invest. 2014;124(6): 2307–14.

63. Mastroianni-Kirsztajn G, Hornig N, Schlumberger W. Autoantibodies in renal diseases – clinical significance and recent developments in serological detection. Front Immunol. 2015;6:221.

64. Schmiedeke TM et al. Histones have high affinity for the glomerular basement membrane. Relevance for immune complex formation in lupus nephritis. J Exp Med. 1989;169(6):1879–94.

65. Johnson RJ, Couser WG. Hepatitis B infection and renal disease: clinical, immunopathogenetic and therapeutic considerations. Kidney Int. 1990;37(2): 663–76.

66. Ponticelli C et al. A randomized trial of methylprednisolone and chlorambucil in idiopathic membranous nephropathy. N Engl J Med. 1989;320(1):8–13.

67. Cattran DC et al. A randomized controlled trial of prednisone in patients with idiopathic membranous nephropathy. N Engl J Med. 1989;320(4):210–5.

68. Ehrenreich T et al. Treatment of idiopathic membranous nephropathy. N Engl J Med. 1976;295(14): 741–6.

69. Donadio Jr JV et al. Idiopathic membranous nephropathy: the natural history of untreated patients. Kidney Int. 1988;33(3):708–15.

70. Falk RJ et al. Treatment of progressive membranous glomerulopathy. A randomized trial comparing cyclophosphamide and corticosteroids with corticosteroids alone. The Glomerular Disease Collaborative Network. Ann Intern Med. 1992;116(6):438–45.

71. Ponticelli C et al. A 10-year follow-up of a randomized study with methylprednisolone and chlorambucil in membranous nephropathy. Kidney Int. 1995;48(5): 1600–4.

# Nonneoplastic Kidney Diseases in the Setting of a Renal Mass

Anthony Chang and Vanesa Bijol

## Abbreviation

CKD    Chronic kidney disease
EM    Electron microscopy
FSGS    Focal segmental glomerulosclerosis
IF    Immunofluorescence
NSS    Nephron-sparing surgery
RCC    Renal cell carcinoma
RN    Radical nephrectomy
PN    Partial nephrectomy
TMA    Thrombotic microangiopathy

## Introduction

In 2014, more than 65,000 patients were newly diagnosed with kidney cancer in the USA. Earlier detection of kidney tumors has steadily increased the incidence by 2 % annually [1] with a notable migration of early-stage kidney cancers over the last two decades, especially in the USA. According to one study, 43 % of kidney cancers were stage I in 1993 and more recently comprise over 60 % of tumors [2]. While surgical resection of low stage tumors offers the best chance for a cure, the preservation of renal function has been recognized in recent years as an important factor for optimal patient outcomes. Early-stage renal cell carcinomas (RCC) that are removed by either partial nephrectomy (PN) or radical nephrectomy (RN) have similar oncologic outcomes, but patients that underwent PN had superior clinical outcomes [3, 4].

Nephron-sparing surgery (NSS) includes cryoablation, thermal and radiofrequency ablation, and PN. Rapid advancements in these procedures and their instrumentation have allowed surgeons and oncologists to gain the upper hand in the fight against kidney cancer. It is also notable that up to 23 % of renal masses are benign and active surveillance is a viable option for poor surgical candidates given the slow growth rate of most tumors (average of 1.3 mm per year) [5]. The 5-year and 10-year disease-free rates for stage I renal cancers approach 100 % and exceed 90 %, respectively [6]. Therefore, given that there are almost 350,000 kidney cancer survivors in the USA, the maintenance of renal health represents an opportunity for additional gains in clinical outcomes.

A. Chang, M.D. (✉)
Department of Pathology, University of Chicago Medical Center, 5841 S. Maryland Ave, Chicago, IL 60637, USA
e-mail: anthony.chang@uchospitals.edu

V. Bijol, M.D.
Department of Pathology, Brigham and Women's Hospital, Boston, MA 02115, USA
e-mail: vbijol@partners.org

© Springer Science+Business Media New York 2016
D.E. Hansel et al. (eds.), *The Kidney*, DOI 10.1007/978-1-4939-3286-3_13

## The Harmful Impact of Chronic Kidney Disease

Chronic kidney disease (CKD) was formerly referred as chronic renal failure, and its harmful effects have only been recognized in the last 10 years. CKD patients are at substantially increased risk for death due to both cardiovascular and non-cardiovascular causes [7]. CKD is categorized into five stages, and stage 3 (glomerular filtration rate of <60 mL/min) or greater CKD will afflict one in seven Americans (>30 years of age) during their lifetime [8]. In the setting of kidney cancer, Huang et al. were among the first to demonstrate that 26 % of kidney cancer patients had CKD even prior to tumor nephrectomy [9]. RN increases the risk of CKD development and progression compared with NSS, which results in inferior outcomes due to the substantial loss of functional nephrons. In 2009, the American Urological Association issued practice guidelines that recommended the use of NSS for T1a (<4 cm) renal masses.

Public awareness of the devastating impact of end-stage kidney disease is low. More than 92,000 Americans died from kidney disease in 2011, which exceeded the number of combined deaths due to breast and prostate cancer, the most common cancers in women and men, respectively [8]. The 1-year mortality rate of a dialysis patient is approximately 20 %, which exceeds most new cancer diagnoses [10]. Despite these data, additional recognition of the tremendous toll from kidney diseases is needed. End-stage renal disease (or stage 5 CKD) portends a 100-fold increased risk for RCC [11], and recently this risk has been identified to a lesser degree for stage 3 or 4 CKD [12]. Therefore, the connection between RCC and any underlying concurrent finding of nonneoplastic kidney diseases in RCC patients is likely to be more than just a coincidence.

The management of CKD is a complex and rapidly evolving topic, which has been extensively addressed by Kidney Disease Improving Global Outcomes (KDIGO) [13] with additional commentary and input [14].

## Renal Pathology

With the improving survival rates of kidney cancer patients due to earlier interventions, proper assessment of the nonneoplastic kidney parenchyma in tumor nephrectomy specimens is emerging as the most important aspect of the evaluation. Overlooking a nonneoplastic kidney disease and missing an opportunity to intervene and delay the progression of CKD can harm patients.

## Processing and Evaluation of the Nonneoplastic Kidney in Tumor Nephrectomy Specimens

The standard protocols for the gross and microscopic evaluation of tumor nephrectomy specimens have been established decades ago. Traditionally, the evaluation has centered around the renal neoplasm and its accurate grading and staging. However, several studies have revealed that 60–88 % of nonneoplastic renal diseases are routinely overlooked and not initially diagnosed by the practicing pathologist [15, 16]. Beginning January 1, 2010, the College of American Pathologist protocols for the evaluation of tumor nephrectomy and nephroureterectomy specimens were modified to require the evaluation of the nonneoplastic kidney parenchyma [17]. All pathologists faithfully sample the nonneoplastic kidney in these specimens, but there is a lot of room for improvement regarding the subsequent microscopic evaluation. In one European study, over 25 % of pathologists did not even look for a nonneoplastic kidney disease [18]. One contributing factor is the increasing complexity and amount of information that is required to function as a competent surgical pathologist. A 2006 survey revealed that nearly 75 % of US pathology residents are not exposed to any nephropathology during their residency training [15], and as a result of this deficiency, the Accreditation Council for Graduate Medical Education will require formal exposure to this subspecialty effective July 1, 2015.

When the specimen is processed, additional tissue can be submitted for immunofluorescence (IF) or electron microscopy (EM) if a glomerular disease is suspected or there is a history of proteinuria. Careful evaluation of the light microscopy will result in the identification of the important subset of cases with significant glomerular alterations that warrant additional ancillary studies with actionable diagnoses. IF [19, 20] and EM [21] can be performed from the formalin-fixed, paraffin-embedded tissue blocks albeit with some limitations, including decreased sensitivity for the former and preservation artifact for the latter. We do recommend ordering special stains (PAS and/or Jones methenamine silver) at the time the specimen is grossly evaluated, so that these histochemical studies may be available along with the H&E slides to remind the pathologist to carefully evaluate the nonneoplastic kidney.

## Algorithm

A systematic evaluation of the four anatomic compartments (glomeruli, tubules, interstitium, vessels) of the kidney should always be performed. For the glomerular evaluation, ischemic glomeruli, which are characterized by fraying of Bowman capsules, should be avoided as the common shrinkage of the glomerular tufts can falsely give the impression of mesangial sclerosis. Therefore, the initial exam of well-preserved glomeruli should determine whether the glomeruli are generally free of histologic abnormalities. If the glomeruli appear normal, overt immune complex-mediated glomerulonephritides can be ruled out. Admittedly, many diseases at early stages would not be identified with this approach, such as early membranous nephropathy, other immune complex-mediated diseases, amyloidosis, or IgA nephropathy. However, the likelihood of their presence in nephrectomy specimens is rather low, particularly in the absence of clinically relevant proteinuria and/or hematuria, or renal failure. We are, therefore, most concerned about not overlooking obvious glomerular alterations that may lead to prompt clinical intervention. To exclude

the presence of focal lesions, such as focal global and segmental glomerulosclerosis, a larger sample should be evaluated; we recommend counting at least 50 glomeruli and assessing the percentage of global and segmental glomerulosclerosis. If there is significant interstitial fibrosis and tubular atrophy, then counting 100 glomeruli may provide a more representative sample to estimate the percentage of sclerosed glomeruli. The diagnosis of any nonneoplastic renal disease should be regarded as an urgent value by the pathologist, and this information should be communicated immediately to the treating physician.

## Artifacts and Pitfalls (Tumor Compression)

It is important to remember that surgical pathology specimens are often sectioned close to 4 μm in thickness, while routine nephropathology specimens are in the 2–3 μm range, which needs to be taken into account when assessing glomerular cellularity. For instance, mesangial hypercellularity is often defined as more than 2 mesangial cell nuclei per mesangial region for a 2 μm thick tissue section, but this criterion increases to more than 3 mesangial cell nuclei per mesangial region for a 3 μm thick tissue section.

Tumor pseudocapsule is created by tumor compression of parenchyma. Generally, the presence of a pseudocapsule is more common in RCC, even when tumors are small in size. In some tumors, such as oncocytomas, pseudocapsule is unusual even with larger tumors [22].

## Diabetic Nephropathy

Diabetes is a well-established independent risk factor for RCC, and approximately 25 % of RCC patients have diabetes [23]. Typically, one third of diabetic patients develop diabetic nephropathy, and most studies have demonstrated that the rate of tumor nephrectomy specimens is 8 % [15, 16] but approaches 20 % in one large study if the earliest changes are included [24]. The glomeruli demonstrate characteristic pathologic features

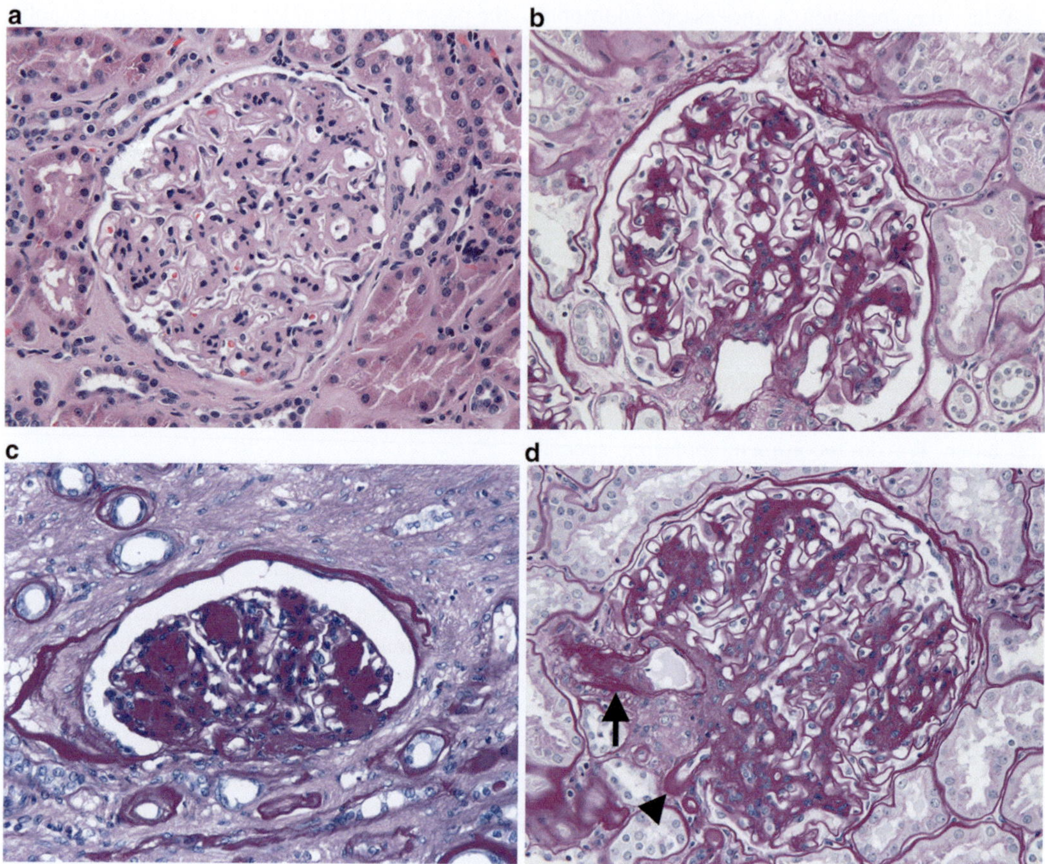

**Fig. 13.1** (**a**) H&E and (**b**) PAS. Diffuse mesangial sclerosis is characterized by increased matrix deposition in mesangial regions and represents one of the earlier changes in diabetic glomerular injury. The periodic acid Schiff (PAS) reveals these mesangial changes much more readily especially at the lower magnifications compared with the H&E slide. (**c**) Nodular mesangial sclerosis with acellular (Kimmelstiel-Wilson) nodules indicates a more advanced phase of diabetic glomerular injury with typically a longer clinical history of diabetes that may also correlate with the presence of proteinuria. This glomerulus was located in an area of tumor compression. (**d**) Arteriolar hyalinosis involving both the afferent (*arrow*) and efferent (*arrowhead*) arterioles is characteristic of diabetic nephropathy, while hypertensive vascular disease preferentially involves the afferent arteriole alone

which begin with mild diffuse mesangial sclerosis (Fig. 13.1a) and can progress to nodular glomerulosclerosis and form acellular (Kimmelstiel-Wilson) nodules (Fig. 13.1b). The finding of diffuse mesangial sclerosis can also impart an appearance of hypercellularity as several mesangial areas may merge together to form one large mesangial region (Fig. 13.1c). Glomerular and tubular basement membrane thickening and arteriolar hyalinosis involving both afferent and efferent arterioles (Fig. 13.1d) are also characteristic. There would be no significant immunofluo-rescence findings, except for dull linear staining of the basement membranes for IgG and albumin. To establish the diagnosis of diabetic nephropathy, the clinical history of diabetes must always be obtained. There are some examples of florid nodular glomerulosclerosis that have been observed in patients without diabetes who have severe hypertension or a heavy cigarette smoking history [25]. Amyloidosis and monoclonal immunoglobulin deposition disease are also common mimics of nodular diabetic glomerulosclerosis and should always be considered in the differential diagnosis.

Approximately 30 million Americans have diabetes, and it is estimated that over 25 % have not yet been diagnosed. Therefore, the pathologist has the unique opportunity to identify some of these undiagnosed patients. We believe that any diagnosis of diabetic nephropathy should trigger direct communication with the treating clinicians and result in nephrology consultation.

## Arterionephrosclerosis/ Hypertensive Nephrosclerosis

Hypertension is another well-established risk factor for RCC and occurs in 25–60 % of RCC patients [26, 27]. As a consequence, the corresponding kidney injury is commonly observed in a significant subset of these patients. However, hypertensive nephropathy consists of a constellation of nonspecific pathologic features, such as global glomerulosclerosis (Fig. 13.2a), interstitial fibrosis, tubular atrophy (Fig. 13.2b), and arteriosclerosis (Fig. 13.2c). In addition, the pathologist may not be able to ascertain whether the patient has hypertension, which can be further confounded by antihypertensive therapy. Therefore, some nephropathologists prefer the use of descriptive terms, such as arterionephrosclerosis or vascular scarring (arteriosclerosis), to describe the pathologic changes without ascribing a definitive etiology.

Regardless of the terminology that is used, it is important to identify the subset of patients at greater risk for CKD progression. Based on the available data, the finding of greater than 20 % global glomerulosclerosis predicts a significant decrease of the glomerular filtration rate after radical nephrectomy [24]. Therefore, this finding should trigger additional nephrology consultation.

## Focal Segmental Glomerulosclerosis

Focal segmental glomerulosclerosis (FSGS) has been identified in 2–9 % of tumor nephrectomy specimens. In this setting, FSGS likely represents a secondary cause due to substantial nephron loss

and hyperfiltration rather than a primary podocyte injury. The identification of hyaline or matrix occluding any of the glomerular capillaries (Fig. 13.3) is sufficient for this diagnosis and typically occurs in the background of arterionephrosclerosis as described in the previous section.

## Thrombotic Microangiopathy

The finding of thrombi in arteries, arterioles, or glomerular capillaries may be consistent with thrombotic microangiopathy (TMA). However, we have observed rare glomerular capillary thrombi adjacent to the tumor resection margin, which likely represent a consequence of surgical manipulation and may not indicate the presence of an underlying thrombotic microangiopathic injury. Some tyrosine kinase inhibitors, such as sunitinib, are increasingly used in RCC patients and can directly affect vascular endothelial growth factor receptors, which can cause TMA. However, these therapeutic drugs are generally given after surgery when indicated and not administered as neoadjuvant therapy.

## Summary

Occasional cases of concomitant membranous nephropathy, IgA nephropathy, or pauci-immune crescentic glomerulonephritis have been reported. In theory, any nonneoplastic kidney disease could occur in the setting of RCC by coincidence.

We recommend that the treating physician should specifically inquire their pathologist about the presence of nonneoplastic kidney diseases, especially when a history of diabetes, hypertension, or proteinuria is present or if the estimated glomerular filtration rate is below 60 mL/min. Clinical practice guidelines have not been established but are needed to aid the treating physicians through these complex medical issues. The evaluation of the nonneoplastic kidney parenchyma is now required by the College of American Pathologist protocols for the evaluation of all tumor nephrectomy and nephroureterectomy

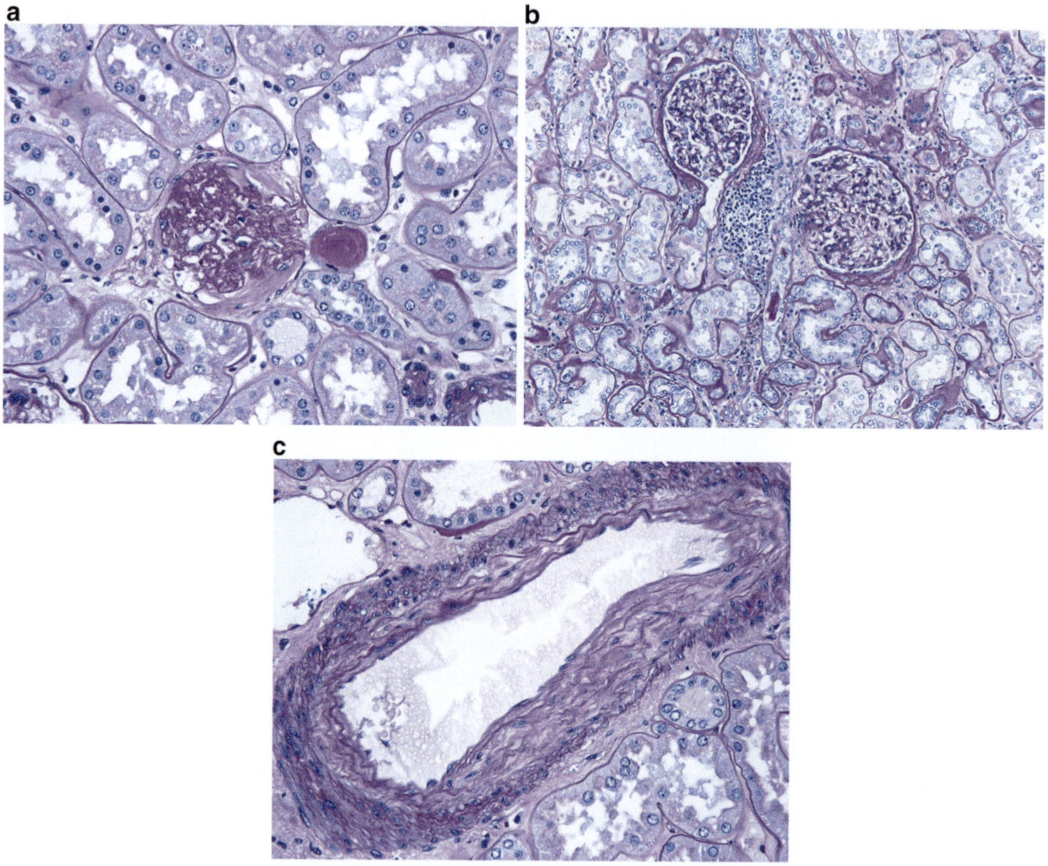

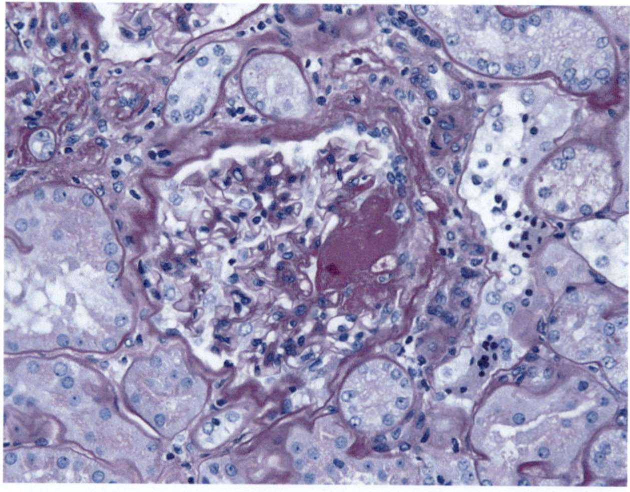

**Fig. 13.2** (**a**) Global glomerulosclerosis or complete scarring of an entire glomerulus is a nonspecific finding that can be observed in any glomerular injury. It is clear that glomerular filtration cannot occur without the presence of any patent capillaries. (**b**) Interstitial fibrosis and tubular atrophy are characterized by thickening, fraying, and wrinkling of tubular basement membranes of atrophic tubules that are separated from each other by interstitial fibrosis. The presence of mild interstitial inflammation in the areas of tubulointerstitial scarring is typical and should not be considered evidence of acute interstitial nephritis. There are also two mildly ischemic glomeruli present. (**c**) Arteriosclerosis is characterized by intimal fibrosis and varying degrees of multilayering of the internal elastic lamina

**Fig. 13.3** Focal segmental glomerulosclerosis is characterized by segmental accumulation of hyaline that fills some of the glomerular capillary lumina

specimens [17]. However, it is unclear whether this modification has resulted in significant practice behavior changes among surgical pathologists since its implementation in 2010. With the number of kidney cancer survivors approaching 350,000 in the USA, significant gains in the clinical outcomes for kidney cancer can be achieved with additional attention on the presence of nonneoplastic kidney diseases and improved coordination between urologists, nephrologists, and pathologists.

# References


1. Patard J-J. Incidental renal tumours. Curr Opin Urol. 2009;19(5):454–8.
2. Pichler M, Hutterer GC, Chromecki TF, Jesche J, Kampel-Kettner K, Pummer K, et al. Renal cell carcinoma stage migration in a single European centre over 25 years: effects on 5- and 10-year metastasis-free survival. Int Urol Nephrol. 2012;44(4):997–1004.
3. Lau WKO, Blute ML, Weaver AL, Torres VE, Zincke H. Matched comparison of radical nephrectomy vs nephron-sparing surgery in patients with unilateral renal cell carcinoma and a normal contralateral kidney. Mayo Clin Proc. 2000;75(12):1236–42.
4. Tan H-J, Norton EC, Ye Z, Hafez KS, Gore JL, Miller DC. Long-term survival following partial vs radical nephrectomy among older patients with early-stage kidney cancer. J Am Med Assoc. 2012;307(15): 1629–35.
5. Jewett MAS, Mattar K, Basiuk J, Morash CG, Pautler SE, Siemens DR, et al. Active surveillance of small renal masses: progression patterns of early stage kidney cancer. Eur Urol. 2011;60(1):39–44.
6. Campbell SC, Novick AC, Belldegrun A, Blute ML, Chow GK, Derweesh IH, et al. Guideline for management of the clinical T1 renal mass. J Urol. 2009; 182(4):1271–9.
7. Go AS, Chertow GM, Fan D, McCulloch CE, Hsu C. Chronic kidney disease and the risks of death, cardiovascular events, and hospitalization. N Engl J Med. 2004;351(13):1296–305.
8. The National Kidney Foundation: News [Internet]. http://www.kidney.org/news/newsroom/factsheets/FastFacts.cfm. Cited 31 Jan 2014.
9. Huang WC, Levey AS, Serio AM, Snyder M, Vickers AJ, Raj GV, et al. Chronic kidney disease after nephrectomy in patients with renal cortical tumours: a retrospective cohort study. Lancet Oncol. 2006;7(9):735–40.
10. Rifkin DE. Doctors without metaphors. Am J Kidney Dis. 2009;54(5):A35–6.
11. Denton MD, Magee CC, Ovuworie C, Mauiyyedi S, Pascual M, Colvin RB, et al. Prevalence of renal cell carcinoma in patients with ESRD pre-transplantation: a pathologic analysis. Kidney Int. 2002;61(6): 2201–9.
12. Lowrance WT, Ordoñez J, Udaltsova N, Russo P, Go AS. CKD and the risk of incident cancer. J Am Soc Nephrol. 2014;25(10):2327–34.
13. Kidney Disease: Improving Global Outcomes (KDIGO) CKD Work Group. KDIGO 2012 clinical practice guideline for the evaluation and management of chronic kidney disease. Kidney Int. 2013;3:1–150.
14. Inker LA, Astor BC, Fox CH, Isakova T, Lash JP, Peralta CA, et al. KDOQI US commentary on the 2012 KDIGO clinical practice guideline for the evaluation and management of CKD. Am J Kidney Dis. 2014;63(5):713–35.
15. Henriksen KJ, Meehan SM, Chang A. Non-neoplastic renal diseases are often unrecognized in adult tumor nephrectomy specimens: a review of 246 cases. Am J Surg Pathol. 2007;31(11):1703–8.
16. Salvatore SP, Cha EK, Rosoff JS, Seshan SV. Nonneoplastic renal cortical scarring at tumor nephrectomy predicts decline in kidney function. Arch Pathol Lab Med. 2013;137(4):531–40.
17. Srigley JR, Amin MB, Delahunt B, Campbell SC, Chang A, Grignon DJ, et al. Protocol for the examination of specimens from patients with invasive carcinoma of renal tubular origin. Arch Pathol Lab Med. 2010;134(4):e25–30.
18. Algaba F, Delahunt B, Berney DM, Camparo P, Compérat E, Griffiths D, et al. Handling and reporting of nephrectomy specimens for adult renal tumours: a survey by the European Network of Uropathology. J Clin Pathol. 2012;65(2):106–13.
19. Nasr SH, Galgano SJ, Markowitz GS, Stokes MB, D'Agati VD. Immunofluorescence on pronase-digested paraffin sections: a valuable salvage technique for renal biopsies. Kidney Int. 2006;70(12): 2148–51.
20. Van der Ven K, Nguyen TQ, Goldschmeding R. Immunofluorescence on proteinase XXIV-digested paraffin sections. Kidney Int. 2007;72(7):896.
21. Nasr SH, Markowitz GS, Valeri AM, Yu Z, Chen L, D'Agati VD. Thin basement membrane nephropathy cannot be diagnosed reliably in deparaffinized, formalin-fixed tissue. Nephrol Dial Transplant. 2007; 22(4):1228–32.
22. Bonsib SM, Pei Y. The non-neoplastic kidney in tumor nephrectomy specimens: what can it show and what is important? Adv Anat Pathol. 2010;17(4): 235–50.
23. Zucchetto A, Dal Maso L, Tavani A, Montella M, Ramazzotti V, Talamini R, et al. History of treated hypertension and diabetes mellitus and risk of renal cell cancer. Ann Oncol. 2007;18(3):596–600.

24. Bijol V, Mendez GP, Hurwitz S, Rennke HG, Nosé V. Evaluation of the nonneoplastic pathology in tumor nephrectomy specimens: predicting the risk of progressive renal failure. Am J Surg Pathol. 2006;30(5):575–84.

25. Markowitz GS, Lin J, Valeri AM, Avila C, Nasr SH, D'Agati VD. Idiopathic nodular glomerulosclerosis is a distinct clinicopathologic entity linked to hypertension and smoking. Hum Pathol. 2002;33(8):826–35.

26. Chow WH, Gridley G, Fraumeni JF, Järvholm B. Obesity, hypertension, and the risk of kidney cancer in men. N Engl J Med. 2000;343(18):1305–11.

27. Choi MY, Jee SH, Sull JW, Nam CM. The effect of hypertension on the risk for kidney cancer in Korean men. Kidney Int. 2005;67(2):647–52.

# Index




© Springer Science+Business Media New York 2016

D.E. Hansel et al. (eds.), *The Kidney*, DOI 10.1007/978-1-4939-3286-3

 MIX
Papier aus verantwortungsvollen Quellen
Paper from responsible sources
FSC® C105338

If you have any concerns about our products,
you can contact us on
ProductSafety@springernature.com

In case Publisher is established outside the EU,
the EU authorized representative is:
Springer Nature Customer Service Center GmbH
Europaplatz 3, 69115 Heidelberg, Germany

Printed by Libri Plureos GmbH
in Hamburg, Germany